Laser Spine Surgery

Junseok Bae • Sang-Ho Lee
Editors

Laser Spine Surgery

Springer

Editors
Junseok Bae
President
Department of Neurological Surgery
Wooridul Spine Hospital
Seoul, Korea (Republic of)

Sang-Ho Lee
Chairman
Wooridul Spine Hospital
Clinical professor of Anatomy
Yonsei University College of medicine
Seoul, Korea (Republic of)

ISBN 978-981-16-2208-3 ISBN 978-981-16-2206-9 (eBook)
https://doi.org/10.1007/978-981-16-2206-9

This Springer imprint is published by the registered company Springer Nature Singapore Pte Ltd.
The registered company address is: 152 Beach Road, #21-01/04 Gateway East, Singapore 189721, Singapore

Preface

Small is Beautiful, Laser Spine Surgery

Minimally invasive spinal surgery is a clear direction for the development of the latest spinal surgery. Small incisions and minimal tissue damage are the basic philosophy. However, accurately treating the pathology is more important. Laser spine surgery is essential for minimally invasive spine treatment in this regard. With the most accurate and detailed "knife of light," we can perform very delicate operations through microscopes and endoscopes. There had been many suspicions about laser spine surgery in the early days. As the effectiveness of laser spine surgery has been proved by the efforts of many researchers, its use is now expanding. Laser is advantageous in various fields of spine surgery, from surgery like simple disk resection or decompression of stenosis to pain intervention such as annuloplasty and adhesiolysis. This book contains the most up-to-date information by integrating the technology of Wooridul Spine Hospital, which has been working for decades as a pioneer in applying laser spine surgery to clinical practice and broadening its indications. We hope that this book will help the reader become aware of laser spine surgery and provide better treatment.

Seoul, Korea

Junseok Bae
Sang-Ho Lee

Contents

Evolution of Spine Surgery as a Request of Endoscopic and Microscopic Laser to Technology

1

Sang-Ho Lee, Seong Kyun Jeong, and Junseok Bae

Abstract

Spine surgery is one of the fastest developing areas of surgery. In the past, a wide field of view was essential to find anatomical landmarks and to access to the lesion, and therefore a wide area of incision was inevitable. However, a wide area of incision may cause extensive tissue damage to important structures, leading to late patient recovery and the development of unnecessary pain after surgery. Since the 1980s, the laser-assisted microscopic surgery allowed for deeper surgery with a smaller incision area of less than 1 inch for a magnified view. In the 1990s, the laser-assisted endoscopic spine surgery became possible with the therapeutic incision range of 0.5–1 cm for the intervertebral disc. Endoscopic or microscopic lasers are essential to perform better surgery with a smaller incision for minimally invasive disc surgery. Minimally invasive spinal surgery using lasers guides patients to return to their daily lives faster and have a quality of life and time economy. Minimally invasive spinal surgery using lasers is already present now, not in the future.

Keywords

Technical developments · Minimally invasive Microscopic surgery · Endoscopic surgery Laser

1.1 Introduction

Spine surgery is one of the fastest developing areas of surgery. In particular, the dramatic development of advanced optical technology, computer diagnostic technology, and advanced laser technology since the 1990s has enabled new methods for more effective and safe treatment in spine surgery. The surgical procedures performed by the great masters of spine surgery in the past are now performed in a more precise, minimally invasive and more developed manner, thanks to the development of the devices and the accumulation of knowledge.

Modern spine surgery began in the late nineteenth century, after the invention of antisepsis and anesthesia. Spine surgery began with decompression surgery, and Dr. Macewen reported the first laminectomy in 1886 [1]. In the twentieth century, there were many advances, especially in the field of spinal fusion. Already in 1891, Dr. Hadra tried cervical wiring [2], and in the twentieth century Dr. Albee [3] and Dr. Hibbs [4] performed posterolateral arthrodesis using decorticated autograft bone. Lately, Dr. Gallie

S.-H. Lee · S. K. Jeong · J. Bae (✉)
Chungdam Wooridul Spine Hospital,
Seoul, Republic of Korea

J. Bae, S.-H. Lee (eds.), *Laser Spine Surgery*, https://doi.org/10.1007/978-981-16-2206-9_1

advanced his technique using C1–2 wiring and autograft implantation [5], which became popular for several decades. In the 1950s, Dr. Harrington introduced a spinal instrumentation system using steel rods and hooks [6], which, combined with the pedicle screws and cages, became the main treatment method for deformity and trauma.

In the past, each spine surgery has been dominated by the operator who has a lot of experience with sophisticated hands. Based on his anatomical knowledge and surgical experience, the surgeon had to accurately detect the lesions and safely remove them or fix important structures in the spine. For this reason, a wide field of view was essential to find anatomical landmarks and to access to the lesion without damaging important structures, and therefore a wide area of incision was inevitable.

However, a wide area of incision causes extensive tissue damage, leading to late patient recovery and the development of unnecessary pain after surgery. Especially in disc diseases, unwanted tissue damage can promote degenerative changes in spinal structures, such as disc or facet joints, and induce spinal instability. It may also contribute to the occurrence of post-discectomy syndrome, post-spinal surgery syndrome (PSSS), or failed back surgery syndrome (FBSS). These facts were the background for the emergence of a surgical technique that minimizes tissue damage, "minimally invasive spinal surgery." Dr. Yaşargil in Switzerland and Dr. Marlis in the USA have contributed to the creation of minimally invasive spinal surgery through research on microscopic neurosurgery since the mid-1970s [7, 8].

Unlike other department of surgery, the spine surgery is almost always performed near neurovascular structures, so safe and effective surgery is possible only when you directly visualize the surgical site. Until the 1970s, the spine surgery performed only with the naked eye or loupe required a wide incision and a large posterior resection for shadowless light to reach every corner of the spinal cavity. Since the 1980s, developed and introduced by Dr. Yaşargil [7] and Dr. Caspar [9], the microscopic surgical technique overcame the limitations by illuminating narrow areas that are difficult to see with the naked eyes and magnifying the affected area 15 times larger. The microscopic surgery allowed for deeper surgery with a smaller incision area of less than 1 inch for a magnified view. Conventional microdiscectomy with a large annulotomy by a scalpel may develop a collapse of the disc height and may associate with post-discectomy back pain. However, laser-assisted microdiscectomy with a small annulotomy can save the disc tissue and maintain the disc height without development of post-discectomy syndrome. The illustrated case is showing a patient who underwent laser-assisted microdiscectomy without post-discectomy syndrome compared to a patient who underwent conventional microdiscectomy which resulted in post-discectomy syndrome (Fig. 1.1). In the 1990s, a ballpoint pen core-sized small lens hanged in a long line can be inserted anywhere in the body, and the captured image can be magnified on a large monitor screen of 17 inches or more. From this time on, the endoscopic spine surgery became possible with the therapeutic incision range of 0.5–1 cm for the intervertebral disc [10]. Endoscopic laser-assisted annuloplasty can treat discogenic back pain. Thanks to this new technological improvement, it became possible to selectively and accurately remove the pathological disc with only a minimum of scars.

To remove the severely herniated disc materials under the endoscope, a laser is essential. LASER is an abbreviation for Light Amplification by Stimulated Emission of Radiation, which is the conversion of any form of energy into the form of electromagnetic radiant energy. A term woven by Gordon Gould in 1959 [11], Theodore Maiman invented the functional laser of this technology in 1960 [12]. Lasers vary in the wavelength of the emitted light, the amount of energy transmitted, the depth of energy permeating the tissue, and so on, depending on the device that generates the laser and the type of laser. Typical types of lasers used in the medical field include KTP ($KTiOPO_4$, potassium titanyl phosphate), Nd:YAG (neodymium:yttrium-aluminum-garnet), CO_2 (carbon dioxide), Ho:YAG (holmium:yttrium-aluminum-garnet), excimer, argon, and dye. The

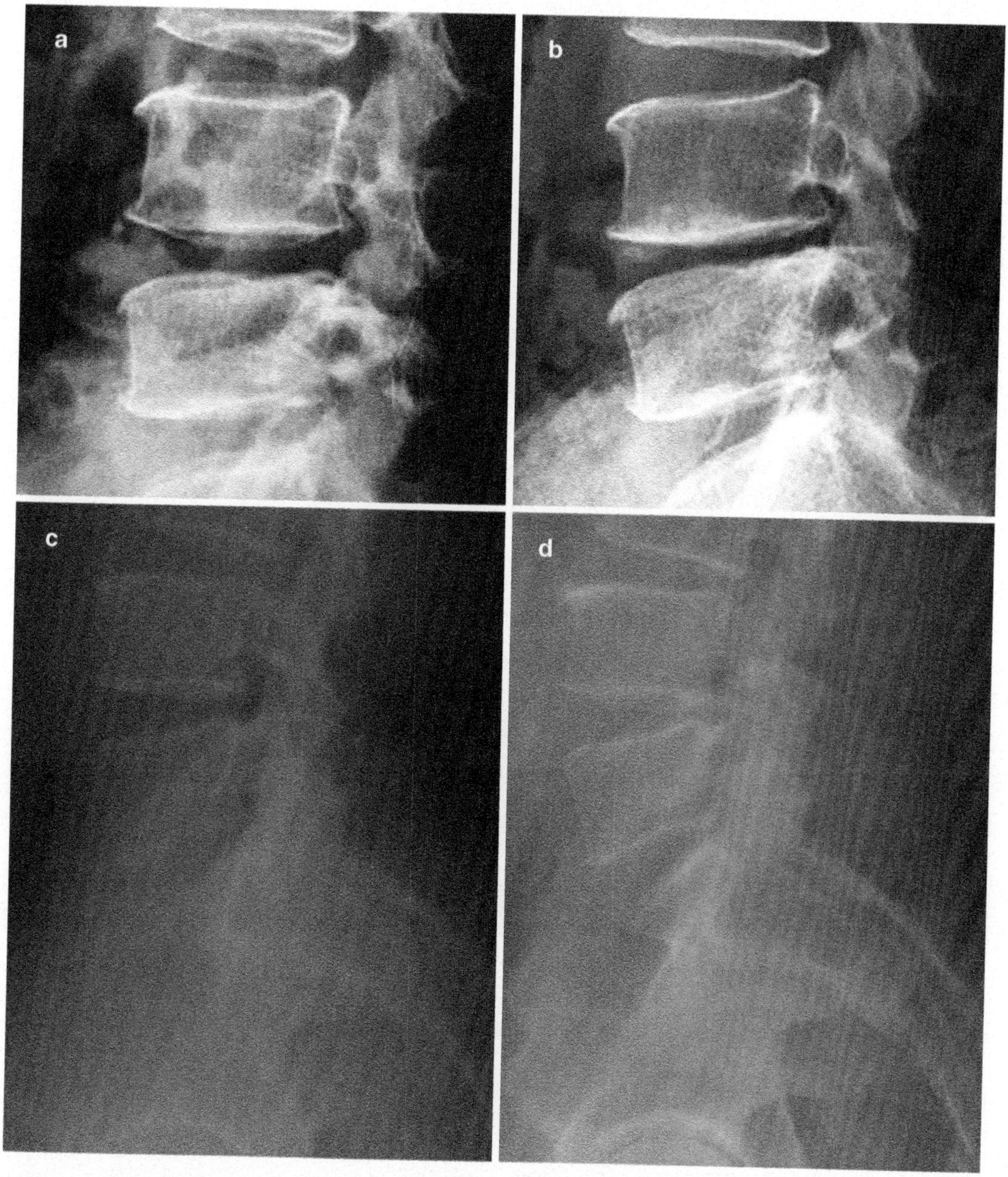

Fig. 1.1 (**a**) Preoperative X-ray image of a patient who underwent conventional discectomy on L4–5 level. (**b**) 2 years and 8 months later, the disc height was significantly decreased to cause lower back pain. (**c**) Preoperative X-ray image of a patient who underwent laser-assisted microdiscectomy on L4–5 level. (**d**) The disc height and the cushioning function had been preserved until 20 years after the laser-assisted microdiscectomy

laser treatment has several effects as follows: (1) a precision excision effect (a sword of light with the thickness of the hair that enters the narrow neural foramen under the endoscope), (2) a pain-blocking effect (blocking the pain nerves that are distributed in the posterior annulus) [13], (3) disc contraction and strengthening effect (contraction of the protruded disc and remodeling of collagen in discal tissue) [14], and (4) hemostatic effect (coagulation). The long-term stability of lasers used in disc surgery was reviewed by the US FDA in 1991 and found to be effective and safe.

The first-generation laser surgery in the field of spine surgery used the Nd:YAG laser and the KTP laser. It was a procedure to shoot a laser at the center of the disc without an endoscope. So, the procedure was less accurate for not looking inside of the discs during the firing, and the posterior part of the disc was remained for concern about nerve damage. Another problem of the procedure was that the transmission range of the lasers was as long as 4–10 mm. The procedure was able to be performed easily but there should be concerns about side effects such as cartilage necrosis. From 1986 to 1995, Dr. Choy and his colleagues used Nd:YAG lasers to 389 people for 9 years and reported a success rate of 75% and side effects of 1% [15]. In 1992, Dr. Davis used a KTP laser for lumbar disc treatment with a success rate of 80% [16].

The second-generation laser disc surgery used the Ho:YAG laser while directly confirming the lesion within the annulus fibrosus through an endoscope by Dr. Sang-Ho Lee, Dr. Hansjörg Leu, and Dr. John Chiu (Fig. 1.2). In 1992, Dr. Gottlob and his colleagues used the first-generation Ho:YAG laser to remove the nucleus pulposus [17]. The Ho:YAG laser had a transmission range of 0.4 mm, which was delicate and safe. Through a bright and clear endoscope, the Ho:YAG laser under irrigation of saline mixed with antibiotics, unlike the first-generation lasers, was a method of selectively shooting only the posterior site of the disc, not the center of the disc. This second-generation laser surgery into intra-annular and subligamentous area of the disc got closer to the lesion, resulting in a 90% success rate [18]. It showed good results for the patients with discogenic back pain. However, since it was not possible to look the neural tissue behind the annulus fibrosus directly, there was a blind spot in the treatment site, and it was difficult to treat large-sized intra-annular subligamentous sequestrated disc and calcified hard disc herniation.

The third-generation laser disc surgery is performed while the endoscope directly visualizes not only the annulus posterior to the disc but also the spinal cavity and the spinal nerves. The Ho:YAG laser in this procedure has evolved into a flexible laser and a side firing, and those were difficult to be performed with the second-generation lasers [19, 20]. It is an epoch-making surgical method that enables effective treatment of blind spots. The endoscopic laser discectomy became very safe and the success rate has increased to around 95% [10, 21, 22]. It can also be applied to the large-sized and sequestrated disc herniation [18, 23].

The third-generation laser disc surgery was simultaneously and collaboratively developed by Dr. Martin Knight in the UK [24]; Dr. Anthony Yeung in the USA [25]; Dr. Sang-Ho Lee, the author; and the spine disc operation team at the

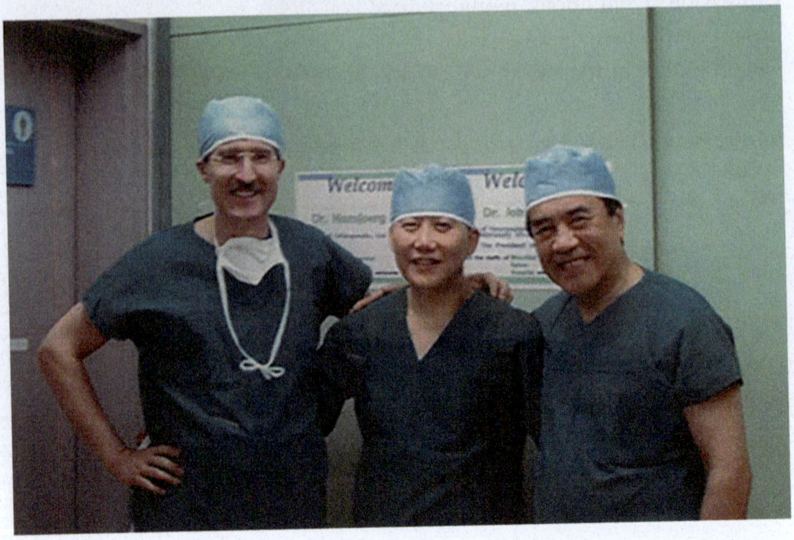

Fig. 1.2 Dr. Hansjörg Leu, Dr. Sang-Ho Lee, and Dr. John Chiu in May 2001

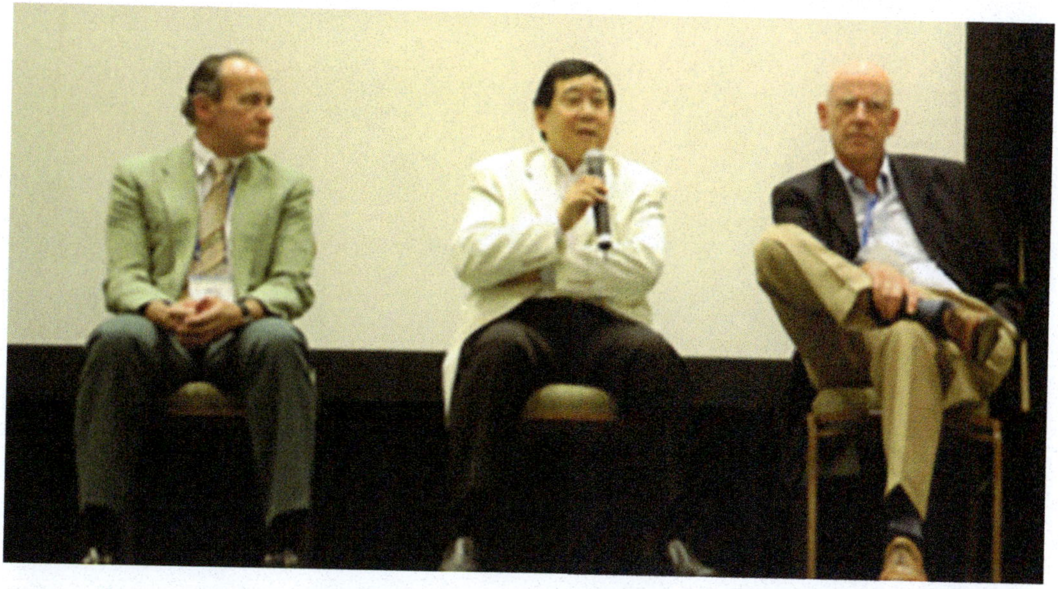

Fig. 1.3 Dr. Martin Knight, Dr. Anthony Yeung, and Dr. Thomas Hoogland (in order from the left)

Wooridul Spine Hospital (WSH) in South Korea [26]. Dr. Martin Knight developed safety in endoscopic laser foraminoplasty and discovered that the main cause of lower back pain is direct touching of the neural structures of foraminal anatomy through communication with his patients during his live surgeries [27]. His endoscopic laser surgery is called the "outside-in technique." Dr. Thomas Hoogland developed the "outside-in" technique with foraminoplasty by a reamer for sequestrectomy [28]. In 1996, Dr. Anthony Yeung developed Yeung Endoscopic Spine System (YESS) by remodeling the German-made Wolf's endoscope for prostate surgery [25]. He also invented the laser-assisted "inside-out technique' in 1997 [29]. From 1991, Dr. Sang-Ho Lee started to remove disc particles, "fragments," using the Ho:YAG laser in combination with endoscopy and called it "intra-annular subligamentous fragmentectomy." During the fragmentectomy, only the fragments are removed, while the normal portion of the nucleus pulposus is preserved because the trajectory is via the annulus fibrosus under the posterior longitudinal ligament and not toward the center of the disc. So, it can save the cushioning function of the disc and its height. At the American Minimally Invasive Surgery Conference held in 2000, Dr. Martin Knight, Dr. Anthony Yeung, and Dr. Sang-Ho Lee introduced their techniques respectively (Fig. 1.3).

Endoscopic laser repairs annular tears, regenerates intervertebral annulus in the disc, and eliminates lower back pain [30]. These endoscopic laser disc surgeries are now widespread worldwide, and in 2018, the US government and academic societies approved medical insurance coverage for endoscopic disc treatment which was initiated by Dr. Parviz Kambin and Dr. Hansjörg Leu with the International Society of Minimally Invasive Spinal Surgery (ISMISS) (Fig. 1.4). At the University of Miami Hospital and the training hospitals of Yale School of Medicine, endoscopic surgery was included in regular spine doctor training program, and in 2019, the North American Spine Society also included this surgery in the formal educational program (Fig. 1.5).

For microscopic surgery as well as endoscopic surgery, lasers are essential to perform better surgery with a smaller incision to preserve the central and anterior disc tissues without a large annulotomy. Lasers are superior to traditional stainless steel surgical instruments such as scalpels, scissors, and forceps. Both hard and soft tissues, including bone, and discs can be precisely

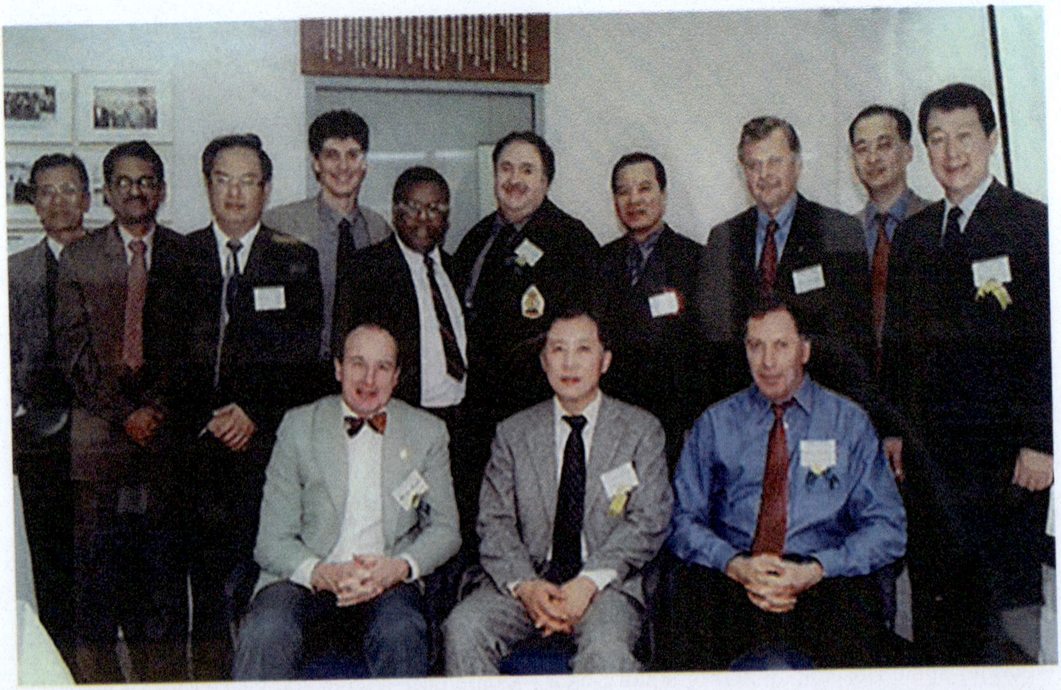

Fig. 1.4 The participants of the Spine Total Care Conference, 2002. Dr. Martin Knight, Dr. Sang-Ho Lee, and Dr. Reuven Gepstein are sitting in the front line (in order from the left)

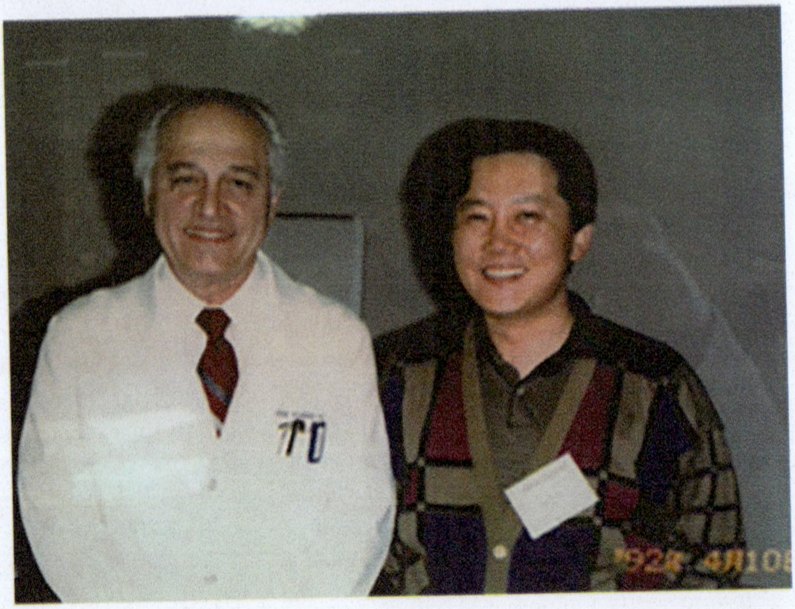

Fig. 1.5 Dr. Parviz Kambin and Dr. Sang-Ho Lee in 1992

cut, removed, well vaporized, and contracted, with much less bleeding during surgery [18, 31]. In addition, almost no edema occurs in the tissue. Laser-based microsurgery can be used for cervical and lumbar disc degeneration, annulus fibrosus surgery, cervical and thoracic posterior longitudinal ligament hypertrophy and ossification [32], cervical spondylosis, and removal of epidural spinal tumors. The low power of milliwatts and delicate energy controllable laser is a powerful weapon capable of accurately and delicately performing difficult operations by accurately aiming and firing under a microscope.

1.2 Summary

The time has come when surgeons who can repair lesions without destruction of normal structures even with a small incision are excellent.

This is thanks to the development of advanced optical technology that allows surgeons to see well even in small incisions, computer-assisted navigation technology that allows surgeons to accurately find lesions without damage to adjacent areas, and advanced laser technology that uses not a stainless steel knife but a very thin knife of light. Minimally invasive spinal surgery using microscopic and endoscopic lasers with saline irrigation with good illumination guides patients to return to their daily lives faster and have a quality of life and time economy [20]. Minimally invasive laser spine surgery is already present now, not in the future.

References

1. Pyogenic infective diseases of the brain and spinal cord: meningitis, abscess of brain, infective sinus thrombosis. Glasgow Med J. 1894;41(1):57–63.
2. Hadra BE. Wiring the spinous processes in Pott's disease. JBJS. 1891;4(1):206–10.
3. Albee FH. Transplantation of a portion of the tibia into the spine for Pott's disease: a preliminary report 1911. Clin Orthop Relat Res. 2007;460:14–6.
4. Hibbs RA. An operation for progressive spinal deformities: a preliminary report of three cases from the service of the orthopaedic hospital. 1911. Clin Orthop Relat Res. 2007;460:17–20.
5. Gallie WE. Fractures and dislocations of the cervical spine. Am J Surg. 1939;46(3):495–9.
6. Harrington PR. The history and development of Harrington instrumentation. Clin Orthop Relat Res. 1973;93:110–2.
7. Yasargil MG, editor. Microsurgical operation of herniated lumbar disc. Berlin, Heidelberg: Springer; 1977.
8. Malis LI. Neurosurgical photography through the microscope. Clin Neurosurg. 1981;28:233–45.
9. Caspar W, editor. A new surgical procedure for lumbar disc herniation causing less tissue damage through a microsurgical approach. Berlin, Heidelberg: Springer; 1977.
10. Lee S-H. Percutaneous cervical discectomy with forceps and endoscopic Ho: YAG laser. Lasers in the musculoskeletal system. Berlin, Heidelberg: Springer; 2001. p. 292–302.
11. Solon LR, Aronson R, Gould G. Physiological implications of laser beams. Science. 1961;134(3489):1506–8.
12. Andrew HR, editor. Theodore Harold Maiman and the invention of laser. New York: Photonics, Devices, and Systems IV; 2008.
13. Lee JH, Lee SH. Clinical and radiographic changes after percutaneous endoscopic cervical discectomy: a long-term follow-up. Photomed Laser Surg. 2014;32(12):663–8.
14. Whipple TL, Caspari RB, Meyers JF. Laser subtotal meniscectomy in rabbits. Lasers Surg Med. 1984;3(4):297–304.
15. CHOY DS. Clinical experience and results with 389 PLDD procedures with the Nd: YAG laser, 1986 to 1995. J Clin Laser Med Surg. 1995;13(3):209–13.
16. Davis J. Early experience with laser disc decompression. A percutaneous method. J Fla Med Assoc. 1992;79(1):37–9.
17. Gottlob C, Kopchok GE, Peng SK, Tabbara M, Cavaye D, White RA. Holmium: YAG laser ablation of human intervertebral disc: preliminary evaluation. Lasers Surg Med. 1992;12(1):86–91.
18. Shin SH, Bae JS, Lee SH, Keum HJ, Jang WS. Transforaminal endoscopic discectomy for hard or calcified lumbar disc herniation: a new surgical technique and clinical outcomes. World Neurosurg. 2020;143:e224–e31.
19. Lee S-H, Gastambide D, editors. Perkutane endoskopische Diskotomie der Halswirbelsäule. Minimal-invasive Verfahren in der Orthopädie und Traumatologie. Berlin: Springer; 2000.
20. Gastambide D, Peyrou P, Lee SH. Discectomia cervicale percutanea. EMC Techniche Chirurgiche Chirurgica Ortopedica. 2005;1(1):1–7.
21. Choi G, Lee SH, Bhanot A, Raiturker PP, Chae YS. Percutaneous endoscopic discectomy for extraforaminal lumbar disc herniations: extraforaminal targeted fragmentectomy technique using working channel endoscope. Spine (Phila Pa 1976). 2007;32(2):E93–9.
22. Choi G, Lee SH, Lokhande P, Kong BJ, Shim CS, Jung B, et al. Percutaneous endoscopic approach for highly migrated intracanal disc herniations by foraminoplastic technique using rigid working channel endoscope. Spine (Phila Pa 1976). 2008;33(15):E508–15.
23. Lee S-H, Ahn Y. Percutaneous endoscopic cervical diskectomy and stabilization. Endoscopic spine surgery and instrumentation. New York: Thieme; 2005. p. 59–65.
24. Knight MT, Vajda A, Jakab GV, Awan S. Endoscopic laser foraminoplasty on the lumbar spine-early experience. Minim Invasive Neurosurg. 1998;41(1):5–9.
25. Yeung AT. Minimally invasive disc surgery with the Yeung Endoscopic Spine System (YESS). Surg Technol Int. 1999;8:267–77.
26. Lee S, Lee S, Park K, Lee I, Sung K, Kim J, et al. Comparison of percutaneous manual and endoscopic

laser diskectomy with chemonucleolysis and automated nucleotomy. Der Orthopade. 1996;25(1):49–55.
27. Savitz MH, Savitz MH, Chiu JC, Yeung AT. The practice of minimally invasive spinal technique. Lima: Wyndham Hall Press; 2005.
28. Schubert M, Hoogland T. Endoscopic transforaminal nucleotomy with foraminoplasty for lumbar disk herniation. Operative Orthopadie Traumatologie. 2005;17(6):641–61.
29. Lewandrowski KU, León JFR, Yeung A. Use of "inside-out" technique for direct visualization of a vacuum vertically unstable intervertebral disc during routine lumbar endoscopic transforaminal decompression: a correlative study of clinical outcomes and the prognostic value of lumbar radiographs. Int J Spine Surg. 2019;13(5):399–414.
30. Ahn Y, Lee SH. Outcome predictors of percutaneous endoscopic lumbar discectomy and thermal annuloplasty for discogenic low back pain. Acta Neurochir. 2010;152(10):1695–702.
31. Lee SH, Ahn Y, Lee JH. Laser-assisted anterior cervical corpectomy versus posterior laminoplasty for cervical myelopathic patients with multilevel ossification of the posterior longitudinal ligament. Photomed Laser Surg. 2008;26(2):119–27.
32. Seokjin K, Junseok B, Sang-Ho L. Transthoracic microsurgical anterior decompression without fusion for ossification of the posterior longitudinal ligament in the thoracic spine. J Neurosurg Spine. 2020;2020:1–9.

Physics and General Principle of Spinal Laser

2

Shin-Jae Kim and Junseok Bae

Abstract

The word LASER stands for Light Amplification by Stimulated Emission of Radiation. The use of laser in spine surgery is not yet more widespread compared to other medical fields. However, there is a great advantage of minimizing damage to surrounding normal structures including nerve tissues when surgery is performed using a laser. Currently, CO_2 laser is used when performing discectomy using a microscope, and holmium YAG (Ho:YAG) laser and neodymium-doped YAG (Nd:YAG) laser are used when performing discectomy using an endoscope. With the diversification of media and the development of laser machines, various types of lasers are being developed, so we look forward to the day when they will be applied to and develop the spine surgery.

Keywords

Laser · CO_2 laser · Holmium YAG laser · Neodymium-doped YAG laser · Percutaneous laser disc decompression · Laser spine surgery

2.1 Introduction

The word LASER stands for Light Amplification by Stimulated Emission of Radiation. Lasers began to develop on the basis of the concept of induced emission mentioned in Albert Einstein's paper on the quantum theory of radiation in 1917. After Theodore H. Maiman first succeeded in the 694 nm ruby laser in 1960, the term laser was established, and there was a great advance in lasers thereafter. Currently, lasers are clinically applied to medical instruments, mainly in dermatology, plastic surgery, otorhinolaryngology, and urology, and are used in various ways. However, the use of laser in spine surgery is not yet more widespread compared to other medical fields. In this chapter, the basic principles of laser and the reason why laser is applied clinically to the spine surgery field will be described. Then, the CO_2 laser, holmium YAG (Ho:YAG) laser, and neodymium-doped YAG (Nd:YAG) laser, which are currently mainly used in spine surgery, will be described briefly.

2.2 Basic Laser Physics

The laser basically consists of four parts: (1) external energy source, (2) medium, (3) optical cavity, and (4) delivery system that delivers the laser to the treatment site (Fig. 2.1).

S.-J. Kim · J. Bae (✉)
Department of Neurosurgery, Chungdam Wooridul Spine Hospital, Seoul, Republic of Korea

J. Bae, S.-H. Lee (eds.), *Laser Spine Surgery*, https://doi.org/10.1007/978-981-16-2206-9_2

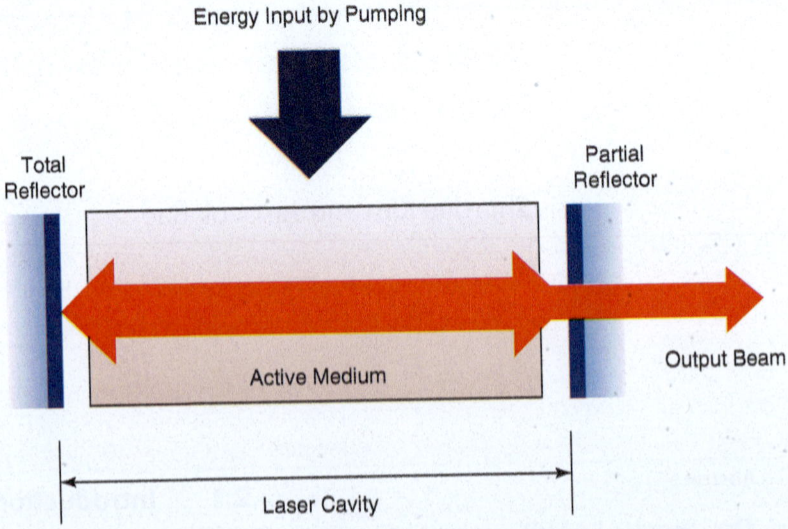

Fig. 2.1 Basic components of a laser

1. Energy source

   To make a laser, there must be several types of external energy sources such as flashlamps, electric currents, and semiconductors. The energy source stimulates atoms of a medium composed of solid, liquid, gas, etc. to emit photons of a certain wavelength, and some of the photons thus formed stimulate other atoms. These actions consist of a chain reaction, and a special light energy amplified in a short time is created.

2. Medium

   As a solid medium, ruby, alexandrite, Nd:YAG, and Nd-glass are currently widely used. Liquid media include dyes such as rhodamine, while gas media include argon, He-Ne, CO_2, excimer, metal, vapor, etc. Recently, semiconductors such as diode lasers are often used. They are contained in an optical cavity called a head or tube. Depending on the medium used, the laser is named, and it has several wavelengths such as ultraviolet, visible, and infrared.

3. Optical cavity

   Since the optical cavity containing the medium has mirrors installed parallel to both ends, it acts to reflect photons emitted from the medium. The reflected photons continuously stimulate the medium, causing a chain reaction. One side of the optical cavity is equipped with a mirror that does not transmit light but only reflects, and the other side is equipped with a partial transmission mirror that transmits only light in a certain direction.

4. Delivery system

   The amplified light is emitted through delivery devices such as articulated arm, fiber optics, micromanipulator, and fiber laser to reach the target. The laser has monochromaticity, uniform collimation, and coherent characteristics with a single wavelength. In addition, it has a characteristic that it can temporarily show strong brightness and focus the force on the lesion to be treated.

A laser medium inside a laser cavity consisted with two mirrors—one highly reflective (HR) and one semitransparent—and an energy source, which can be electricity, radio frequency, flashlamp, or laser light. The laser medium consists of atoms, which contain electrons that orbit the nucleus in a stable state. When the energy from the energy source is pumped into the laser medium, the electrons are excited to a higher-energy orbit. By nature, excited electrons are compelled to return to their stable states. As this occurs, the electrons release energy in the form of a light particle called a photon. A released photon sets off a chain reaction, called stimulated emission, in which the photon (as an energy source) excites atoms it encounters, causing them to release photons as well. When stimulated emission is established between two mirrors, the effect is amplified. Photons that escape via the semitransparent mirror produce a coherent, collimated, monochromatic laser beam.

Currently, there are many types of lasers so far, but basically they are in common with the principle of selective photopyrolysis (using an appropriate amount of laser of an appropriate wavelength to destroy only a specific tissue while preserving surrounding tissues). Most medical lasers are designed to control power and pulse length. In general, the length of the pulse is as important as the wavelength or output of the laser. The laser is operated in continuous or pulsed mode. Continuous mode irradiates a continuous beam, which may cause burns if the heat dissipation time is exceeded. Pulse types are classified into long pulse, short pulse, or Q switch mode, and Q switch accumulates energy between each pulse for instantaneous output of high energy.

2.3 The Utility of Laser Application in Spinal Surgery

The advantages of laser in spinal surgery are as follows:

1. Minimizing pain: Pain is caused by injury where there are nerve receptors. By using laser, the surgeon can minimize injury of the normal structures.
2. Minimizing recovery time: Recovery time is impacted by complications that occur during the procedure, like large incisions, open blood vessels, and unintended injury to vital organs. The surgeon can minimize the contributions to these complications (cauterize vessels, control energy around vital organs).
3. Reducing procedure time: Procedure time increases when there are access issues, bleeding that has to be managed, preparation required to protect vital organs, and a constant exchange of multiple instruments to cut, coagulate, and retrieve. Laser can improve access, control bleeding, control energy around vital organs, and combine surgical function.

2.4 The Principle of the Laser in the Treatment of PLDD

Percutaneous laser disc decompression (PLDD) is a type of surgery that relieves pain by inserting a laser probe into the intervertebral disc space by an endoscope or shooting the laser directly by the microscope and applying laser energy to achieve decompression and nerve control [1, 2]. PLDD is a minimally invasive procedure aiming to significantly reduce the patient's pain and recover from neurological deficit [3]. A certain amount of heat is sent by a laser with an absorbed energy coefficient adjusted for soft disc tissue, allowing the water to evaporate from the disc without additional thermal damage, achieving decompression, and creating a stable inner disc scar. With the development of laser technology, lasers using many new media have been developed. However, until now, the use of laser in the spine field is very limited. Currently, CO_2 laser is used for discectomy using a microscope, and Ho:YAG laser is mainly used for PLDD using an endoscope [4, 5]. Figure 2.2 compares the wavelengths of the three lasers. Laser absorption and tissue penetration power is compared in Fig. 2.3. Since the degree of penetration is different for each laser, the types of lasers that can be applied as surgical devices are limited. For example, Ho:YAG laser ablates soft tissue such as disc material and hard tissue such as osteophytes [6]. Therefore, the low penetration of the Ho:YAG laser makes it the ideal instrument for the laser spine surgery.

2.5 CO_2 Laser

The carbon dioxide (CO_2) laser was first introduced in 1964 by Patel and has been widely used in the next two decades as an incision tool in many surgical fields, including neurosurgery [7]. In 1984, it was approval by the US Food and Drug Administration (FDA), making the medical use of lasers more common. Currently, the CO_2 laser is considered an indispensable part of diagnostic and therapeutic equipment. The CO_2

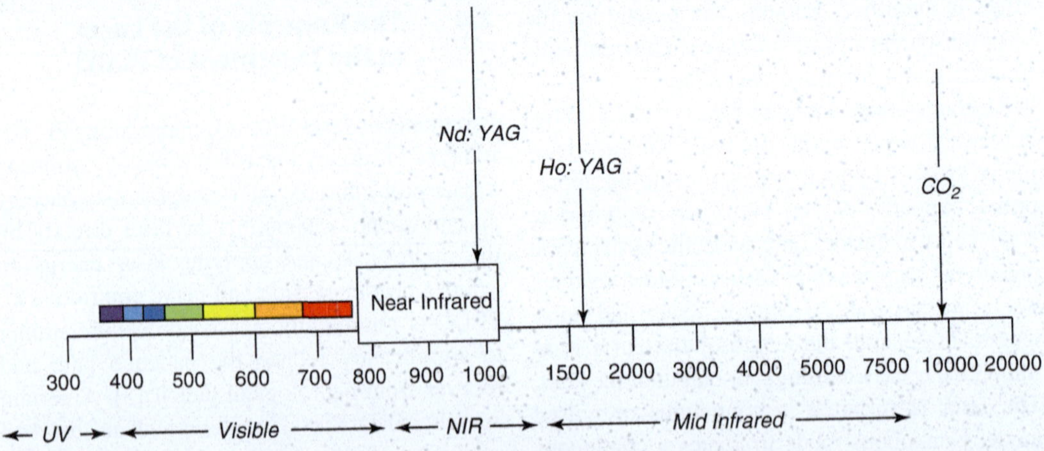

Fig. 2.2 Wavelength of three lasers (CO_2, Ho:YAG, Nd:YAG)

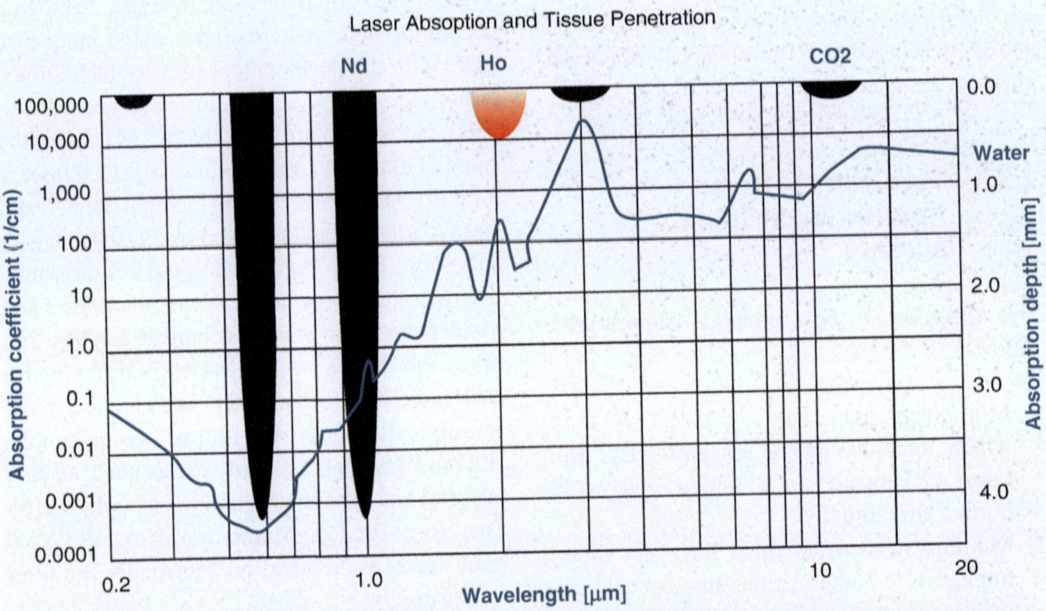

Fig. 2.3 Laser absorption and tissue penetration power of three lasers (CO_2, Ho:YAG, Nd:YAG)

laser produces an infrared beam light with the principal wavelength bands centering at 10,600 nanometers (Fig. 2.4). Collisional energy transfer between the nitrogen and the carbon dioxide molecule has sufficient efficiency to induce oscillatory excitation of the carbon dioxide to induce the desired population inversion necessary for laser operation [8]. The CO_2 laser machine is docked with the microscope to elaborately irradiate the laser beam on the micro field (Fig. 2.5).

CO_2 lasers are attracting attention as cutting tools. They can seal lymphatic and blood vessels less than 0.5 mm, and it can reduce intraoperative bleeding and postoperative swelling. CO_2 lasers emit longer wavelengths than those transmitted by other types of lasers. The penetration depth of CO_2 laser (0.03 mm) is very safe (Fig. 2.6). Coagulation of small blood vessels and sealing of lymphatic, small peripheral nerves have been reported in experimental studies using CO_2 lasers. This sealing alleviates postoperative pain.

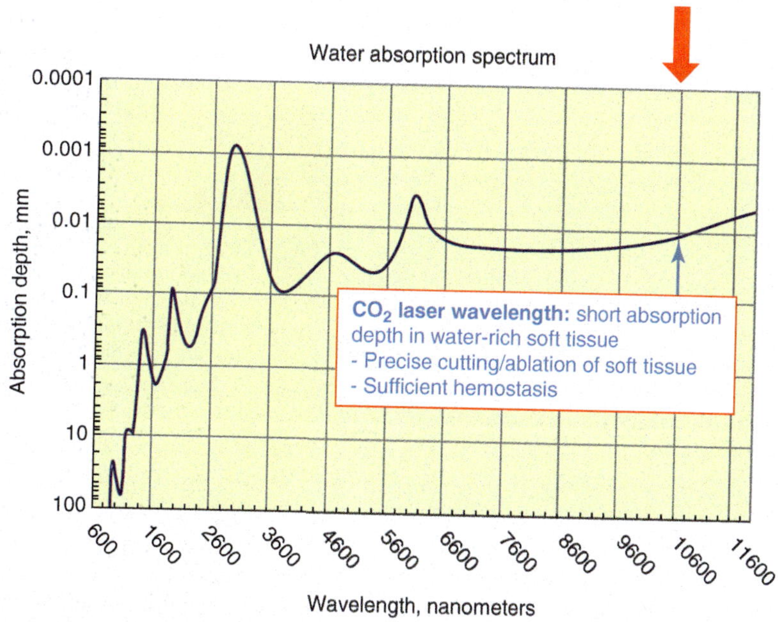

Fig. 2.4 Water absorption spectrum of CO_2 laser

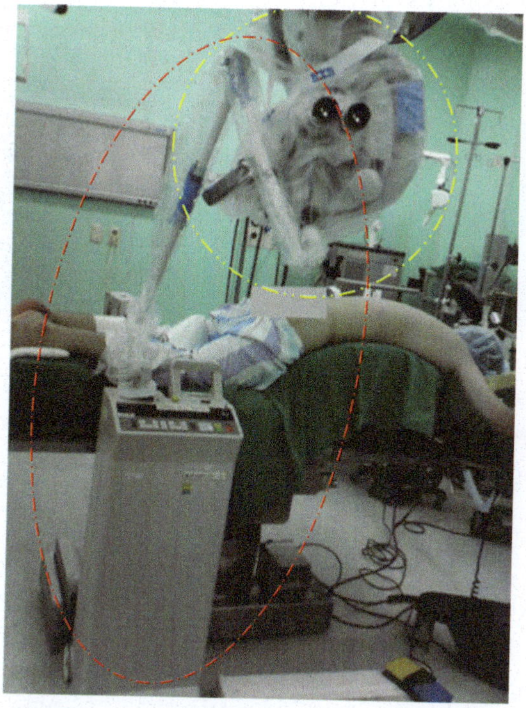

Fig. 2.5 CO_2 laser device docked with the microscope

The CO_2 laser also reduces intraoperative bleeding and postoperative swelling, providing more comfort for patients and facilitating the postoperative wound healing process. The boundary between the tissue subject to heat damage and the surrounding intact tissue is very well defined. The CO_2 laser can evaporate through the surrounding tissue without physical force, sealing blood vessels and minimizing bleeding. Therefore, it is useful when bloodless observation is required during surgery. It can also sterilize wounds caused by hot evaporation of tissue lesions. The downside is that the equipment is expensive, the operator takes time to get used to, and the sophisticated operation is technically difficult. So, more repetitions are required to gain the necessary experience and practice. There is a risk of fire if the laser is used improperly. It can also damage the cornea. Therefore, it is necessary to protect the eyes of the surgeon and the patient. The gases released by the vaporization of tissues contain excess CO_2 or viral particles, which can be harmful to the human body.

2.6 Holmium:YAG (Ho:YAG) Laser

Currently, Ho:YAG is the most commonly used laser for ablation therapy. The Ho:YAG laser has been accepted as the safest laser because of its low tissue penetration [9]. The near-infrared

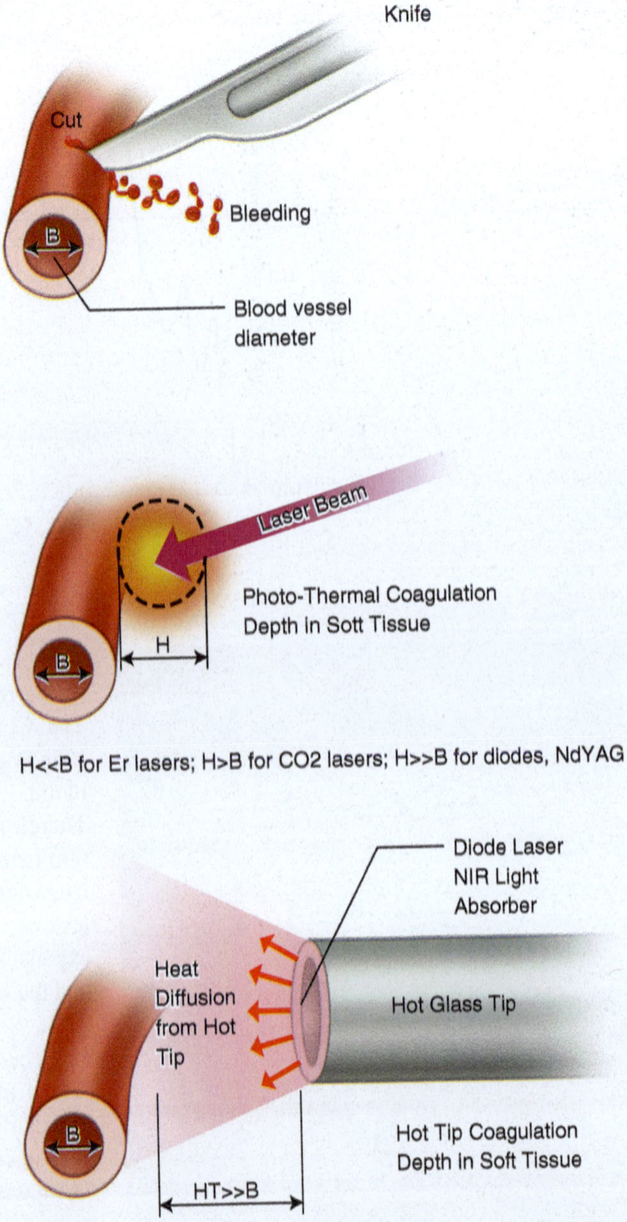

Fig. 2.6 The penetration depth of CO_2 laser compared with scalpel

(2100 nm) (Fig. 2.7) Ho:YAG laser has wavelengths that are substantially absorbed by water, an advantage for endoscopic ablation of soft tissue while protecting deeper structures. Endoscopy has been steadily developed for the treatment of patients with lumbar disc herniation since Kambin and Schaffer first introduced it. The 7 mm inner diameter percutaneous endoscope, which is currently mainly used, can obtain a wider endoscopic field of view, and the introduction of the Ho:YAG laser has dramatically improved the spinal endoscopic procedure.

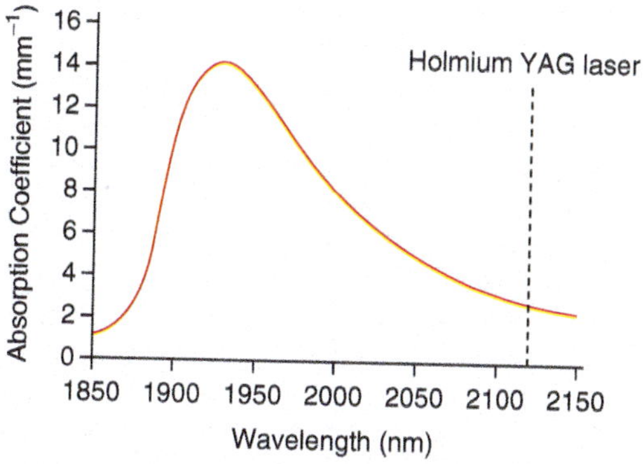

Fig. 2.7 Wavelength and absorption coefficient of Ho:YAG laser

Ho:YAG laser is mainly used for endoscopic treatment such as intervertebral disc herniation. With the continuous physiological saline permeation, it is possible to penetrate the tissue of 0.3 mm under and effectively excise, remove, or vaporize it. The risk of damage to the surrounding normal tissue and nervous tissue is extremely low, and it is transmitted through an optical fiber cable. The effect is enhanced in a water medium, which concentrates the energy within an air bubble formed where the laser contacts the tissue.

2.7 Neodymium-Doped YAG (Nd:YAG) Laser

The Nd:YAG laser, which was introduced earlier than was the Ho:YAG laser, was not used for deep tissue penetration. However, the Nd:YAG laser can also provide shallow tissue penetration by adjusting its wavelength just like the Ho:YAG laser [10]. The advantages of using the Nd:YAG laser include easier laser control, a smaller manufacturing fee, and equivocal effectiveness [11]. To the best of our knowledge, there has been no report on the use of a 1414 nm Nd:YAG laser for intraspinal use. The purpose of this study was to investigate the efficacy and safety of epiduroscopic laser ablation with the 1414 nm Nd:YAG laser. Nd:YAG is a crystal that is used as a lasing medium for solid-state lasers. At an earlier stage of development are lasers based on Ho:YAG and erbium YAG. Again these offer outputs at longer wavelengths of 1.6 and 2.9 micrometer, respectively.

2.8 Summary

The concept of laser-based PLDD in spine surgery has not yet been widely known. However, there is a great advantage of minimizing damage to surrounding normal structures including nerve tissues when surgery is performed using a laser. Currently, CO_2 laser is used when performing discectomy using a microscope, and Ho:YAG laser and Nd:YAG laser are used when performing discectomy using an endoscope. With the diversification of media and the development of laser machines, various types of lasers are being developed, so we look forward to the day when they will be applied to and develop the spine surgery.

References

1. Ahn Y, Lee U. Use of lasers in minimally invasive spine surgery. Expert Rev Med Devices. 2018;15(6):423–33.
2. Boult M, Fraser RD, Jones N, Osti O, Dohrmann P, Donnelly P, et al. Percutaneous endoscopic laser discectomy. Aust N Z J Surg. 2000;70(7):475–9.
3. Radcliff K, Vaccaro AR, Hilibrand A, Schroeder GD. Lasers in spine surgery. JAAOS. 2019;27(17):621–32.
4. Casper GD, Hartman VL, Mullins LL. Results of a clinical trial of the holmium:YAG laser in disc decompression utilizing a side-firing fiber: a two-year follow-up. Lasers Surg Med. 1996;19(1):90–6.
5. Casper GD, Mullins LL, Hartman VL. Rapid communication: laser-assisted disc decompression: a clinical trial of the holmium: YAG laser with side-firing fiber. J Clin Laser Med Surg. 1995;13:27–32.
6. Hafez M, Coombs R, Zhou S, McCarthy I. Ablation of bone, cartilage, and facet joint capsule using Ho:YAG laser. J Clin Laser Med Surg. 2002;20(5):251–5.
7. Dumitras DC. CO_2 laser: optimisation and application. Măgurele: National Institute for Laser Plasma and Radiation Physics; 2012.
8. Witteman WJ. The CO_2 laser. Berlin: Springer; 2013.
9. Moon BJ, Lee HY, Kim KN, Yi S, Ha Y, Shin DA. Experimental evaluation of percutaneous lumbar laser disc decompression using a 1414 nm Nd:YAG laser. Pain Phys. 2015;18:E1091.
10. Jayasree R, Gupta AK, Bodhey NK, Mohanty M. Effect of 980-nm diode laser and 1064-nm Nd:YAG laser on the intervertebral disc—in vitro and in vivo studies. Photomed Laser Surg. 2009;27(4):547–52.
11. Marguet CG, Sung JC, Springhart WP, L'esperance JO, Zhou S, Zhong P, et al. In vitro comparison of stone retropulsion and fragmentation of the frequency doubled, double pulse Nd:YAG laser and the holmium:YAG laser. J Urol. 2005;173(5):1797–800.

3 Setting Up Lasers in Spine Surgery

Shih Min Lee and Junseok Bae

Abstract

Laser spine surgery has made numerous advances over the past few decades. This has helped many patients to be free from pain. Through laser surgery in spinal disease treatment, surgeries have been carried out with advantages at lumbar radiculopathy, lumbar discogenic back pain, recurrent herniation of lumbar disc, cervical foraminotomy, removal of ossification of the posterior longitudinal ligament (OPLL), and lumbar discal cyst. This has advantages such as reduction of intraoperative bleeding, reduction of edema after surgery, clean incision window, and reduction of postoperative inflammation.

Although operating room (OR) settings for laser surgery are similar to conventional open approaches in many respects, additional equipment such as laser machine, microscope, endoscope, video monitor, C-arms, and O-arms require additional space and must be arranged to optimize the flow of work.

This chapter reviews the general concept of OR layout, laser machine, setting of machine, and equipment placement to help many physicians who want to know how to use the laser machine in their field and it will be some guidance when they perform the setting of laser in their operating room.

S. M. Lee · J. Bae (✉)
Department of Neurosurgery, Chungdam Wooridul Spine Hospital, Seoul, Republic of Korea

Keywords

Operating room setting · Laser machine · CO_2 laser · Holmium:YAG laser

3.1 General Operating Room Layout

The basic design of an operating room begins with a rectangular space of ~20 × 20 feet, although a larger size of around 30 × 30 feet would be preferable to take a wider variety of laser procedures such as open microscopic surgery or endoscopic procedures. The room should have adequate ventilation channels with temperature control and adequate storage space for surgical utility items. To prevent the growth of unwanted infectious organisms, the laminar airflow system should be required.

3.2 Laser Spine Surgery Equipment

The arrangement of equipment in the operating room is a very important step for operation. Several equipment which are required for laser spine surgery are as follows which are also mentioned for other endoscopic spinal procedures or minimally invasive spinal surgeries:

J. Bae, S.-H. Lee (eds.), *Laser Spine Surgery*, https://doi.org/10.1007/978-981-16-2206-9_3

- Operating table: A radiolucent table is essential for successful spinal surgery even for laser surgery.
- Laser machine:
  - Holmium:YAG laser
  - Nd:YAG laser
  - Carbon dioxide laser
- Fluoroscope: C-arm or O-arm.
- Radiofrequency generator.
- Microscope.
- Endoscopy cart: This cart contains a video monitor, a light source, a recording device, and an irrigation pump.
- Motorized high-speed drill console.
- Anesthesia table: This is equipped with infusion pump, emergency medications and pulse monitor, and oxygen saturation, blood pressure, and electrocardiographic monitor.
- Irrigation fluid stand for endoscopic procedures.
- Computer console for easy access of the patient's information such as radiographic images.

Several equipment should be arranged to suit for optimal flow work of the entire surgical team. The surgical table should be located in the middle of the operating room and be able to verify the radiographic images during surgery by enabling radiolucent transmission. The operating table should be tailored to the convenience of the surgeon by allowing sufficient bending and up-and-down motion. Then, anesthesia machines and microscopes are placed above the patient's head. The anesthesia machine should be held in a position where motion is not required during surgery, and it is important that the connection to the intubation tube is never lost by keeping it not too far from the patient.

For the open microscopic surgical approach, the position of the microscope should be adjusted so that the arm can be easily entered in the surgical field. The arms should be set to bend sufficiently so that microscopic surgical vision can be seen from various cranial or caudal angles. And for endoscopic procedures, the endoscopic cart is positioned at the foot end alongside an irrigation fluid stand and laser machine. The laser machine should be located on the head or leg of the patient according to the surgical posture and should be connected to the surgical microscope or endoscope in a sterile manner to be used during surgery (Figs. 3.1 and 3.2).

3.3 Positioning

It is the most important step before performing a surgery; thus, special caution is needed when determining the patient's surgical position. Exact positioning for surgery would allow the surgeon to achieve pathology, reduce intraoperative bleeding, and reduce skin injury. To reduce skin injury related to the surgical positioning, sufficient paddings at pressure point of each joint are essential.

- Prone position

  Prone position is probably the most commonly used position in spinal surgery. Since it allows direct approach to the posterior midline and lateral pathology, it is also used at the laser spine surgery of the thoracolumbar area.

  After intubation and general anesthesia are done, the surgical team determines the position of surgery. When turning the patient from supine position to prone position, the arms are placed sticking to their body and are rotated along the sagittal plane without any resistance of the shoulder joint. The arms are placed at the armboard 90 degrees at the elbow to minimize risk of brachial plexus injury. All pressure points must be carefully padded with special attention paid to the eyes.
- Supine position

  Supine position is not often used in laser surgery areas but is used for endoscopic cervical disc removal or cervical ossification of the posterior longitudinal ligament (OPLL) removal through anterior cervical approach. When doing the supine position, a shoulder roll should be placed between the neck and both shoulders to make the extension position of the cervical spine. If necessary, both arms should be retracted gently for getting the radiological images before and during the sur-

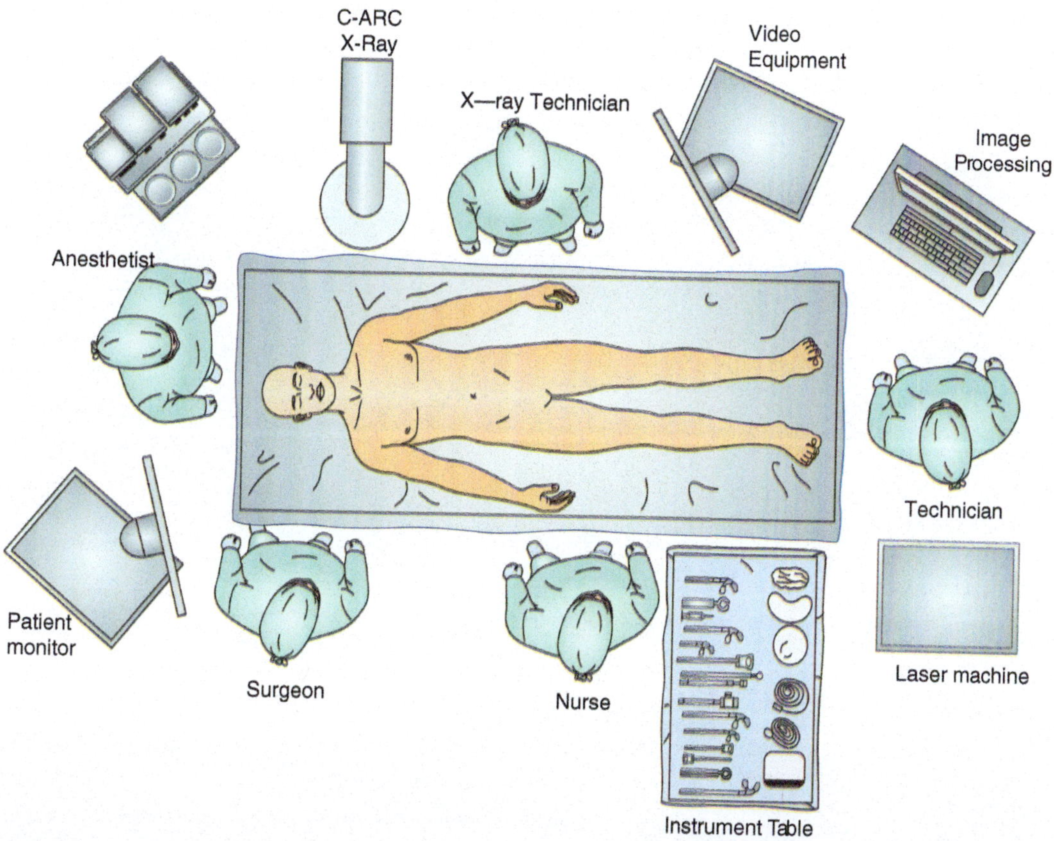

Fig. 3.1 Visual representation of optimal operating suite layout

gery to ensure where the disease levels are. After the surgical position is done, place the sufficient pads on the joints, such as the heel or elbow, to reduce the pressure applied to the skin.

3.4 Laser Machine

For decades, spinal surgery has made constant progress in the field of minimally invasive surgery. Minimally invasive spine surgery has made great advances in its application, from minimally invasive microscopic spinal surgery to endoscopic spinal surgery.

In the process, laser machines that are used for herniated disc removal, tumor removal, or soft tissue incision have expanded along the mainstream of medical advances. There are many kinds of laser machines which are used in medicine, but according to the medium type of lasers, carbon dioxide lasers using gas and neodymium-doped-yttrium-aluminum-garnet (Nd:YAG) or holmium-yttrium-aluminum-garnet (Ho:YAG) lasers using solids have become widely used in spinal surgery areas. The application of these lasers has been chosen according to the method of surgery, and the choice of the machine depends on which lasers surgeons use. There are two categories according to the method of surgery: (1) open microscopic surgery using carbon dioxide laser and (2) endoscopic surgery using mainly Ho:YAG laser (Fig. 3.3).

1. **Open microscopic surgery**

The carbon dioxide laser has been used in many areas as an incision tool since it was announced by Patel in 1964, which was approved by the Food and Drug Administration in the

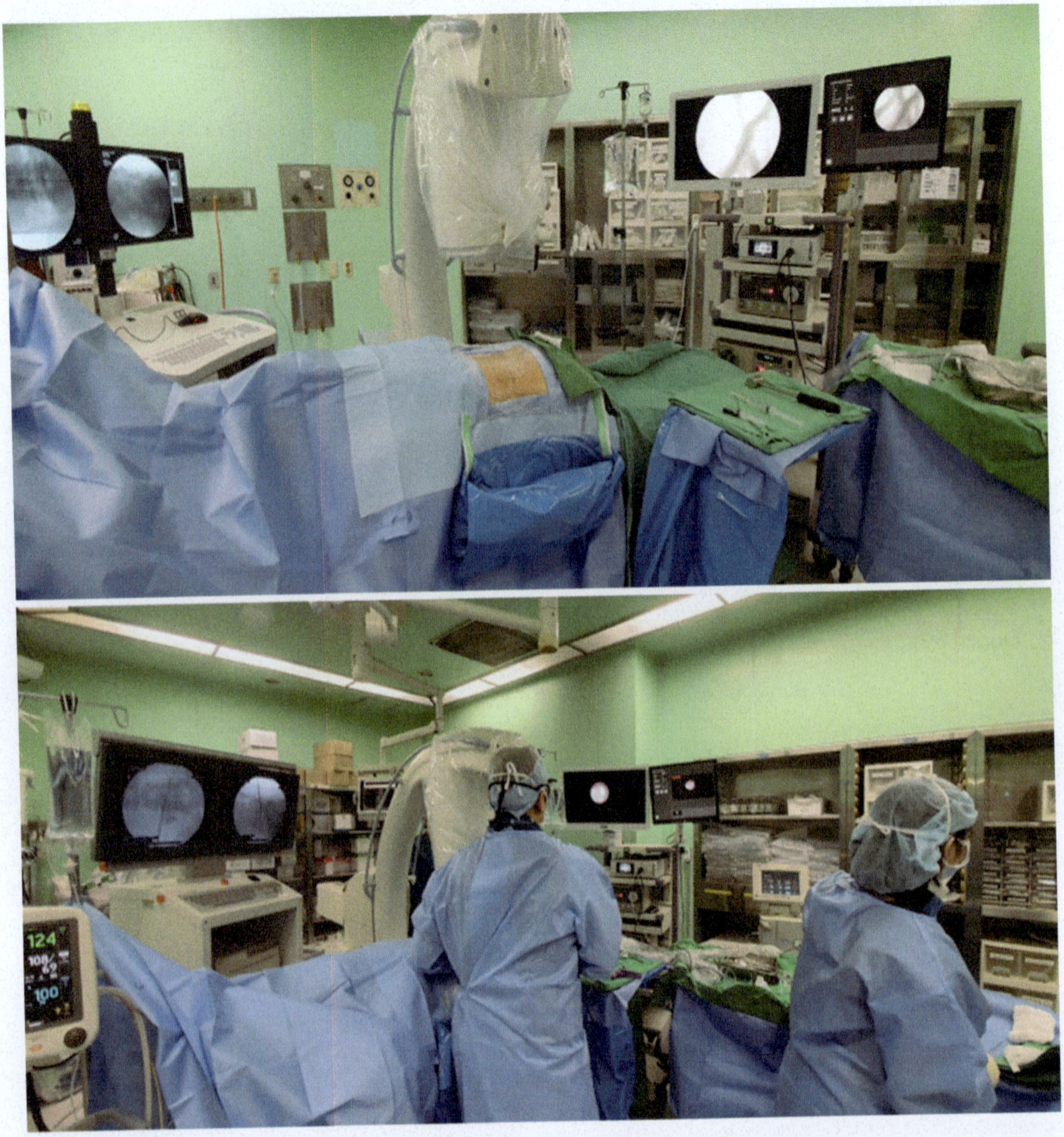

Fig. 3.2 The actual scene during surgery

United States in 1984 and became more commonly used. The carbon dioxide laser shows that lymphatic tissue and blood vessels could be sealed to a thickness smaller than 0.5 mm, reducing intraoperative bleeding or postoperative edema. The carbon dioxide laser machines are mainly used in open microscopic spine surgeries, and the beam of laser devices can be used in microscopic operative view to make precise incision through microscopic attachment that connects the laser machine to the surgical microscope (Fig. 3.4). Before using the laser machine, it is necessary to accurately check whether it is firmly fixed to the floor and the aiming beam has a round and sharp shape. Because surgery requires very gentle manipulation, slight shaking of the machine or scattering of laser aiming beam may cause damage to surrounding tissues. The laser beam can be

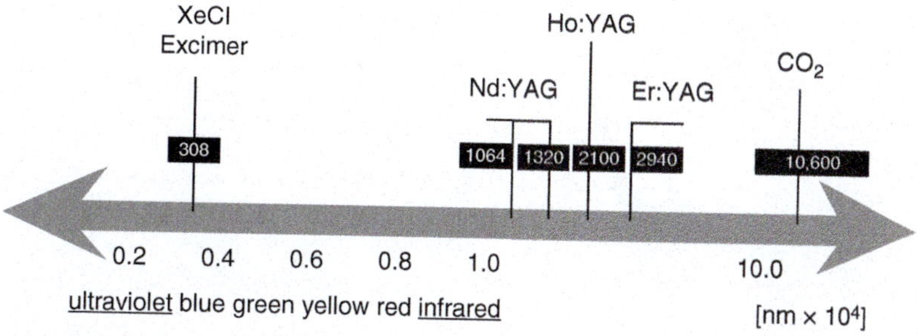

Fig. 3.3 Lasers used in spine surgery and their respective wavelengths. Er:YAG, erbium:yttrium-aluminum-garnet; Ho:YAG, holmium:yttrium-aluminum-garnet; Nd:YAG, neodymium:yttrium aluminum garnet; XeCL excimer, xenon chlorine excimer

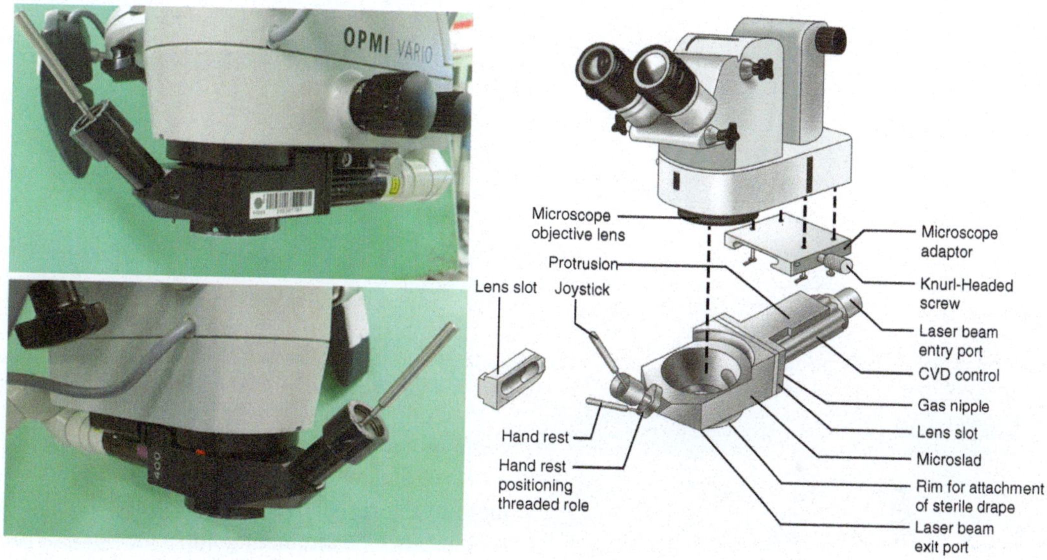

Fig. 3.4 Laser controller and microscope were connected

oriented using a joystick attached to a microscope (Figs. 3.5 and 3.6). The power of the laser beam can be increased to 60 watts depending on the setting of the laser machine, but due to the nature of the spinal surgery, set the power to 20–30 watts. It may cause thermal damage or direct neural injury to the surrounding tissue. The machine makes continuous laser beams that have the character of short-period, high-peak power which transmit the energy to the target tissue with vaporization. Finally, it makes the surgery with lesser retraction injury and shorten surgical dissection time.

2. **Endoscopic surgery**

Ho:YAG laser which is commonly used at endoscopic procedures can transmit energy to tissues like carbon dioxide lasers to minimize damage to surrounding tissues. However, unlike CO_2 lasers, it enables the fiber-optic delivery so that it is suitable for endoscopic laser and has the advantage of enabling laser transmission in liquid-filled spaces for treatment. Many studies have been published that Ho:YAG laser is more efficacious than conventional methods.

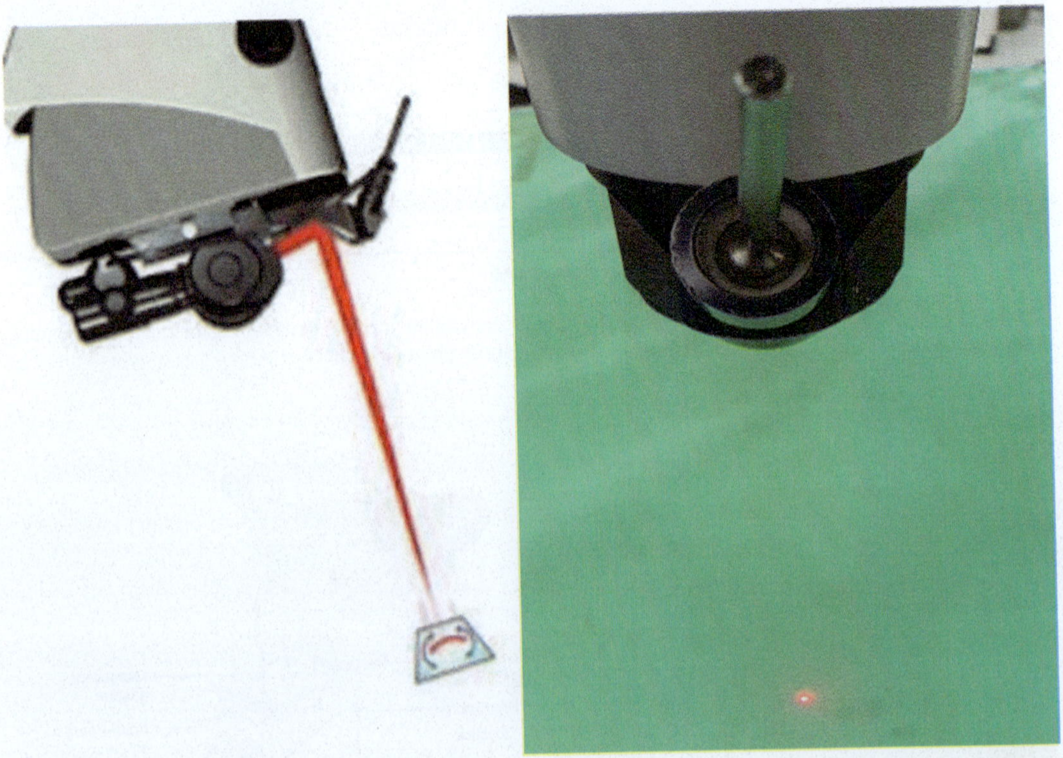

Fig. 3.5 Joystick allows intuitive control

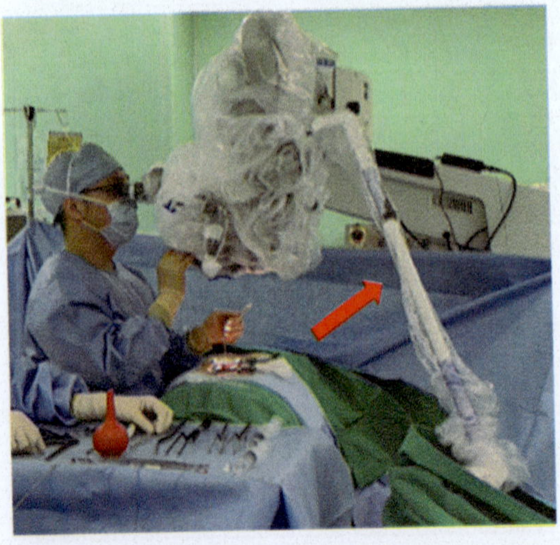

Fig. 3.6 CO_2 laser was connected to the microscope (red arrow). Joystick is being used during surgery

After the draping with sterile manners, the circulating nurse receives from the scrub nurse the cables to the motorized instruments and connects them to the respective control unit of the endoscopic cart. The circulating nurse then passes the camera to the scrub nurse who directs it into the sterile plastic sleeve. And the laser probe is also connected to the base unit in a similar fashion (Fig. 3.7).

The laser tip of endoscopic Ho:YAG is a 90-degree side-firing laser tip fiber with 360-degree rotation capabilities. It provides precise aiming of the beam and easy using and also provides safety with lower risk of anterior structural injury such as large vessels anterior to the vertebral body (Fig. 3.8).

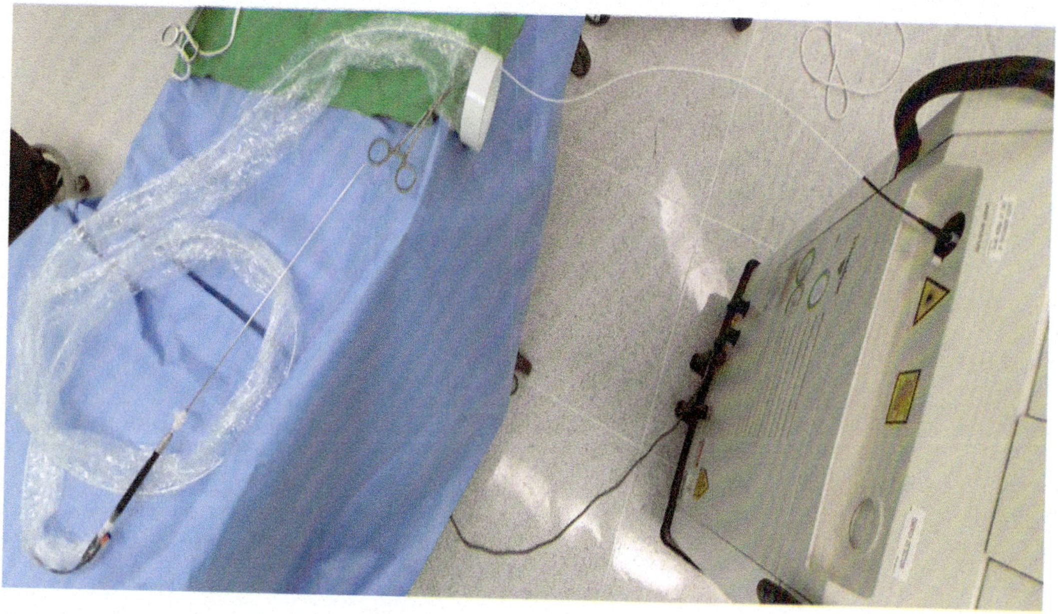

Fig. 3.7 Laser probe was connected to the base unit

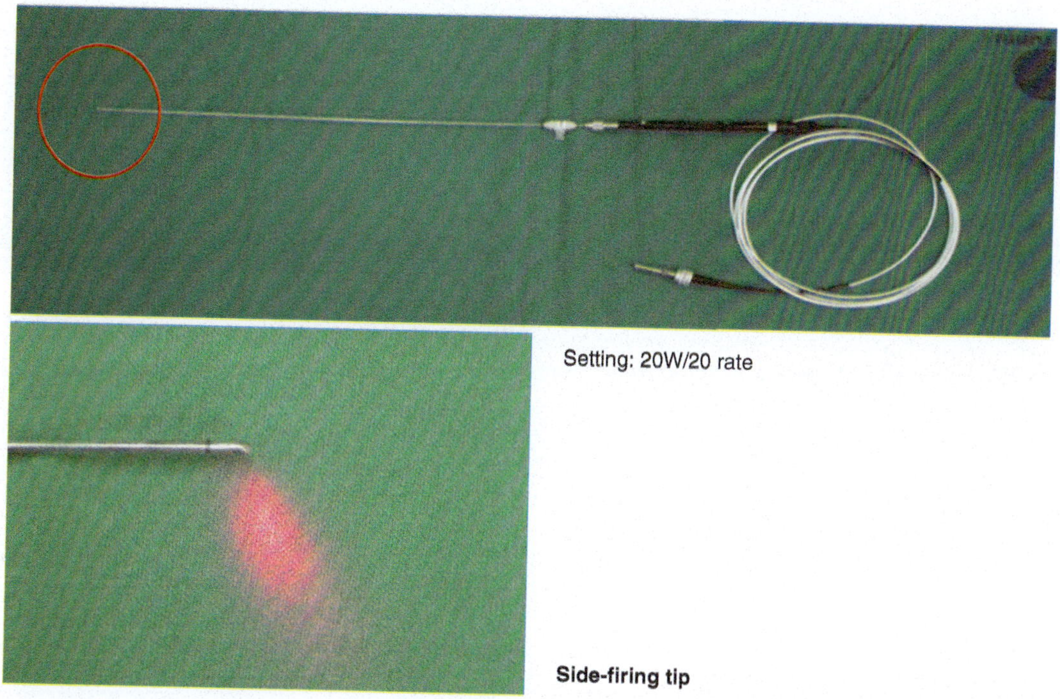

Fig. 3.8 Side-firing laser tip

Anesthetic Consideration of the Laser Spine Surgery

4

Jisang Kim, Gyu Dae Shim, and Junseok Bae

Abstract

It is important to comprehend the anesthetic considerations of laser spine surgery for an exquisite and safe procedure. The type of anesthesia for laser spine surgery is determined by several factors: approach and length of surgery, patient health, and preference of the patient and surgeon. Preoperative evaluation should focus on assessment of the airway and the respiratory, cardiac, and neurologic system. Endoscopic procedures using laser are performed under local anesthesia with sedation, which is favored by both patients and surgeons. There are some considerations for the safe practice of monitored anesthesia care by experienced anesthesiologists.

Keywords

Anesthesia for laser spine surgery · Preoperative evaluation · Intraoperative management · Postoperative care · Awakened sedation

J. Kim · J. Bae (✉)
Department of Neurosurgery, Chungdam Wooridul Spine Hospital, Seoul, Republic of Korea

G. D. Shim
Department of Anesthetic Pain Medicine, Chungdam Wooridul Spine Hospital, Seoul, Republic of Korea

4.1 Introduction

The progression of laser technology in medical use enabled the progression of spine surgery. Considerable advancement in laser technology made spinal surgeries more effective and safe. Hereby, we cannot help emphasizing the importance of anesthesia. It is essential to comprehend the anesthetic considerations of laser spine surgery for an exquisite and safe procedure.

Laser spine surgery includes microscopic and endoscopic procedures. The type of anesthesia for laser spine surgery is determined by several factors: approach and length of surgery, patient health, and preference of the patient and surgeon.

Regarding the traditional microscopic procedure, laser spine surgery is commonly performed under general anesthesia. Patients presenting for spine surgery under general anesthesia are a diverse population undergoing a wide variety of operative procedures and present diverse challenges to the anesthesiologists.

In today's era, when minimally invasive procedures such as endoscopic discectomy have been performed commonly, anesthesiologists must be aware of the various anesthetic techniques for endoscopic spine surgery. Endoscopic procedures with holmium (Ho):YAG or neodymium (Nd):YAG present anesthetic considerations that are distinct from traditional open surgeries. Sedation techniques in combination with local anesthesia can not only reduce hospital day but

J. Bae, S.-H. Lee (eds.), *Laser Spine Surgery*, https://doi.org/10.1007/978-981-16-2206-9_4

also improve patient comfort, safety, and satisfaction during surgery.

In this chapter, preoperative evaluation and intraoperative management will be discussed, which are followed by consideration of awakened sedation with local anesthesia.

4.2 Anesthetic Considerations for General Anesthesia

Preoperative evaluation for laser spine surgery must take into account the medical condition as well as the surgical procedures including the duration and surgical approach.

1. Airway evaluation
   The potential for difficulty in airway management should always be considered, particularly in patients with a cervical or upper thoracic spine problem. A careful assessment should be made for the previous difficulty in intubation, distorted airway anatomy, restriction of neck movement, and the stability of the cervical spine. The anesthesiologist needs to discuss preoperatively the stability of the spine with the surgeon.
2. Pulmonary evaluation
   Patients scheduled for laser spine surgery may have conditions that affect pulmonary function. Elderly patients with degenerative spinal diseases have a risk of pulmonary dysfunction. Depending on the situation and type of procedure, the patient is subjected to various clinical and laboratory tests ranging from bedside pulmonary function evaluation to pulmonary function tests, arterial blood gas analysis, and chest radiograph.
3. Cardiac evaluation
   Cardiac function may be compromised by underlying medical conditions, neuromuscular disorder, rheumatoid arthritis, and the result of the pathology for which spine surgery is being performed. Preoperative cardiac evaluation should take into account both patient factors and the invasiveness of the surgery. Most spine surgery is performed in the prone position, which is associated with a reduction of the cardiac index compared to the supine position. Pulmonary hypertension and congestive heart failure are highly associated with perioperative adverse events after spine surgery, and surveillance for these conditions should be performed in the preoperative cardiac evaluation. It should include an electrocardiography and echocardiography to assess left ventricular function and pulmonary arterial pressures.
4. Neurologic evaluation
   It is not uncommon that patients suffering from spine pathology may present with various grades of neurological deficits ranging from weakness and atrophy of specific muscle groups to paraplegia and quadriplegia. A thorough neurological examination and careful documentation of preexisting neurological deficits are essential. The extent of neurological dysfunction may impact the intubation technique and the choice of neuromuscular blockade.

4.2.1 Monitoring

Standard monitoring used for all patients having general anesthesia includes blood pressure, pulse oximetry, electrocardiogram, end-expired carbon dioxide, and temperature monitoring (Fig. 4.1). Employing a more advanced monitoring technique depends on the patient's medical condition, the expected length of surgery, and the anticipated blood loss. Patients undergoing lengthy procedures that have the potential for large volume shifts and those who have a complicated medical history or hemodynamic instability, invasive blood pressure, central venous pressure, and urine output are monitored. Placement of a pulmonary artery catheter may be required for a patient with severe cardiac or respiratory disease.

4.2.2 Induction

The choice of induction technique, intravenous or inhalation, is guided primarily by the patient's

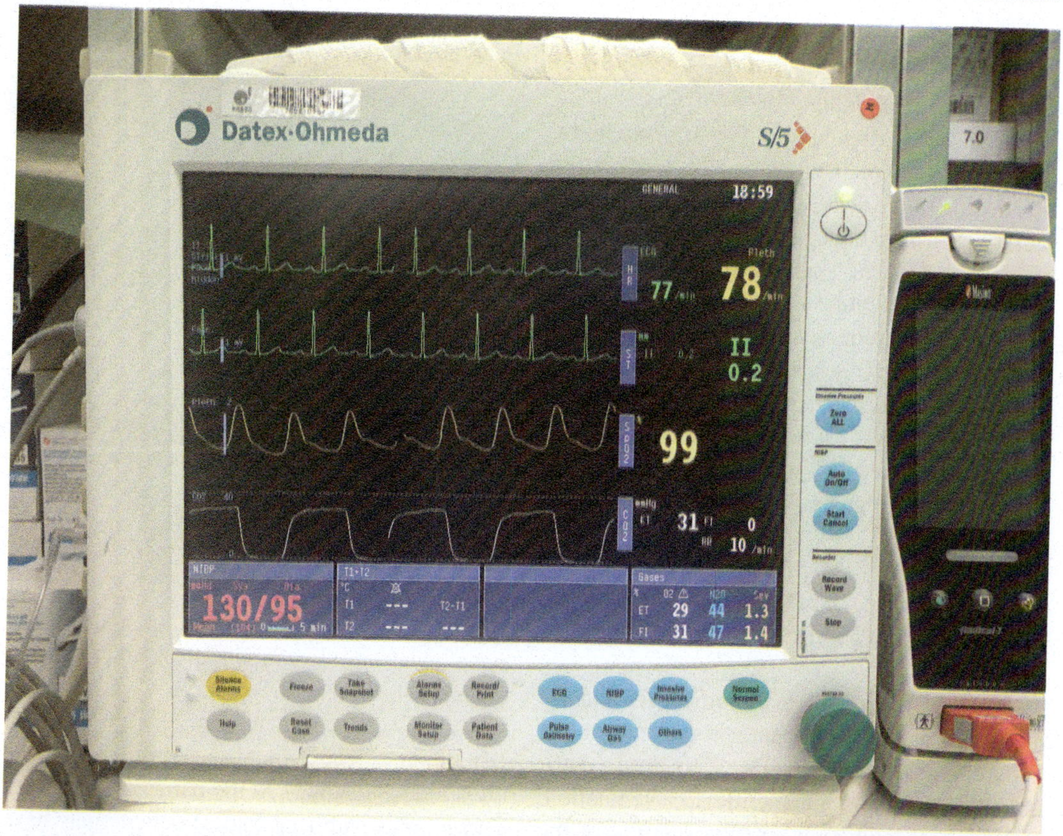

Fig. 4.1 Standard American Society of Anesthesiologists (ASA) monitors applied to the patient include a pulse oximeter, electrocardiography, noninvasive blood pressure device, and a temperature monitor. In addition, the ASA monitoring standards include measurement of end-tidal carbon dioxide, inspired oxygen concentration, and the use of low oxygen concentration and ventilator disconnect alarms

condition and by consideration of the ease with which the trachea may be intubated. Unless there are concerns over the stability of the cervical spine or airway maintenance, intravenous induction is suitable for all but the sickest patients. Any standard technique of intubation is acceptable; the choice is generally determined by the expertise of the clinician and the availability of an airway device. Consider using a wire-reinforced tube to avoid tube kinking and occlusion while turning the patient from supine to prone position. It also allows maximal banding to remove it from the surgical field and prevent compression from cervical surgical procedures.

4.2.3 Positioning

Patient position for laser spine surgery varies depending on the level of the spine to be operated upon and the nature of the planned surgery. A major problem during spine surgery is the maintenance of basic cardiovascular monitoring techniques during the positioning of the patient. This period may represent stress to circulatory integrity, and it is very difficult to prevent an almost total monitoring "blackout" as anesthetized patients are turned from the supine to prone position, which is the most frequently used position in spine surgery.

The goals of positioning are the avoidance of injury to the eyes, peripheral nerves, and bony prominences and maintenance of low venous pressure at the surgical site. While positioning, particular attention should be focused on the positioning of the neck, arms, and eyes to protect pressure-sensitive areas. Patients who have a lateral approach to the spine may be positioned in the lateral decubitus position and require a heightened level of sensitivity to positioning. Regardless of how well a patient is positioned at the start of a procedure, ongoing vigilance concerning position is essential because a patient's situation may change after movement during wakeup test or manipulation of the operating table.

4.2.4 Airway Management

The strategy for airway management for general anesthesia for laser spine surgery depends on the expected degree of difficulty with mask ventilation, supraglottic airway device ventilation, endotracheal intubation, and the stability of the cervical spine. Patients undergoing cervical spine procedures require special consideration for airway management, and they have a high incidence of difficult intubation. The risk of neurologic injury is also more when endotracheal intubation has been attempted in patients suffering from cervical spine disease. In the presence of a recognized unstable cervical spine, a variety of intubation techniques in experienced hands have consistently been shown to be safe and not associated with increased risk of neurologic injury. But there are no outcome studies that support one technique over another. Results of studies of cervical motion and intubation characteristics of different intubation maneuvers suggest potential advantages with fiberoptic laryngoscopy (Fig. 4.2), use of video laryngoscope, and use of inline stabilization for decreasing cervical spine motion during intubation [1, 2]. The use of a rigid color is of no benefit during airway management.

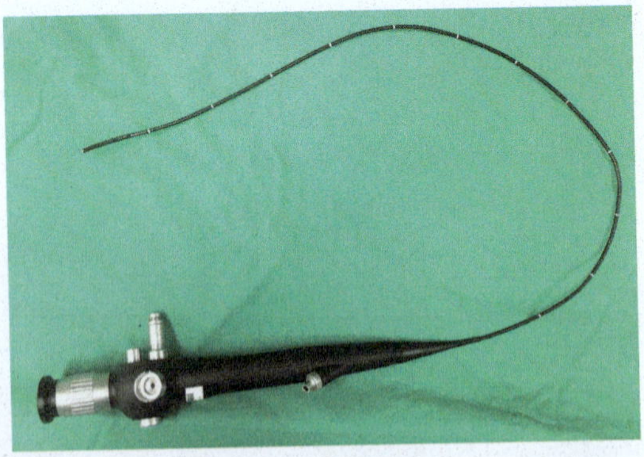

Fig. 4.2 Fiberoptic bronchoscopes are used to facilitate endotracheal intubation via either the nasal or oral route, in the positioning of endotracheal and endobronchial tubes and bronchial blocking devices

4.2.5 Maintenance

A propofol-based intravenous or inhalational technique using a low minimum alveolar concentration of isoflurane or sevoflurane with a remifentanil infusion is generally chosen for laser spine surgery. The maintenance dose of anesthetics is altered as many of the patients with spinal cord injuries and neurological deficits may have altered pharmacokinetics due to muscle wasting, increased volume of distribution, and decreased serum albumin.

The type, duration, and extent of surgery may guide the approach to fluid administration and replacement. It is well agreed that dextrose-containing solution should be avoided because of the risk of worsening neurosurgical outcome in the presence of hyperglycemia during spinal cord ischemia.

4.2.6 Transfusion Management

Major spine surgery can result in significant and occasionally massive blood loss. Surgical procedures involving significant bone work at multiple levels may be associated with large intraoperative blood loss and a higher requirement for transfusion of blood and blood products. Strategies that reduce the risk of allogeneic transfusion include preoperative autologous donation, acute normovolemic hemodilution, perioperative cell salvage techniques, and pharmacologic interventions. Each is similarly effective when used alone to decrease the requirement for transfusion of homologous blood products during major spine procedures as compared to routine transfusion without the use of any autologous blood products. But when combined, strategies decreased the quantity not only of allogeneic red cells transfused but also of other blood products in those patients undergoing reconstructive spinal surgery. Induced hypotension is no longer recommended for patients having spine surgery [3, 4]. Blood loss can be minimized by careful operative positioning, good surgical technique, controlled hypotensive anesthesia, and the use of agents such as antifibrinolytics. The operative position which minimizes abdominal compression has been reported to result in less blood loss and a lower rate of transfusion requirement as compared to the position in which some degree of abdominal compression may occur. In spine surgery, both tranexamic acid and epsilon-aminocaproic acid have been shown to reduce estimated blood loss, the need for transfusion, and the total amount of transfusion when compared to controls [5, 6].

4.2.7 Extubation

The timing of extubation is an important consideration. Retrospective studies have shown a correlation between operative duration, intravascular volume replacement, obesity, and the number of levels of spinal surgery and the decision to delay extubation at the end of surgery [7, 8]. Airway and facial edemas commonly occur during long procedures in the prone position and with the administration of large volumes of intravenous fluid. The patient with significant airway edema is at risk for airway obstruction after extubation. Some select patients may require postoperative care in an intensive care setting. If there is any question about the adequacy of the airway after removal of the endotracheal tube, a conservative approach to extubation should be employed. It is desirable to leave the endotracheal tube in place until the patient is fully awake, responding to the command, and able to manage his/her airway.

4.2.8 Postoperative Care

Postoperative care is individualized for each patient. The preoperative status, surgical procedures, intraoperative complications, and pain tolerance are to be considered in planning postoperative management. Most spinal surgery is painful and good postoperative analgesia is important. Multimodal pain management has been recommended for spine surgery patients. A combination of continuous local anesthetic infiltration or regional anesthesia plus opioids, ketamine, and NSAIDs can be used. Oral or intravenous acetaminophen has also been shown to decrease opioid consumption after major surgery. Adjuvant gabapentin may well also have a role in the multimodal analgesic approach.

4.2.9 Postoperative Complications

In the early postoperative phase, potential complications of spinal surgery include fluid volume deficit, neurologic injury or deficit, dural tear with cerebral spinal fluid leakage, anemia, urinary retention, ileus, atelectasis/pneumonia, and venous thrombosis. Complications specific to anterior cervical procedures include dysphagia, hoarseness, and airway obstruction from edema. Late complications of spine surgeries include skin breakdown, wound infection, spinal instability (after wide lumbar decompressive procedures not accompanied by fusion), hardware failure, pseudoarthrosis, epidural fibrosis, transitional syndrome, and more rarely, arachnoiditis.

Visual loss after spinal surgery is a rare but devastating complication of increasing concern to both surgeons and patients with a reported incidence of 0.017 to 0.1% [9–11]. The major causes of visual loss include ischemic optic neuropathy (ION), central retinal artery occlusion, and retinal vein occlusion. While corneal abrasion is the most common eye injury after spine surgery, it rarely leads to permanent vision problems. ION is a rare (incidence 0.028%) but potentially devastating and untreatable complication of spine surgery particularly that performed with the patient in the prone position. Independent risk factors for the development of ION include male sex, obesity, anemia, use of the Wilson frame (the head lower than the heart), longer anesthetic time, greater estimated blood loss, and lower percent of colloid in the non-blood fluid replacement. All patients undergoing spine surgery should be informed about the low but definite risk of this condition, and every attempt should be made during surgery to maintain stable hemoglobin and mean arterial pressure and to avoid overhydration.

4.3 Awakened Sedation

The endoscopic procedure using the Ho:YAG or Nd:YAG laser is a minimally invasive technique that requires a small skin incision and performed under local anesthesia with or without sedation. Awakened sedation allows a patient to undergo painful procedures with less anxiety by inducing decreased levels of consciousness but not requiring intubation as the patient ventilates spontaneously. A combination of a sedative and an opioid analgesic is most commonly used for this purpose.

The American Society of Anesthesiologists has defined monitored anesthesia care (MAC) as a specific anesthesia service performed by a qualified anesthesia provider, for a diagnostic or therapeutic procedure [12]. MAC is a distinguishable way of sedation from awakened sedation. During the awakened sedation, the surgeon supervises or personally administers the sedative and/or analgesic medications that can alleviate patient anxiety and limit pain during a diagnostic or therapeutic procedure. In MAC, by contrast, the qualified anesthesiologist is focused exclusively and continuously on the patient for any attendant airway, hemodynamic, and physiologic derangements. Further, an anesthesiologist of MAC must be prepared to intervene to rescue a patient's airway from a sedation-induced compromise and convert to general anesthesia. MAC allows for the safe administration of a maximal depth of sedation over that provided during awakened sedation [13].

Comprehensive preoperative patient evaluation is important for a patient undergoing MAC during the minimally invasive endoscopic procedure. Before surgery, the anesthesiologist should review previous medical records of the patient for underlying medical problems; sedation, anesthesia, and surgery history; the history of or sensitivity to anesthesia or sedation; current medications; extremes of age; psychotropic drug use; use of nonpharmaceutical; and family history. Preprocedural laboratory testing is also needed. A preoperative visit should be made by the anesthesiologist responsible for the procedure. The anesthesiologist must evaluate whether the patient is suitable for MAC. And the patient should receive information relating to the benefits and risks of sedatives and analgesics, preprocedural instruction, and medication usage.

Intraoperative monitoring during MAC should be the same as that for general anesthesia. Patients given sedatives or analgesics in unmonitored settings may be at increased risk of complications. It is necessary to monitor ventilation and oxygenation by observation of qualitative clinical signs, capnography, and pulse oximetry as well as hemodynamic measurements including blood pressure, heart rate, and electrocardiography. The patient's level of consciousness should be assessed by the response of patients, including spoken responses to commands or other forms of bidirectional communication during procedures.

After connected to the monitoring equipment, the patient is given 0.5 mg of midazolam intravenously at the start of anesthesia, and continuous infusion of remifentanil is started at the rate of 0.1 μg/kg/min (Fig. 4.3). Another bolus of 0.5 mg of midazolam is administered just before the incision. Regarding the sedative agent, mid-

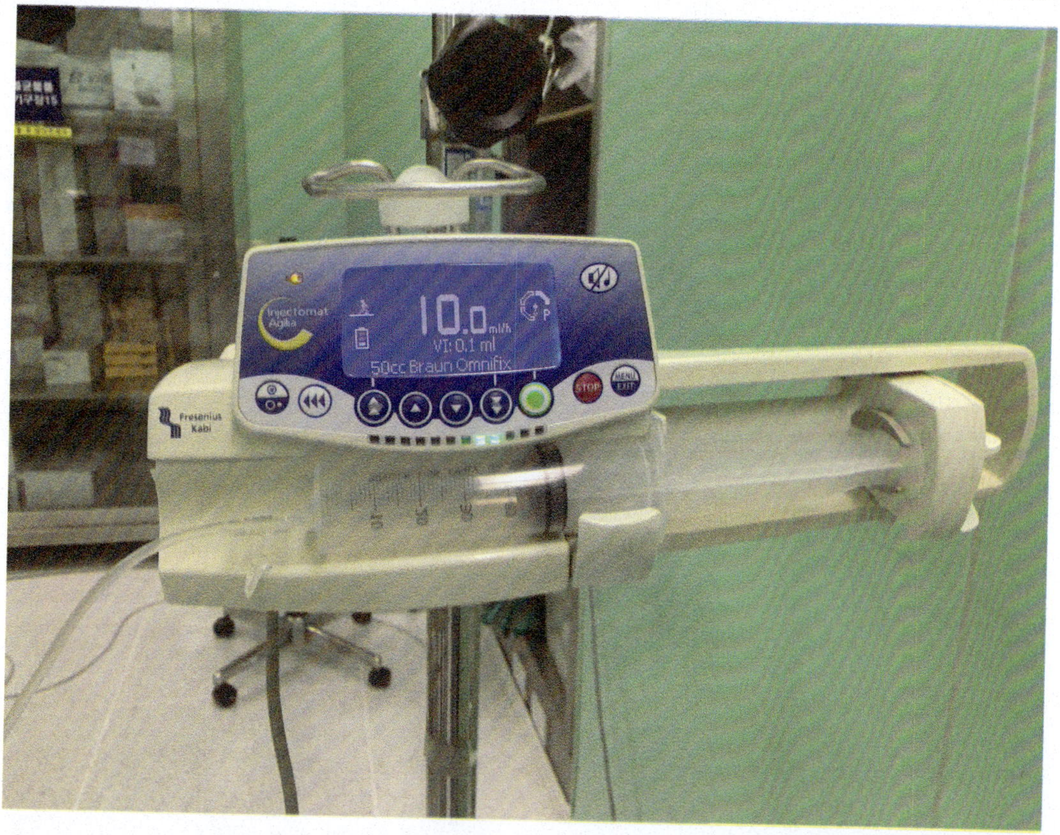

Fig. 4.3 An infusion pump is used to deliver remifentanil continuously in awakened sedation

azolam is favored than propofol which may reduce blood pressure during the procedure. Midazolam has a greater amnesic effect than propofol and can be reversed by flumazenil in case of unintended deep sedation. Supplemental oxygen is administered with a nasal cannula at 5 L/min. During the procedure, the infusion of remifentanil should be stopped immediately if a decrease in oxygen saturation is noted.

After awakened sedation, the patients should be observed and monitored in an appropriately staffed and equipped area until they recover to their baseline level of consciousness and are no longer at increased risk for cardiorespiratory depression. Continuous monitoring of oxygenation is recommended as well until the patients are no longer at risk for hypoxemia. Ventilation and circulation should be checked every 5–15 min until the patients are suitable for discharge. Discharge of the patients should be authorized by the anesthesiologist and surgeon.

References

1. Cohn AI, Zornow MH. Awake endotracheal intubation in patients with cervical spine disease: a comparison of the Bullard laryngoscope and the fiberoptic bronchoscope. Anesth Analg. 1995;81(6):1283–6. https://doi.org/10.1097/00000539-199512000-00027.
2. Watts AD, Gelb AW, Bach DB, Pelz DM. Comparison of the Bullard and Macintosh laryngoscopes for endotracheal intubation of patients with a potential cervical spine injury. Anesthesiology. 1997;87(6):1335–42. https://doi.org/10.1097/00000542-199712000-00012.
3. Walsh M, Devereaux PJ, Garg AX, Kurz A, Turan A, Rodseth RN, et al. Relationship between intraoperative mean arterial pressure and clinical outcomes after noncardiac surgery: toward an empirical definition of hypotension. Anesthesiology. 2013;119(3):507–15. https://doi.org/10.1097/ALN.0b013e3182a10e26.
4. Tse EY, Cheung WY, Ng KF, Luk KD. Reducing perioperative blood loss and allogeneic blood transfusion in patients undergoing major spine surgery. J Bone Joint Surg Am. 2011;93(13):1268–77. https://doi.org/10.2106/JBJS.J.01293.
5. Li G, Sun TW, Luo G, Zhang C. Efficacy of antifibrinolytic agents on surgical bleeding and transfusion

requirements in spine surgery: a meta-analysis. Eur Spine J. 2017;26(1):140–54. https://doi.org/10.1007/s00586-016-4792-x.
6. Soroceanu A, Oren JH, Smith JS, Hostin R, Shaffrey CI, Mundis GM, et al. Effect of Antifibrinolytic therapy on complications, thromboembolic events, blood product utilization, and fusion in adult spinal deformity surgery. Spine. 2016;41(14):E879–86. https://doi.org/10.1097/BRS.0000000000001454.
7. Kwon B, Yoo JU, Furey CG, Rowbottom J, Emery SE. Risk factors for delayed extubation after single-stage, multi-level anterior cervical decompression and posterior fusion. J Spinal Disord Tech. 2006;19(6):389–93. https://doi.org/10.1097/00024720-200608000-00002.
8. Anastasian ZH, Gaudet JG, Levitt LC, Mergeche JL, Heyer EJ, Berman MF. Factors that correlate with the decision to delay extubation after multilevel prone spine surgery. J Neurosurg Anesthesiol. 2014;26(2):167–71. https://doi.org/10.1097/ana.0000000000000028.
9. Patil CG, Lad EM, Lad SP, Ho C, Boakye M. Visual loss after spine surgery: a population-based study. Spine. 2008;33(13):1491–6. https://doi.org/10.1097/BRS.0b013e318175d1bf.
10. Shen Y, Drum M, Roth S. The prevalence of perioperative visual loss in the United States: a 10-year study from 1996 to 2005 of spinal, orthopedic, cardiac, and general surgery. Anesth Analg. 2009;109(5):1534–45. https://doi.org/10.1213/ane.0b013e3181b0500b.
11. Stevens WR, Glazer PA, Kelley SD, Lietman TM, Bradford DS. Ophthalmic complications after spinal surgery. Spine. 1997;22(12):1319–24. https://doi.org/10.1097/00007632-199706150-00008.
12. Anesthesiologists ASo. Position on monitored anesthesia care 2018. Available from https://www.asahq.org/-/media/sites/asahq/files/public/resources/standards-guidelines/position-on-monitored-anesthesia-care.pdf.
13. Anesthesiologists ASo. Distinguishing monitored anesthesia care ("MAC") from moderate sedation/analgesia (conscious sedation) 2018. Available from http://asahq.org/~/media/Sites/ASAHQ/Files/Public/Resources/standards-guidelines/distinguishing-monitored-anesthesia-care-from-moderate-sedation-analgesia.pdf.

Transforaminal Endoscopic Lumbar Discectomy for Paramedian Disc Herniation with Ho:Yag Laser

5

Sang-Ha Shin

Abstract

The main advantage of endoscopic surgery is that it minimizes skin incision, preserves bone and muscle tissue as much as possible, and has less bleeding than incision surgery. Laser has been used in various medical fields since it was discovered in 1958. The authors describe the method of discectomy using Ho:YAG laser after transforaminal approach in paramedian disc herniation and intend to review literature.

Keywords

Lumbar · Endoscopic · Discectomy · Foraminoplasty · Transforaminal

5.1 Introduction

Surgical treatment for degenerative disc disease has been developed from conventional open decompression to minimally invasive spine surgery [1–3]. Among them, endoscopic spine surgery is one of the main minimally invasive spine surgery techniques. After Kambin et al. reported on minimal access surgery in lumbar disc herniation in 1983, endoscopic discectomy has rapidly gained worldwide popularity, due to increased need by patients [4]. This procedure is widely performed by interventional pain physicians as well as by spine surgeons because it requires no general anesthesia or admission to a hospital.

The main advantage of endoscopic surgery is that it minimizes skin incision, preserves bone and muscle tissue as much as possible, and has less bleeding than incision surgery [5]. This makes it possible to quickly return to normal life after surgery. Recent advances in tools for endoscopic treatment such as optics, high-resolution cameras, light sources, high-speed burrs, irrigation pumps, lasers, etc. and new technological advances can provide successful surgical results in patients with spinal disc disease.

Laser has been used in various medical fields since it was discovered in 1958 by Schawlow and Townes [6]. In spinal surgery, Ascher and Heppner first used a CO_2 laser for spinal disc decompression, and it has since been applied to a wider variety of surgery [7]. Ho:YAG laser is mainly used in endoscopic disc treatment. Gottlob et al. performed disc removal in 1992 using a Ho:YAG laser, and now side-firing lasers are popularly used [8]. Side-firing Ho:YAG laser directly removes soft tissue, reduces intradiscal pressure, cuts fibrotic anchorage, and can be used

Supplementary Information The online version of this chapter (https://doi.org/10.1007/978-981-16-2206-9_5) contains supplementary material, which is available to authorized users.

S.-H. Shin (✉)
Department of Neurosurgery, Chungdam Wooridul Spine Hospital, Seoul, Republic of Korea
e-mail: burrhoer@wooridul.co.kr

J. Bae, S.-H. Lee (eds.), *Laser Spine Surgery*, https://doi.org/10.1007/978-981-16-2206-9_5

for annulus shrinkage and tightening, so it is very helpful in endoscopic treatment. In this chapter, transforaminal endoscopic lumbar discectomy will be described in case of paramedian disc herniation using Ho:YAG laser.

5.2 Indication

Endoscopic lumbar spine surgery is largely divided into an interlaminar approach and a transforaminal approach [9]. In this chapter, we will describe the indications for a transforaminal approach to disc herniation located in the central and subarticular zones. For successful outcome, proper patient selection is the most important. Patient with radicular leg pain which originated from soft lumbar disc herniation without lateral stenosis is a good indication for transforaminal endoscopic lumbar disc discectomy. In addition, clinically positive straight leg raising test, leg pain more severe than back pain, and no improvement in conservative treatment are targeted for endoscopic treatment. Due to the technological advancement of endoscopic treatment, it is applied to endoscopic treatment in patients with calcified or hard disc herniation, which was considered a contraindication until recently, or in patients with herniated discs with spinal canal stenosis [10, 11].

Relative contraindications are when extensive migrated disc or calcified disc is shown, iliac crest is high at L5/S1 level, multiple levels are involved, spinal stenosis is accompanied, spondylolisthesis is accompanied, and conjoined nerve root is shown.

5.3 Surgical Technique

5.3.1 Anesthesia and Position

Transforaminal endoscopic decompression can be performed under local anesthesia. But it is recommended to have an anesthesiologist for sedation and pain control. Midazolam or fentanyl may be given intravenously to relieve pain and sedation during procedure. The degree of sedation is controlled to respond to the physician's verbal command during the procedure. The patient is placed on the prone position under the guidance of fluoroscope (Fig. 5.1).

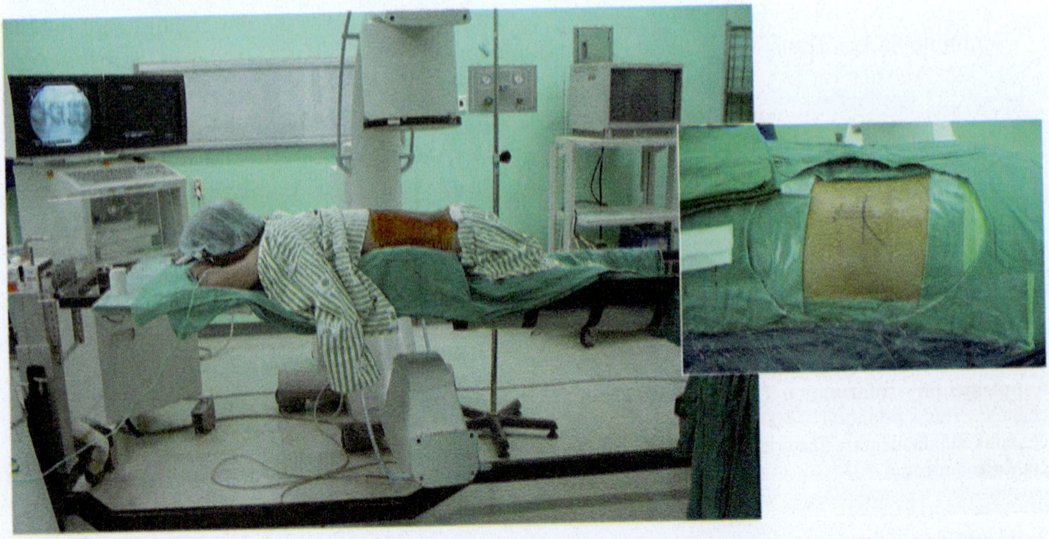

Fig. 5.1 Position. Patients are most often placed in a prone position in radiolucent table with fluoroscopic guidance

5.3.2 Special Surgical Instrument

A fluoroscope is used to access the target, and decompression is performed using an endoscope. A laser or bipolar coagulator and forceps of various shapes can be used to remove the disc (Fig. 5.2). An endoscopic laser is a very useful device for accurate removal of ligamentum flavum, disc material, and bony tissue (Fig. 5.3). Migrated disc herniation, calcified disc herniation, or spinal stenosis requires a foraminoplastic approach. Therefore, manual bone reamers, manual bone drills, or electrical endoscopic drills for foraminoplasty may be necessary (Fig. 5.4).

5.3.3 Surgical Step

Preoperative MRI should be carefully checked to determine the appropriate skin entry point and approaching angle. The distance from the midline to the skin entry point can be calculated in the axial image of the MRI, usually 10–14 cm (Fig. 5.5). An access angle of about 30° is recommended for removal of the disc in the subarticular zone. After determining the proper approach angle and skin entry point, insert an 18-gauge spinal needle using a fluoroscope. In the anterior-posterior fluoroscopic view, the tip of the needle is directed into the disc space, and in lateral view, the tip of the needle points toward the inferior portion of the superior articular process. After touching the superior articular process, insert the needle into the foramen. The epidurogram is then performed using radiocontrast dye. Epidurograms can be used to identify the lateral margin of the thecal sac, which can help access disc space safely. In addition, 2–3 ml of lidocaine 0.5% may be administered after the epidurogram, which may reduce patient's pain during the procedure (Fig. 5.6).

The needle is then inserted into the disc space. The discogram confirms the extent of the herniated disc and observes whether concordant pain is caused (Fig. 5.7). And a guidewire is inserted into the epidural space through the needle. Insert the serial dilatator and obturator along the guidewire and insert the working cannular along it. After that, decompression is performed by inserting an endoscope. Initially, internal disc decom-

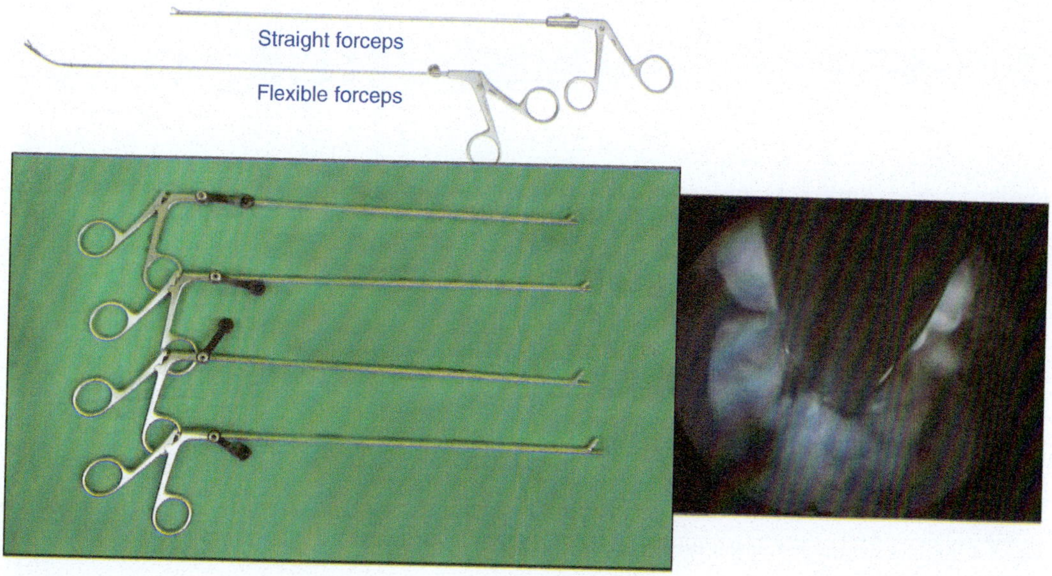

Fig. 5.2 Various sized and shaped forceps

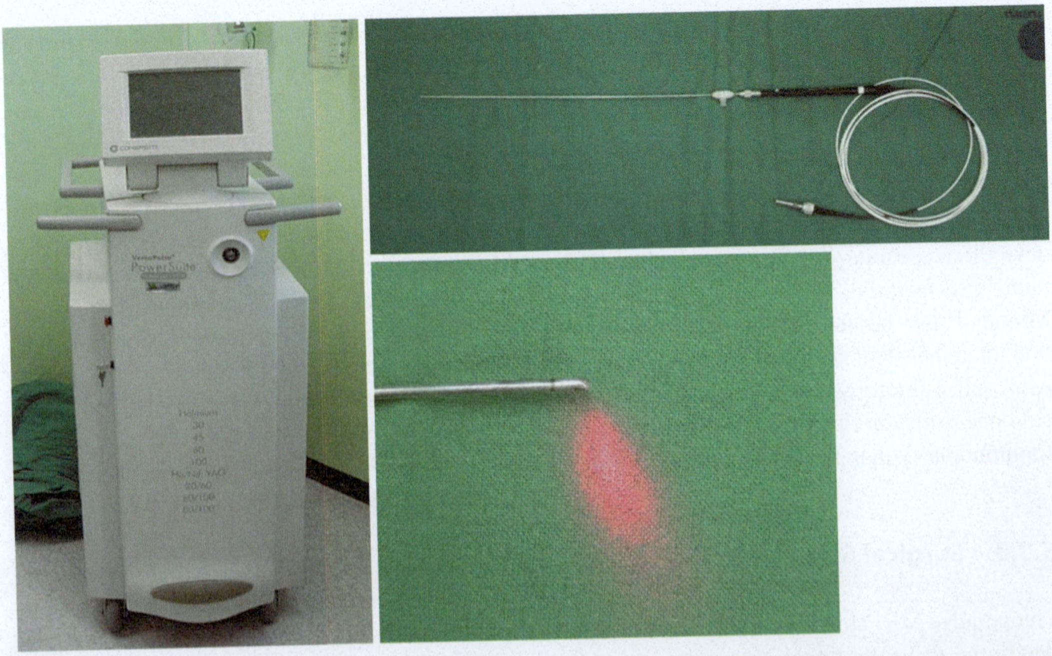

Fig. 5.3 Laser system. Side-firing laser tip. Ho:YAG laser

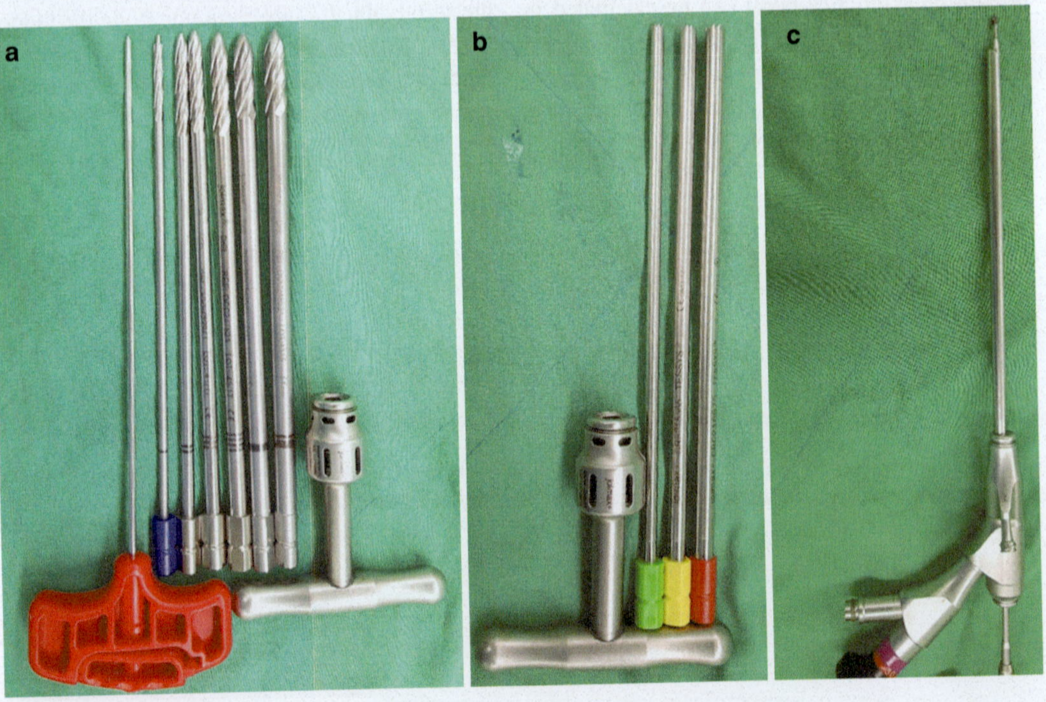

Fig. 5.4 Special surgical instrument used for foraminoplasty. (**a**) Manual bone drill. (**b**) Manual bone reamer. (**c**) Electrical endoscopic drill

pression is performed using a laser. As the intradiscal-working cavity widens, the angle of the endoscope can become more horizontal. With levering technique, the surgeon can examine the full undersurface of the annulus even to the contralateral side. Generally, the soft hernia mass is anchored by the fibrotic annular fissure. So, the annular anchorage should be loosened by the laser or cutters. After doing that, the hernia mass can be easily removed by the endoscopic forceps.

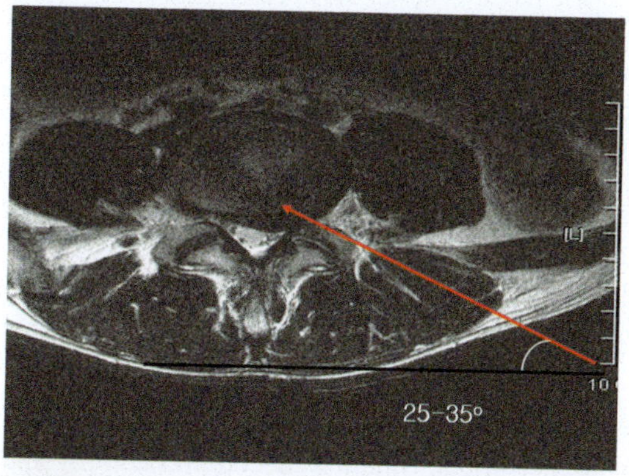

Fig. 5.5 Preoperative planning using axial MRI

The surgeon can see the "anatomical layers" through endoscopic overview: traversing root, PLL, and remained nucleus (Fig. 5.8). Finally, we must remove both epidural and intradiscal fragments because the remained intradiscal fragment may cause reherniation after the procedure. The soft disc herniation can be treated with this technique (Fig. 5.9).

When accompanied by lateral recess stenosis, foraminoplasty is required, and endoscopic drill or bone reamer is used for this. The inferior part of the superior articular process undercuts the medial pedicular line on the fluoroscopic anteroposterior image by using a serial bone reamer or endoscopic drill (Fig. 5.10a, b). Then, a working cannula and an endoscope are inserted along the reamed hole. Laser can be used to remove remnant osseous fragments and the ligamentum flavum to expose the traversing nerve root and extruded disc (Fig. 5.10c, d). The disc herniation with spinal stenosis can be treated with this technique (Fig. 5.11).

A calcified disc is defined as calcification within the disc space, excluding the disc at the

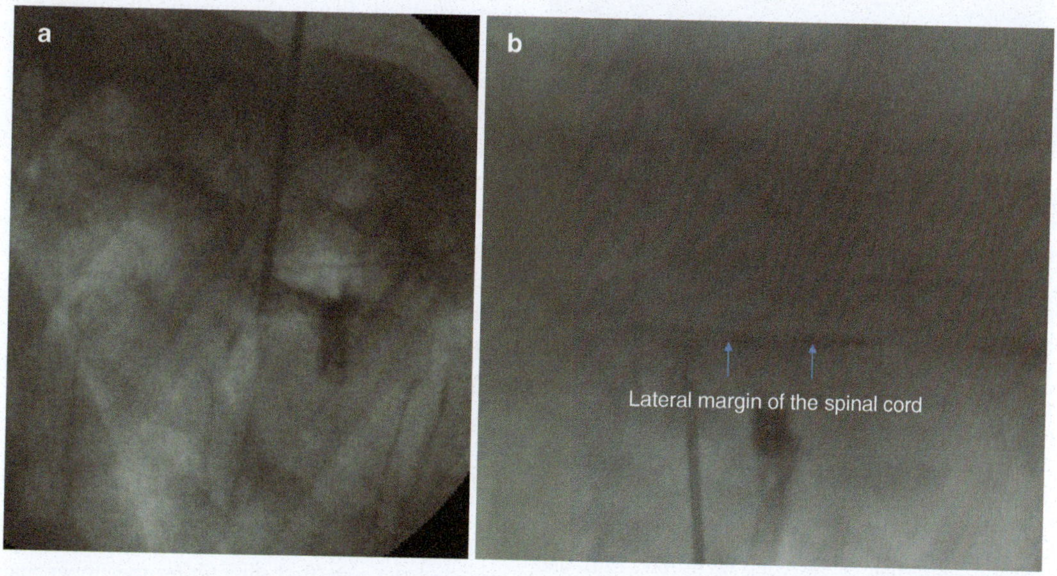

Fig. 5.6 Epidurogram. (**a**) Lateral fluoroscopic view. Tip of the needle is located in epidural space. (**b**) Anterior-posterior view. The lateral margin of the spinal cord can be identified

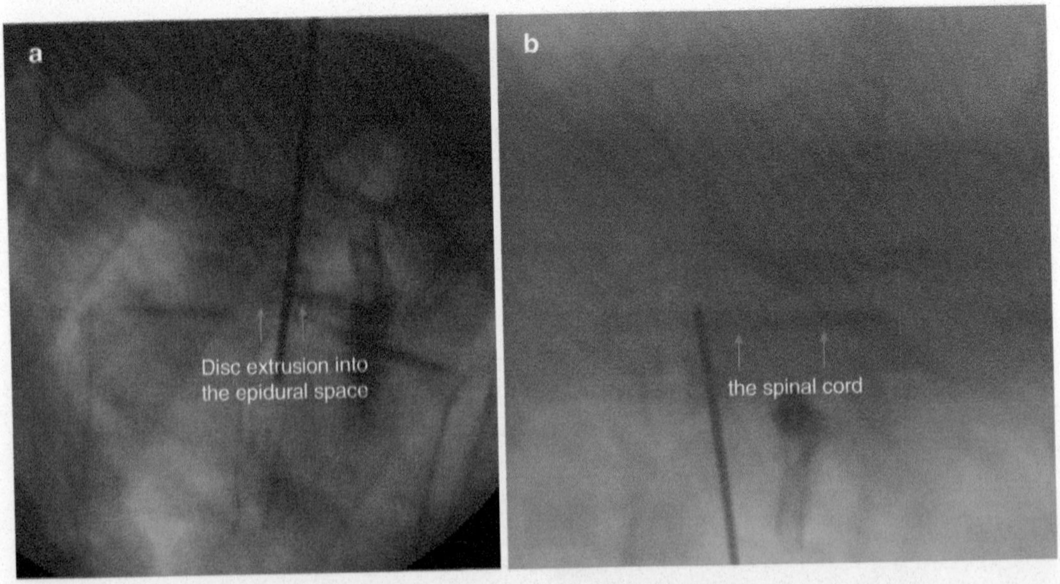

Fig. 5.7 Discography. (**a**) Lateral fluoroscopic view. Extent of the disc herniation can be confirmed. (**b**) Anterior-posterior view. Tip of the needle is located in the disc space beyond the lateral margin of the spinal cord

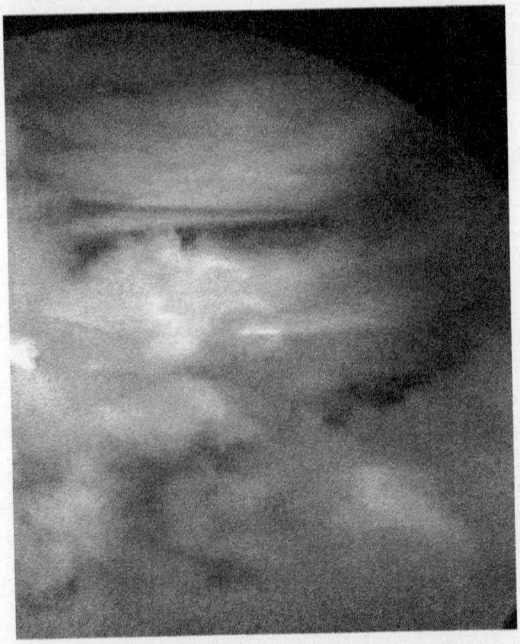

Fig. 5.8 Anatomical layers through endoscopic overview. Confirmation of traversing nerve root, PLL, and remained nucleus

periphery of the disc space. The approach angle was approximately 30° in the horizontal section of the axial image (Fig. 5.12a, b). After landing the working cannula into the disc using a transforaminal route, internal decompression of the degenerated disc is first performed to secure the empty space (Fig. 5.12c). Unlike soft disc herniation, calcified disc herniation usually does not fall into the decompressed intradiscal space even after internal decompression. The decompressed intradiscal space provides a wide field of view for epidural dissection and allows the calcified disc to be dropped into the decompressed space after dissection, to facilitate removal. After internal decompression, the working cannula is pulled back and placed in the epidural space. At this moment, the herniated disc can be visible in the endoscopic view, but the traversing nerve root may be difficult to observe because of the dorsal lifting by the herniated disc. By using the levering technique, the traversing nerve root can be identified after moving the working cannula to the dorsal side. Then, at the discal level, dissection is performed between the traversing nerve root and the calcified disc along the upper and lower endplates by using a probe (Fig. 5.12d). If epidural bleeding occurs during the dissection, the visual field may become cloudy, and care should be taken for hemostasis. Pain may be induced when the nerve is touched, and pain con-

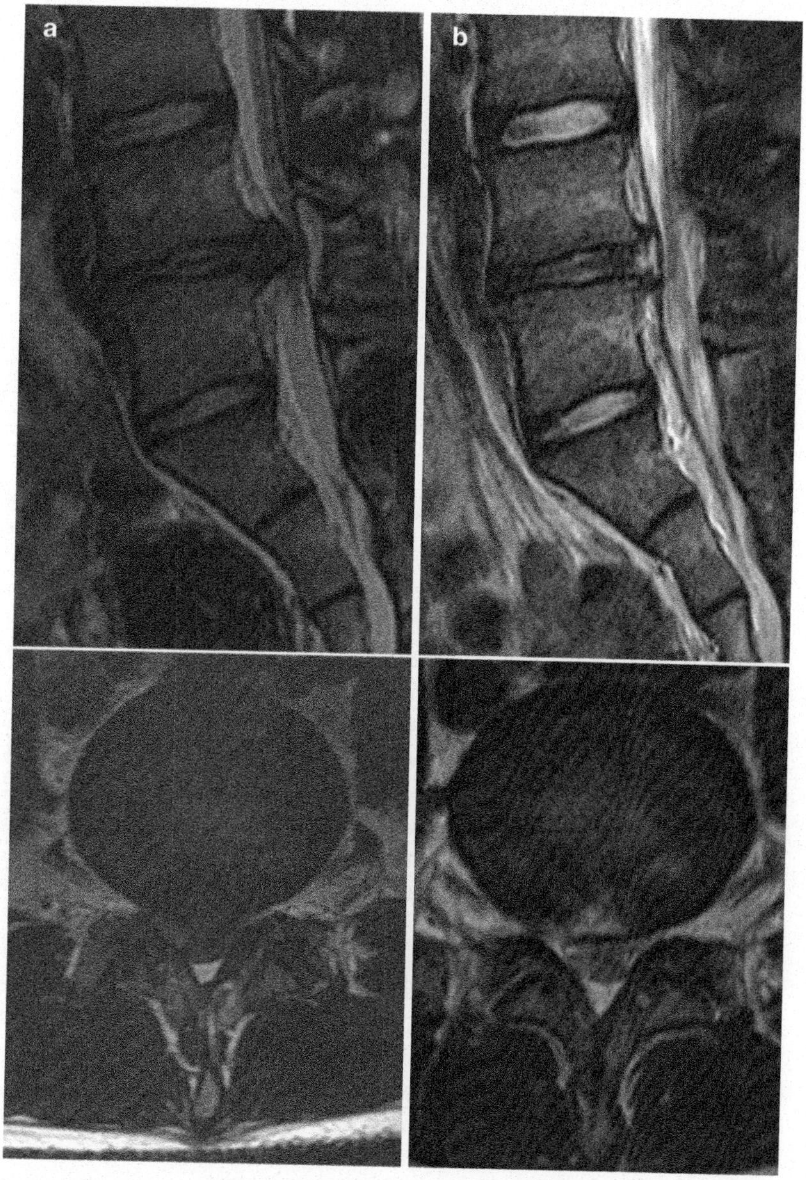

Fig. 5.9 Illustrative case of soft disc herniation. (**a**) Preoperative MR images showing a large centrally herniated disc. (**b**) Postoperative MR images showing a complete decompression

trol may be required using intravenous analgesics. The calcified disc and traversing nerve root are separated through dissection from the annular window to the central zone. The annulus is then cut from the annular window of the foraminal zone to the central zone by using endoscopic scissors (Fig. 5.12e). The calcified disc is then dropped into the decompressed intradiscal space, and the distal part of the herniated disc is cut using a laser or bipolar coagulator, and then removed using forceps (Fig. 5.12f). The calcified disc can be successfully removed without foraminoplasty by using this technique (Fig. 5.13).

For hard discs, a foraminoplastic approach is required to reach the migrated portion. If the approach angle is 30°, the target is difficult to reach without significant resection of the facet joint. In this study, foraminoplasty was performed through the extreme lateral approach to reach the target. The access angle approaches approximately 15° in the horizontal plane of the axial image. The distance from the midline to the

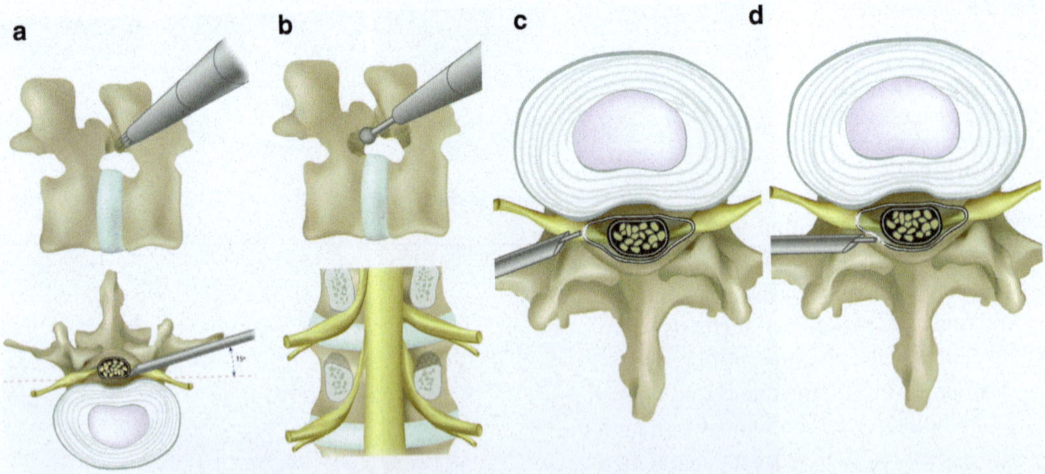

Fig. 5.10 Schematic illustrations of endoscopic lateral recess decompression. (**a**) Extreme lateral transforaminal approach with foraminoplasty. (**b**) Partial upper pediculectomy of the lower pedicle following vertical foraminal widening. (**c**) Removal of the ligamentum flavum in the lateral portion of the spinal canal using side-firing laser. (**d**) Removal of the ligamentum flavum in the dorsal portion of the spinal canal using side-firing laser

skin entry point was calculated via axial MRI evaluation. The distance is approximately 13–17 cm, which is farther than the distance of a typical transforaminal approach. The craniocaudal skin entry point was determined parallel to the disc space because it provides the best working mobility vertically during dissection.

The lateral edge of the superior articular process is approached using an 18-gauge introducer needle in the prone position under local anesthesia. The inferior part of the superior articular process undercuts the medial pedicular line on the fluoroscopic anteroposterior image by using a serial bone reamer or endoscopic drill (Fig. 5.14a). Then, a working cannula and an endoscope are inserted along the reamed hole (Fig. 5.14b). Laser and drill can be used to remove remnant osseous fragments and the ligamentum flavum to expose the traversing nerve root and extruded disc (Fig. 5.14c, d). Internal decompression of the degenerated disc in the disc space is first performed to secure the intradiscal space in which the herniated disc can be dropped later (Fig. 5.14e). In the epidural space, a probe can be used to dissect between the traversing nerve root and the hard disc (Fig. 5.14f). The laser probe is inserted between the hard disc and the traversing nerve root, the opening site of the side-firing laser is directed to the hard disc, the closing site is directed to the nerve, and the laser is used to thin the hard disc (Fig. 5.14g). Endoscopic scissors are then used to break the hard disc (Fig. 5.14h). Forceps are used to pull the broken hard disc down into the decompressed disc space and remove it (Fig. 5.14i). Hard disc herniation can be successfully removed using the foraminoplastic approach through the abovementioned technical method (Fig. 5.15, Video 5.1).

5.4 Literature Review

Choi et al. evaluated the predisposing factors for refractory postoperative back pain after percutaneous endoscopic lumbar discectomy and annuloplasty (PELDA) [12]. The authors stated that the relief of leg pain was common with PELDA, but that the relief of back pain was much less predictable. In their prospective study of 58 patients with leg and back pain from lumbar disc herniation, the authors analyzed PELDA outcomes by dividing patients into two groups: "unfavorable"

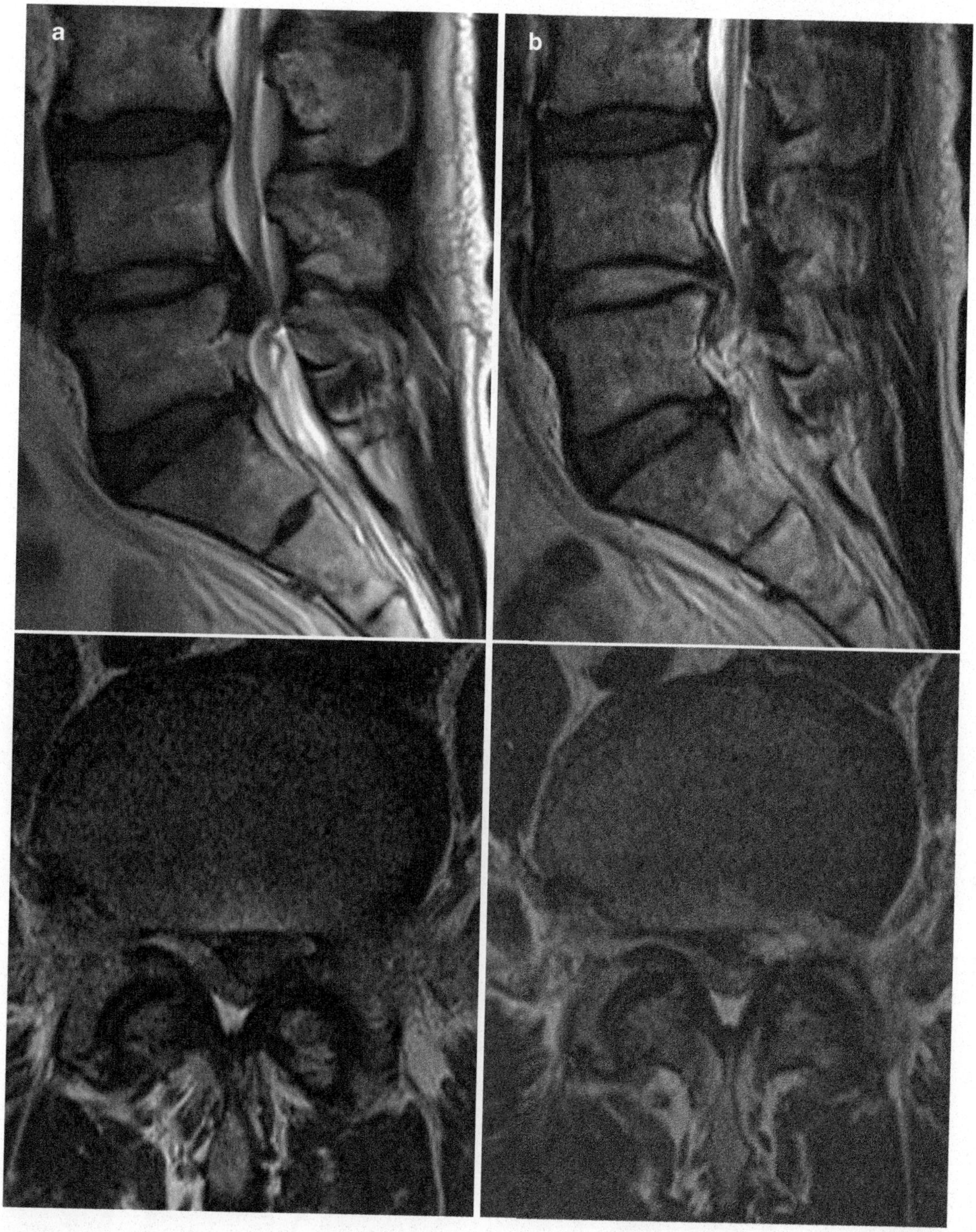

Fig. 5.11 Illustrative case of disc herniation accompanying lateral recess stenosis. (**a**) Preoperative MR images showing downward migrated disc herniation with lateral recess stenosis. (**b**) Postoperative MR images showing decompression of the left lateral recess with removal of the herniated disc compressing the neural structures

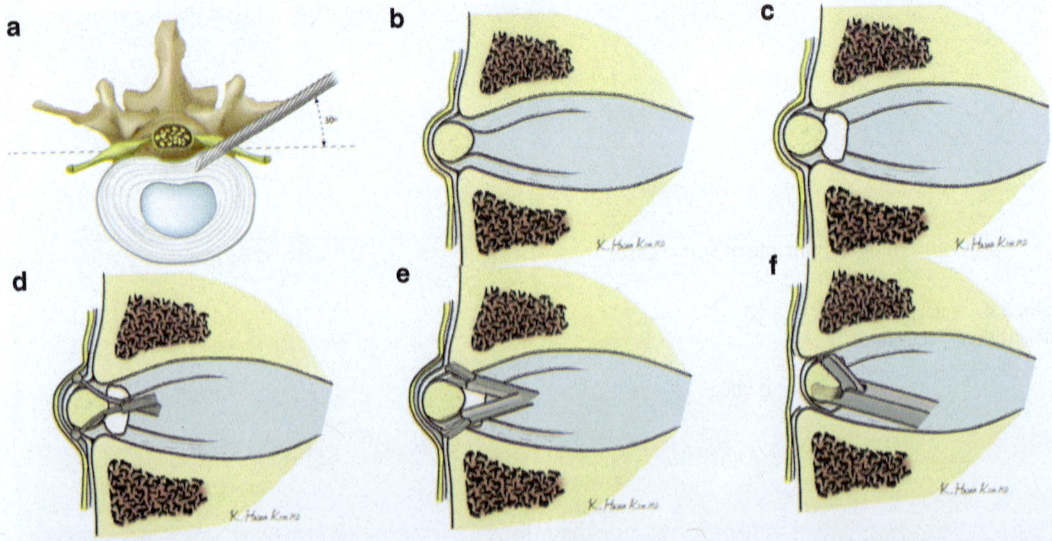

Fig. 5.12 Schematic illustrations of endoscopic discectomy for calcified disc herniation. (**a**) Conventional transforaminal approach. (**b**) Approach to the disc space. (**c**) Internal decompression of degenerated disc. (**d**) Dissection between the traversing nerve root and calcified disc. (**e**) Cutting annulus along both upper and lower endplates using side-firing laser and scissor. (**f**) Removal of calcified disc using forceps

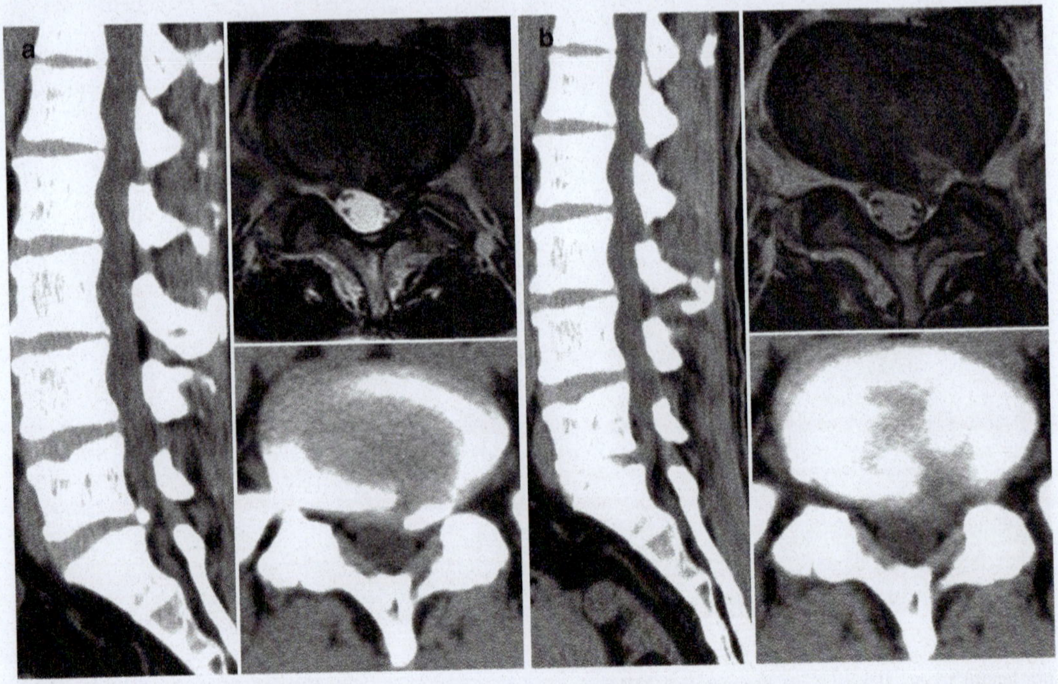

Fig. 5.13 Illustrative case of calcified disc herniation. (**a**) Preoperative CT and MR images showing a calcified disc herniation. (**b**) Postoperative CT and MR images showing decompression of the calcified disc

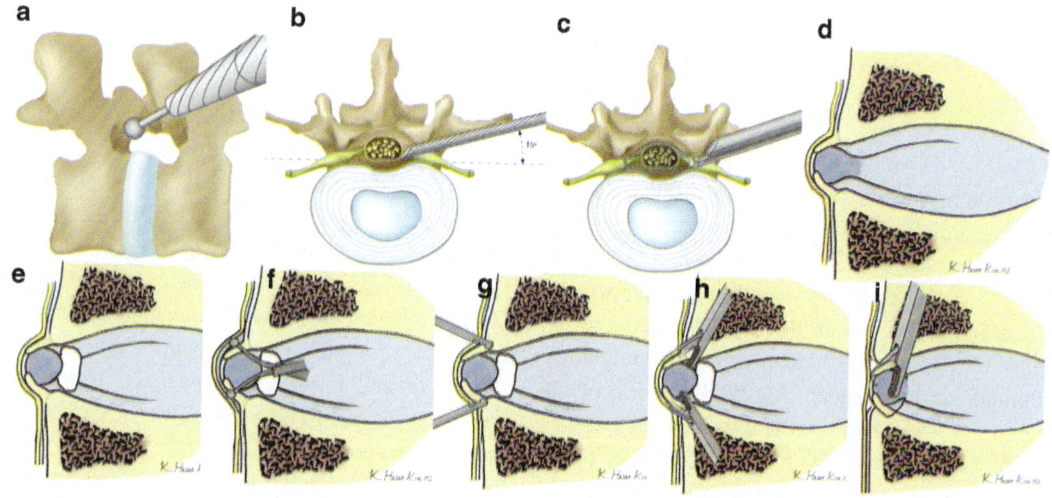

Fig. 5.14 Schematic illustrations of endoscopic discectomy for hard disc herniation. (**a, b**) Extreme lateral transforaminal approach. (**c**) Removal of the ligamentum flavum. (**d**) Approach to the disc space. (**e**) Internal decompression of degenerated disc. (**f**) Dissection between the traversing nerve root and hard disc. (**g**) Breakage of the hard disc using side-firing laser. (**h, i**) Removal of hard disc

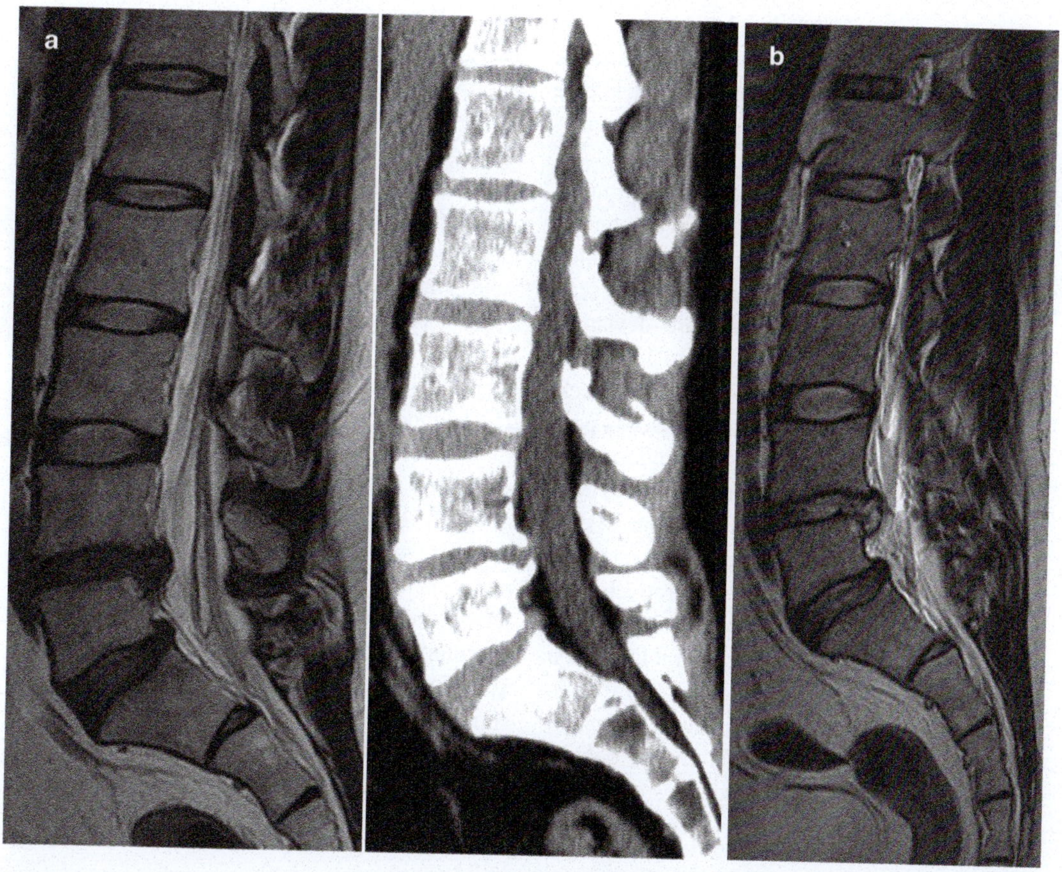

Fig. 5.15 Illustrative case of hard disc herniation. (**a**) Preoperative CT and MR images showing hard disc herniation. (**b**) Postoperative CT and MR images showing decompression of the hard disc

and "favorable." Patients were defined as having unfavorable outcomes if the percentage improvement of back pain assessed by a visual analog scale (VAS) was <50% or the postoperative Oswestry Disability Index (ODI) was >20% at 24 months postoperatively. The mean VAS and ODI scores for back pain improved significantly from 6.6% and 55.9% preoperatively to 2.5% and 12.7% at the 24-month follow-up. The surgical satisfaction rate was 78.4% at the final follow-up, and 34.6% patients had unfavorable outcomes. Patients with advanced disc degeneration of the operative levels had significantly worse outcomes than those with mild disc degeneration (odds ratio = 6.316; 95% confidence interval = 1.25–31.86; $P < 0.05$). The severity of postoperative back pain was negatively correlated with surgical satisfaction (correlation coefficient = −0.564; $P = 0.00$). The authors concluded that PELDA had the ability to improve both back and leg pain due to direct decompression and thermal ablation of the annular defect, both noted that inferior patient satisfaction due to persistent back pain was common in patients with advanced degenerative disc disease.

Shin et al. described the details of the transforaminal endoscopic lumbar discectomy technique for hard or calcified disc and reported the clinical results [11]. The preoperative visual analog scale score for leg pain (mean ± standard deviation) was 7.09 ± 1.74. The score improved to 2.55 ± 1.35 at 1 week postoperatively, 1.88 ± 1.29 at 4 weeks postoperatively, and 1.58 ± 1.0 at 26 weeks postoperatively ($P < 0.01$ for all). The preoperative Oswestry Disability Index (mean ± standard deviation) was 55.4 ± 23.04, which improved to 30.89 ± 13.64 at 1 week postoperatively, 23.08 ± 11.64 at 4 weeks postoperatively, and 16.42 ± 9.76 at 26 weeks postoperatively ($P < 0.01$ for all). Two patients developed a dural laceration. Both patients were discharged after several hours of observation. None of the patients had postoperative infection, epidural hematoma, or delayed neurological deterioration. And they concluded that transforaminal endoscopic discectomy could be an effective treatment method for a selected group of patients with hard or calcified lumbar disc herniation.

Manchikanti et al. studied the evidence for automated and laser discectomy of contained herniated lumbar disc compared with traditional microdiscectomy techniques [13, 14]. They performed a PubMed and EMBASE literature search from 1966 to September 2012 and manual searches on automated percutaneous mechanical lumbar discectomy for their management of chronic low back pain and lower extremity pain. Using the quality assessment and clinical relevance criteria of the Cochrane Musculoskeletal Review Group for interventional techniques for randomized trials, and the criteria developed by the Newcastle-Ottawa scale criteria for observational studies, the authors classified the level of evidence as "good," "fair," and "limited" or "poor" based on the quality of evidence scale developed by the US Preventive Services Task Force (USPSTF). Primary outcome measures were pain relief, as well as functional improvement, improvement of psychological status, level of opioid intake, and speed of return to work. Short-term effectiveness was defined as lasting for <1 year, whereas long-term effectiveness was defined as lasting for >1 year. The authors identified 19 randomized trials, and observational studies met the inclusion criteria for methodologic quality assessment. These studies comprised a total of 5.515 patients, 4.412 (80%) of which showed clinical improvements for 1 year or longer. The authors also reported limited evidence for short- and long-term pain relief for automated percutaneous mechanical lumbar discectomy based of USPSTF criteria. Manchikanti et al. concluded that there was currently limited evidence for automated percutaneous mechanical lumbar discectomy, mainly due to the paucity of controlled randomized trials. However, they did report adequate pain relief with the procedures, which was similar to that observed after conventional open techniques. The authors arrived at a similar conclusion with a review of the Dekompressor system, using similar literature review techniques.

5.5 Postoperative Consideration

A neurological examination of the patient should be done immediately following the procedure. Neurological examination should confirm whether the symptom is improved and whether motor deficit has occurred. In addition, postoperative MR can be used to check for complete decompression of the lesion. The patient may be discharged after several hours of observation. At discharge, oral antibiotics are considered to prevent procedure-related infection.

References

1. Choi G, Lee S, Deshpande K, et al. Working channel endoscope in lumbar spine surgery. J Neurosurg Sci. 2014;58:77–85.
2. Cong L, Zhu Y, Tu G. A meta-analysis of endoscopic discectomy versus open discectomy for symptomatic lumbar disk herniation. Eur Spine J. 2016;25:134–43.
3. Ruan W, Feng F, Liu Z, et al. Comparison of percutaneous endoscopic lumbar discectomy versus open lumbar microdiscectomy for lumbar disc herniation: a meta-analysis. Int J Surg. 2016;31:86–92.
4. Kambin P, Gellman H. Percutaneous lateral discectomy of the lumbar spine a preliminary report. Clin Orthopaed Relat Res. 1983;174:127–32.
5. Shin S-H, Hwang B-W, Keum H-J, et al. Epidural steroids after a percutaneous endoscopic lumbar discectomy. Spine. 2015;40:E859–E65.
6. Schawlow AL, Townes CH. Infrared and optical masers. Phys Rev. 1958;112:1940.
7. Ascher PW, Heppner F. CO_2-laser in neurosurgery. Neurosurg Rev. 1984;7:123–33.
8. Gottlob C, Kopchok GE, Peng SK, et al. Holmium:YAG laser ablation of human intervertebral disc: preliminary evaluation. Lasers Surg Med. 1992;12:86–91.
9. Ruetten S, Komp M, Merk H, et al. Full-endoscopic interlaminar and transforaminal lumbar discectomy versus conventional microsurgical technique: a prospective, randomized, controlled study. Spine. 2008;33:931–9.
10. Shin S-H, Bae J-S, Lee S-H, et al. Transforaminal endoscopic decompression for lumbar spinal stenosis: a novel surgical technique and clinical outcomes. World Neurosurg. 2018;114:e873–e82.
11. Shin S-H, Bae J-S, Lee S-H, et al. Transforaminal endoscopic discectomy for hard or calcified lumbar disc herniation: a new surgical technique and clinical outcomes. World Neurosurg. 2020;143:e224–e31.
12. Choi K-C, Kim J-S, Kang B-U, et al. Changes in back pain after percutaneous endoscopic lumbar discectomy and annuloplasty for lumbar disc herniation: a prospective study. Pain Med. 2011;12:1615–21.
13. Manchikanti L, Falco F, Benyamin RM, et al. An update of the systematic assessment of mechanical lumbar disc decompression with nucleoplasty. Pain Phys. 2013;16:SE25.
14. Manchikanti L, Singh V, Calodney AK, et al. Percutaneous lumbar mechanical disc decompression utilizing Dekompressor®: an update of current evidence. Pain Phys. 2013;16:SE1–24.

Transforaminal Endoscopic Lumbar Discectomy for Foraminal Disc Herniation with Ho:Yag Laser

6

Sang Soo Eun

Abstract

Foraminal disc herniations present the unique surgical challenge for exiting nerve root retraction and decompression. Severe radiating pain arises from impingement of existing nerve root ganglion by foraminal disc herniation. In this chapter, we describe rotate-to-retract technique for endoscopic decompression of foraminal disc herniations.

Keywords

Foraminal disc · Disc herniation · PELD · Transforaminal · Rotate-to-retract technique · Dorsal root ganglion

6.1 Introduction

Posterolateral endoscopic lumbar decompression (PELD) is fast becoming the procedure of choice for surgical management of lumbar disc herniations [1–7]. Endoscopic discectomy techniques have produced surgical results similar to those of other discectomy techniques while offering various advantages like avoidance of general anesthesia, preservation of paravertebral soft tissues, faster rehabilitation, and better clinical results overall [1–7]. Cases of foraminal disc herniation (FDH) present a unique surgical challenge for exiting nerve root retraction and decompression [8–11]. Irrespective of the surgical technique used, the clinical outcome can be significantly affected by both, technique of exiting nerve visualization/retraction and adequacy of decompression [8–11]. Use of appropriate exiting nerve retraction and visualization technique is paramount to adequate decompression [8–11]. In this chapter, we will introduce the "rotate-to-retract technique," for safe retraction and decompression of the exiting neural structures during PELD in cases of FDH.

6.2 Indications

- Symptomatic foraminal soft disc herniation without calcification that does not respond to conservative treatment

6.2.1 Surgical Technique

The procedure was performed under local anesthesia with mild sedation. The patient was positioned prone. A standard lumbar endoscopic instrument set (TESSYS, Joimax GmbH, Germany) was used. The surgical steps were as follows:

S. S. Eun (✉)
Department of Orthopedics, Chungdam Wooridul Spine Hospital, Seoul, Republic of Korea

J. Bae, S.-H. Lee (eds.), *Laser Spine Surgery*, https://doi.org/10.1007/978-981-16-2206-9_6

1. The skin entry point and trajectory of the endoscope was planned based on the axial magnetic resonance (MR) images. The surgeon preferred to use a more direct trajectory toward the herniation resulting in the skin entry point about 7–8 cm from the midline with a steep angle of approach (Fig. 6.1).
2. The path of the endoscope was infiltrated with local anesthesia.
3. An 18-G spinal needle was inserted under fluoroscopy guidance along the preplanned trajectory.
4. Epidurography was performed to confirm the location of the neural structures.
5. After confirmation of correct needle tip position, a guide wire was introduced via the spinal needle, followed by an obturator and a beveled working cannula (Fig. 6.1).
6. The whole procedure was performed under fluoroscopy guidance. After satisfactory positioning of the working channel, a 25° endoscope was introduced.
7. To safely approach the foraminal disc, rotate-to-retract technique was employed:

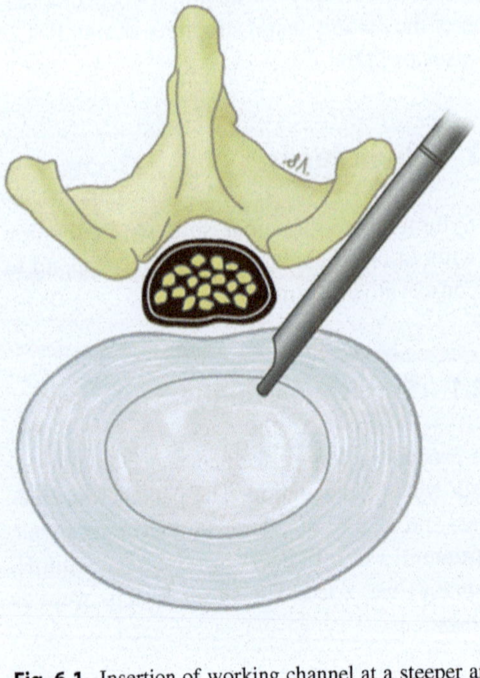

Fig. 6.1 Insertion of working channel at a steeper angle than usual PELD

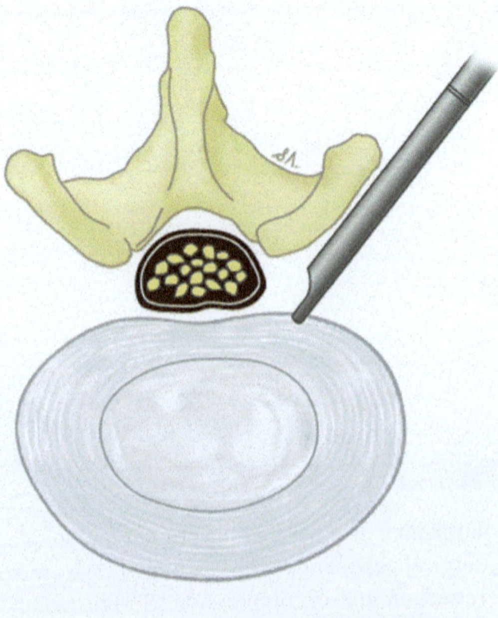

Fig. 6.2 Working cannula is retrieved until its tip is outside the disc

   (a) The working cannula was retrieved until its tip was outside the disc (Fig. 6.2).
   (b) The working cannula was rotated such that the tip and opening of the bevel was on the cranial side (Fig. 6.3).
   (c) It was then rotated clockwise, which resulted in spontaneous retraction of the exiting nerve root (Fig. 6.4).
   (d) The working channel was placed in the most lateral part of Kambin's triangle with its bevel tip retracting the exiting root (Fig. 6.5).
   (e) By rotating the opening of the working channel to the lateral side, endoscopic forceps could be used to grasp the extraforaminal disc herniation underneath the exiting root (Fig. 6.6).
8. The rest of the discectomy was performed and concluded in the standard manner. Laser is used to release PLL in central and extraforaminal area (Fig.6.7). Foraminal disc on axillar side of exiting root can be removed by laser with protection of working channel. Do not beam laser directly on ganglion of nerve.

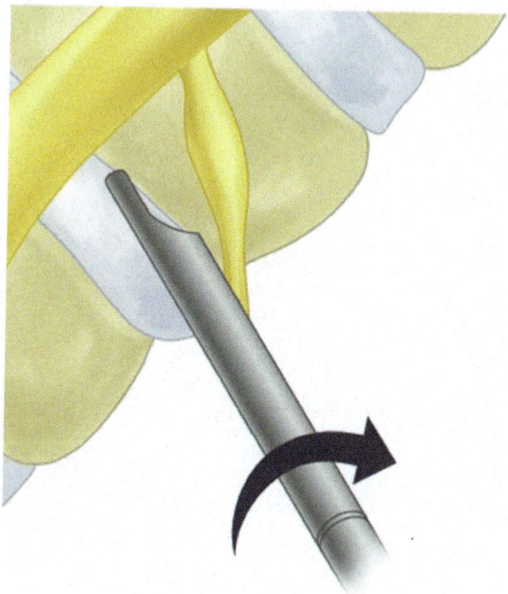

Fig. 6.3 Working cannula is rotated such that the tip and opening of bevel is on the cranial side

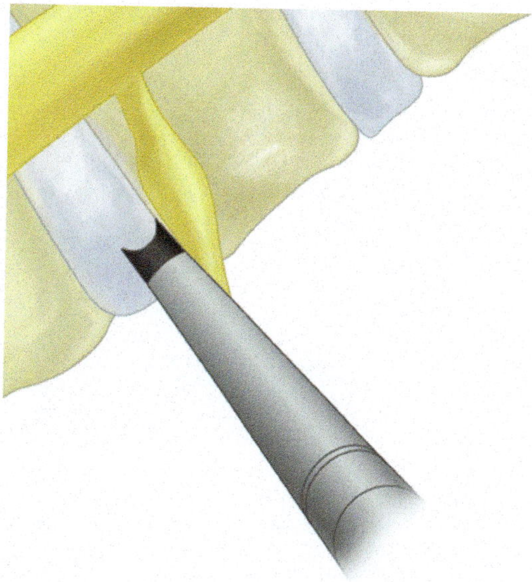

Fig. 6.5 Working channel is placed most lateral part of Kambin's triangle and bevel is retracting exiting root

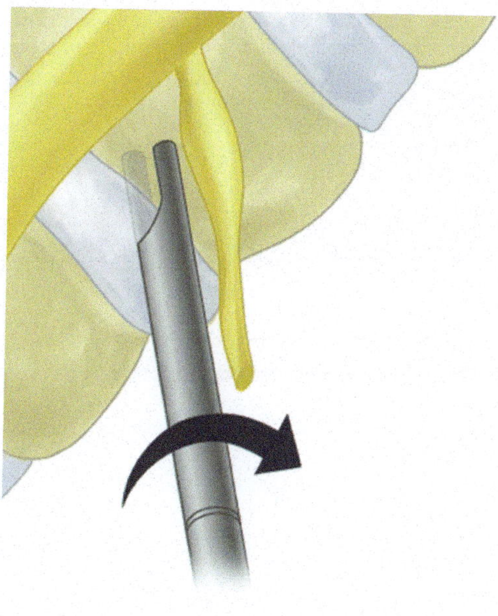

Fig. 6.4 Working cannula is rotated clockwise

9. Intraoperatively, exiting nerve root decompression could be assessed by direct inspection with endoscope (Fig. 6.8).

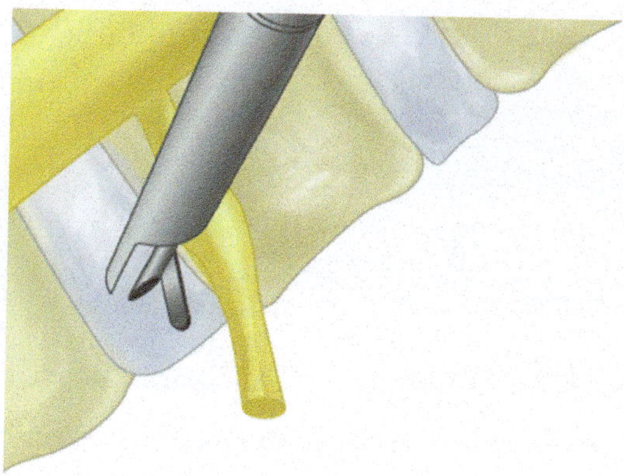

Fig. 6.6 Rotate the opening of working channel to lateral side and forceps can grasp extra-foraminal disc underneath exiting root

Compared with central disc herniations, foraminal disc herniation discectomies (microscopic/endoscopic) have a reportedly higher postoperative incidence of remnant radicular pain and paresthesia [12]. The authors postulate that the inferior outcomes of FDH discectomies can be attributed to DRG (dorsal root

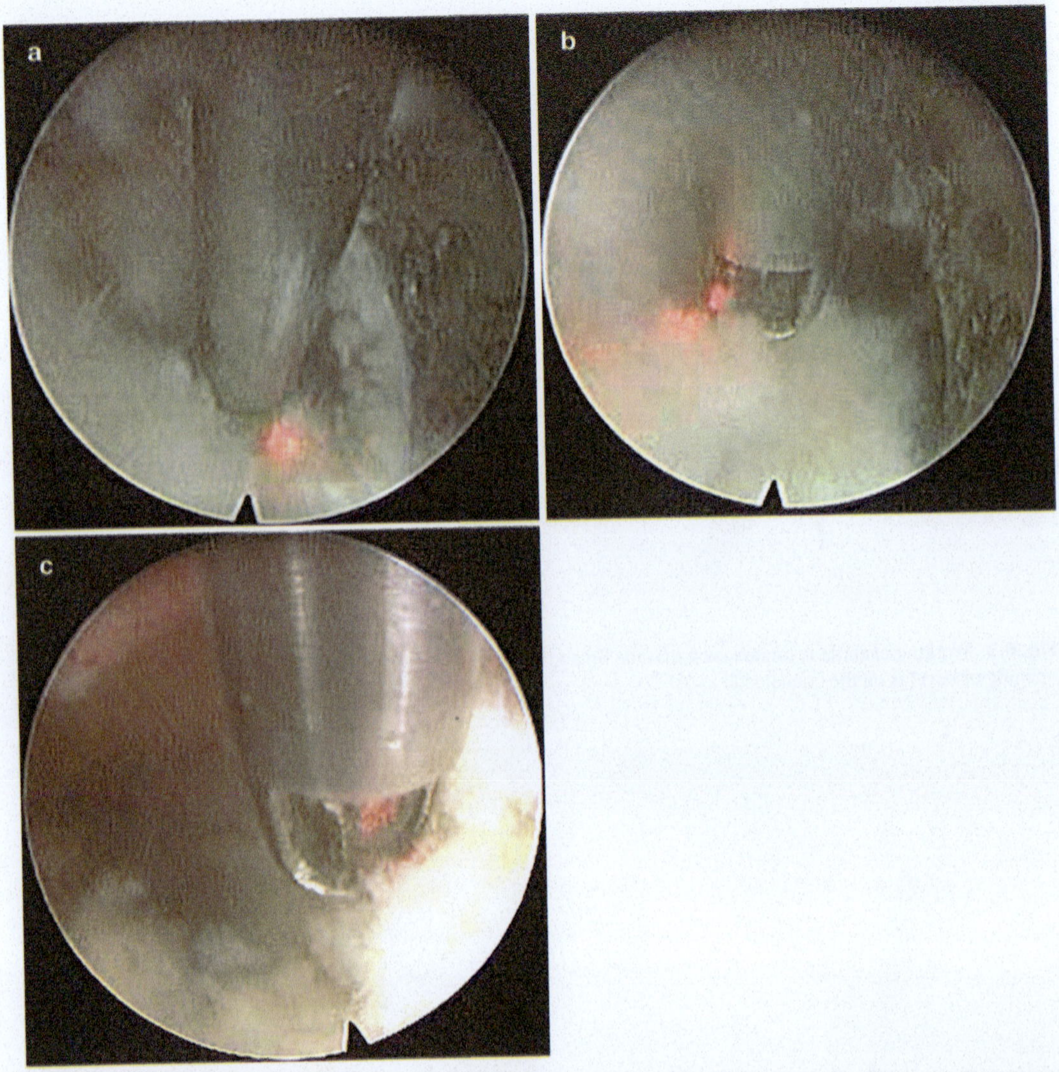

Fig. 6.7 Laser probe is inserted to release extra-foraminal area PLL. Exiting root is protected with bevel of working channel

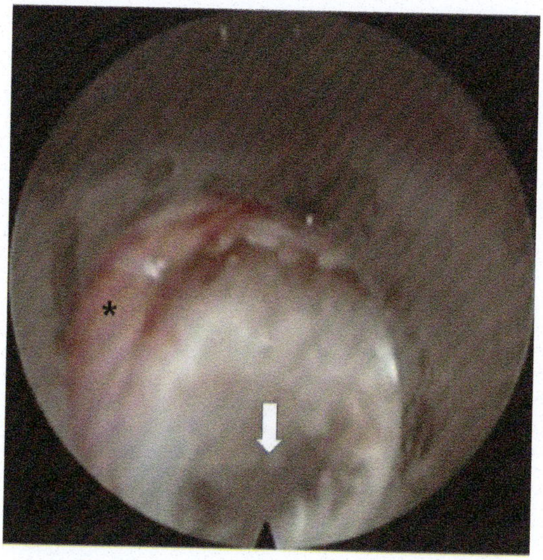

Fig. 6.8 Endoscopic image showing exiting nerve root (*) and disc space (arrow) after decompression

ganglion) manipulation. Furthermore, removal of FDH can result in disc height decrement, segmental instability, and foraminal stenosis [7, 11] (Fig. 6.9).

The rotate-to-retract technique is a simple-easy-to-learn maneuver involving the use of beveled end of the working cannula to safely retract the exiting nerve root in its axilla, permitting complete removal of the pathological disc material.

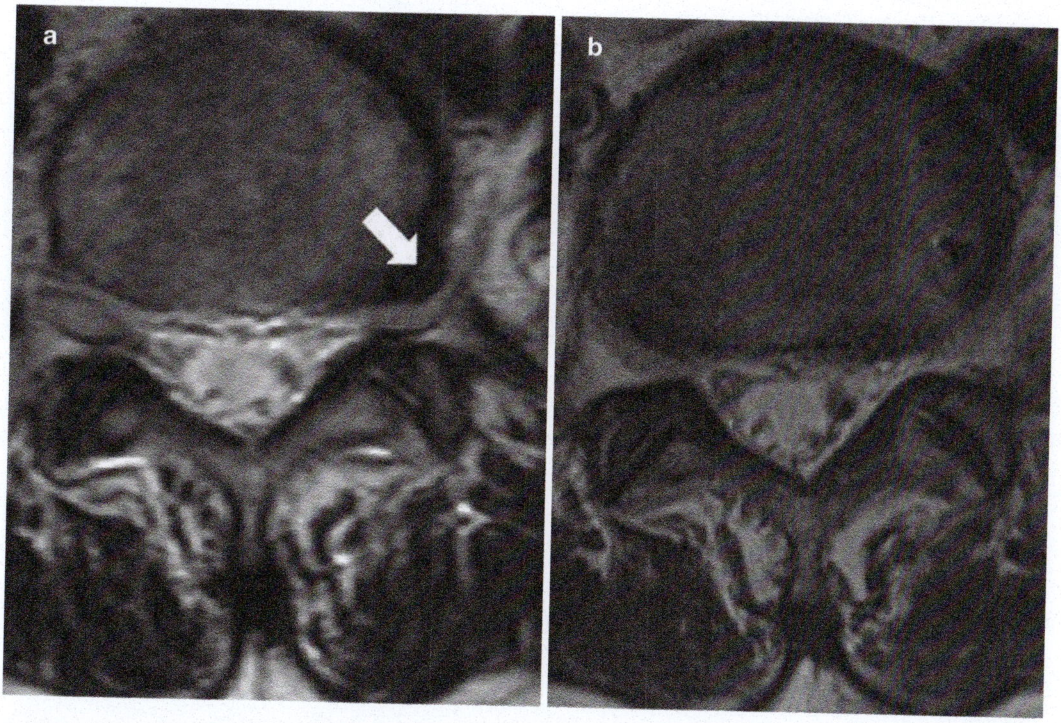

Fig. 6.9 A. Pre-op axial MRI showing left-side extra-foraminal disc herniation (white arrow) at L5–S1 level. B. Post-op axial MRI showing removal of extra-foraminal disc herniation

References

1. Hirano Y, Mizuno J, Numazawa S, Itoh Y, Watanabe S, Watanabe K. Percutaneous endoscopic lumbar discectomy (PELD) for herniated nucleus pulposus of the lumbar spine: surgical indications and current limitations. Jpn J Neurosurg. 2017;26(5):346–52.
2. Du J, Tang X, Jing X, Li N, Wang Y, Zhang X. Outcomes of percutaneous endoscopic lumbar discectomy via a translaminar approach, especially for soft, highly down-migrated lumbar disc herniation. Int Orthop. 2016;40(6):1247–52.
3. Peng CWB, Yeo W, Tan SB. Percutaneous endoscopic discectomy. J Spinal Disord Tech. 2010;23(6):425–30.
4. Kim M-J, Lee S-H, Jung E-S, Son B-G, Choi E-S, Shin J-H, Sung J-K, Chi Y-C. Targeted percutaneous transforaminal endoscopic diskectomy in 295 patients: comparison with results of microscopic diskectomy. Surg Neurol. 2007;68(6):623–31.
5. Telfeian AE, Veeravagu A, Oyelese AA, Gokaslan ZL, MD. A brief history of endoscopic spine surgery. Neurosurg Focus. 2016;40(2):E2.
6. Dasenbrock HH, Juraschek SP, Schultz LR, Witham TF, Sciubba DM, Wolinsky J-P, Gokaslan ZL, Bydon A. The efficacy of minimally invasive discectomy compared with open discectomy: a meta-analysis of prospective randomized controlled trials. J Neurosurg Spine. 2012;16(5):452–62.
7. Pan L, Zhang P, Yin Q. Comparison of tissue damages caused by endoscopic lumbar discectomy and traditional lumbar discectomy: a randomised controlled trial. Int J Surg. 2014;12(5):534–7.
8. Epstein NE. Management of far lateral lumbar disc herniations. Schmidek and Sweet's operative neurosurgical techniques. 2012, 2012 1871–1882.
9. Jang J-S, An S-H, Lee S-H. Transforaminal percutaneous endoscopic discectomy in the treatment of foraminal and extraforaminal lumbar disc herniations. J Spinal Disord Tech. 2006;19(5):338–43.
10. Choi G, Lee S-H, Bhanot A, Raiturker PP, Chae YS. Percutaneous endoscopic discectomy for extraforaminal lumbar disc herniations. Spine. 2007;32(2):E93–9.
11. Lew SM, Mehalic TF, Fagone KL. Transforaminal percutaneous endoscopic discectomy in the treatment of farlateral and foraminal lumbar disc herniations. J Neurosurg. 2001;94(2 Suppl):216–20.
12. Maio K, Yoshida M. Clinical outcomes of microendoscopic discectomy for extraforaminal lumbar disc herniation. In: Dezawa A, Chen PQ, Chung JY, editors. State of the art for minimally invasive spine surgery. Tokyo: Springer; 2005.

7 Endoscopic Lumbar Foraminotomy with Ho:Yag Laser

Han Joong Keum and Kang Seok Moon

Abstract

Lumbar foraminal stenosis has been identified as a common cause of radicular symptoms and can lead to persistent pain after prolonged treatment. A facet-preserving microdecompression technique using a paraspinal approach has been considered the gold standard for the surgical treatment of lumbar foraminal or far lateral stenosis but has been associated with postoperative leg pain or dysesthesia. More recently, authors have reported the use of a technique known as endoscopic foraminal discectomy with or without foraminotomy for the treatment of foraminal stenosis. Recent advancement in endoscopic devices as well as the use of a side-firing, holmium:yttrium-aluminum-garnet (Ho:YAG) laser has further the surgeon to treat foraminal stenosis more quickly and with less complications.

Supplementary Information The online version of this chapter (https://doi.org/10.1007/978-981-16-2206-9_7) contains supplementary material, which is available to authorized users.

H. J. Keum (✉) · K. S. Moon
Department of Neurosurgery, Chungdam Wooridul Spine Hospital, Seoul, Republic of Korea

Department of Neurosurgery, Seoul Gimpo Airport Wooridul Spine Hospital, Seoul, Republic of Korea
e-mail: hanj@wooridul.co.kr

Keywords

Endoscopic · Foraminal stenosis · Foraminotomy · Laser · Lumbar

7.1 Introduction

Lumbar foraminal stenosis has been identified as a common cause of radicular symptoms and is unfortunately readily overlooked or unrecognized, leading to persistent pain after prolonged treatment. Surgical options for treatment of lumbar foraminal stenosis consist of total facetectomy with or without fusion and facet-preserving microforaminotomy. Total facetectomy offers decompression of the whole nerve root course but often leads to segmental instability and is usually supplemented by fusion techniques [1, 2]. A facet-preserving microdecompression technique using a paraspinal approach enables direct access to a foraminal or far lateral lesion with minimal violation of the facet joint and less postoperative back pain [3–5]. This technique has been considered the gold standard for the surgical treatment of lumbar foraminal or far lateral stenosis. However, excessive manipulation of the dorsal root ganglion has been associated with postoperative leg pain or dysesthesia [6–8].

More recently, various minimally invasive techniques have been developed for the treatment of lumbar foraminal stenosis. Many authors have reported the use of a technique known as endo-

J. Bae, S.-H. Lee (eds.), *Laser Spine Surgery*, https://doi.org/10.1007/978-981-16-2206-9_7

scopic foraminal discectomy with or without foraminotomy [9–11]. However, the application of these minimally invasive techniques has been limited to foraminal soft disc herniation or concurrent mild foraminal stenosis. Moreover, the practical application of this technique has been limited by its steep learning curve. Recent advancement in endoscopic devices, such as reamers, drills, and Kerrison rongeurs, has paved the way for more intricate and sophisticated manipulation of the intervertebral foramen. This had led to a more widespread application of endoscopic lumbar foraminotomy with a safer approach to the stenotic foramen and a more thorough decompression of hard bony stenosis [12–15]. Also, the use of a side-firing, holmium:yttrium-aluminum-garnet (Ho:YAG) laser during this procedure has further enabled the surgeon to treat foraminal stenosis more quickly and with less complications [16, 17].

7.2 Indications

Patients with lumbar foraminal to extraforaminal stenosis causing radiculopathy and without symptom relief after conservative management (medication, physical therapy, transforaminal nerve root blocks) should be considered for endoscopic lumbar foraminotomy.

7.3 Surgical Procedure

The patient is placed in a prone position on a radiolucent table after use of local anesthesia and with conscious sedation. The patient is injected with midazolam (0.05 mg/kg) intramuscularly and fentanyl (0.8 μg/kg) intravenously as a premedication. Additional medication can be administered during the procedure according to the condition of the patient. The appropriate skin entry point is predetermined after checking the patient's waist size and preoperative imaging studies and confirmed through intraoperative fluoroscopy. The approximate entry point should be between 8 and 12 cm from the midline.

An 18-gauge spinal needle is inserted after administering 2% lidocaine for local anesthesia under fluoroscopic guidance. The needle is placed at the caudal surface of the superior articular process (SAP) to avoid injury to the exiting root and then is replaced by a guidewire. Serial dilators are inserted through the guidewire and placed in the foraminal area to gently retract the exiting root and provide a guide into the foraminal area. Then, a bevel-ended working cannula is introduced over the dilator and placed on the undersurface of the SAP. The working cannula can be slightly more retracted if the patient complains of excessive pain which may be caused by compression of the exiting root. After confirming the working cannula placement under fluoroscopic guidance, an endoscope is introduced through the working cannula and the surgeon can confirm adequate placement through endoscopic visualization and can begin foraminal decompression (Fig. 7.1).

The first step in foraminal decompression is bone resection of the hypertrophied SAP and part of the pedicle. This can be described as the foraminal unroofing process as this step provides direct foraminal decompression as well as creates a larger safe working space for more precise decompression inside the foramen (Fig. 7.2). The hypertrophied bone can be effectively resected by the bone trephines using fluoroscopy or endoscopic burrs under direct endoscopic guidance. Bone trephines can reduce operation time, but endoscopic drilling is much safer and effective as it is performed under direct visualization. Various types of endoscopic burrs can be used for effective foraminotomy. Removal of the bone is performed from caudal to cranial and from outside to inside the stenotic foramen until the ligamentum flavum and fibrotic soft tissues appear. After bony decompression, the foraminal structures such as the foraminal ligament, ligamentum flavum, perineural fat covering the exiting nerve root, shoulder osteophytes, and the disc surface should be visible through the endoscope. The working cannula and endoscope can then be advanced further into the widened foraminal area for more sophisticated decompression. The bevel of the working cannula can be used as a useful nerve root retractor by rotating the cannula.

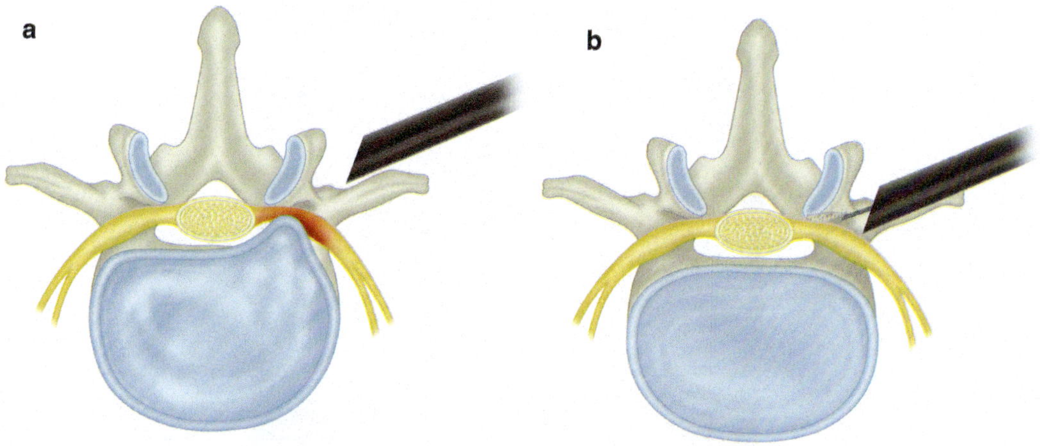

Fig. 7.1 Schematic view of endoscopic lumbar foraminotomy. (**a**) The working channel is placed on the undersurface of the superior articular process (SAP). (**b**) Foraminal decompression is done using forceps, punches, and laser

After completion of foraminal unroofing, further decompression is done by removing any offending soft tissues and adhesions using various mechanical instruments and side-firing Ho:YAG laser (Fig. 7.2b, c). On the dorsal side of the foramen, any hypertrophied ligamentum flavum compressing the nerve root can be removed using endoscopic punches and side-firing laser. On the ventral side, an extruded disc fragment, if any, may be removed using pituitary forceps and the side-firing laser. A contained, redundant disc and surrounding soft tissue adhesions can be reduced and lysed using endoscopic punches and dissecting probes. Bipolar radiofrequency is used concordantly to shrink the disc, dissect neural adhesions, and control epidural bleeding. Ventral ligaments and shoulder osteophytes can also be evaporated using the side-firing laser.

When complete decompression is achieved, the exiting nerve root and dural sac can be defined and mobilized (Fig. 7.2d). A flexible, curved tissue dissector is then used to probe and confirm neural decompression under endoscopic visualization. The end point of the procedure should not only be exposure of the nerve root but also complete release and mobilization of the neural tissues. Then, a bipolar coagulator and hemostatic agent are used for hemostasis, the endoscope is withdrawn, and a sterile dressing is applied with a subcutaneous suture.

7.4 Role of Ho:Yag Laser in Endoscopic Foraminotomy

Holmium:yttrium-aluminum-garnet (Ho:YAG) laser is a side-firing laser that is used in a pulsed mode. The Ho:YAG laser has the benefit of less thermal conduction to the surrounding tissues and for this reason is called a cold laser. This is the most frequently used laser in endoscopic procedures. The side-firing laser beam can treat any remote or corner site, which can be difficult to approach, and can ablate or coagulate a specific lesion while protecting normal tissues. The Ho:Yag laser can directly remove any offending ligamentum flavum, can safely dissect fibrotic scar tissue, and can evaporate shoulder osteophytes. The power setting of the laser is usually 40 to 60 watts for soft tissue ablation and can be increased to 80 watts for bone ablation [17].

7.5 Case Illustration

7.5.1 Case 1

A 56-year-old male patient presented with right leg radiating pain and walking difficulty which had persisted for several years. On magnetic resonance (MR) imaging, foraminal stenosis was seen

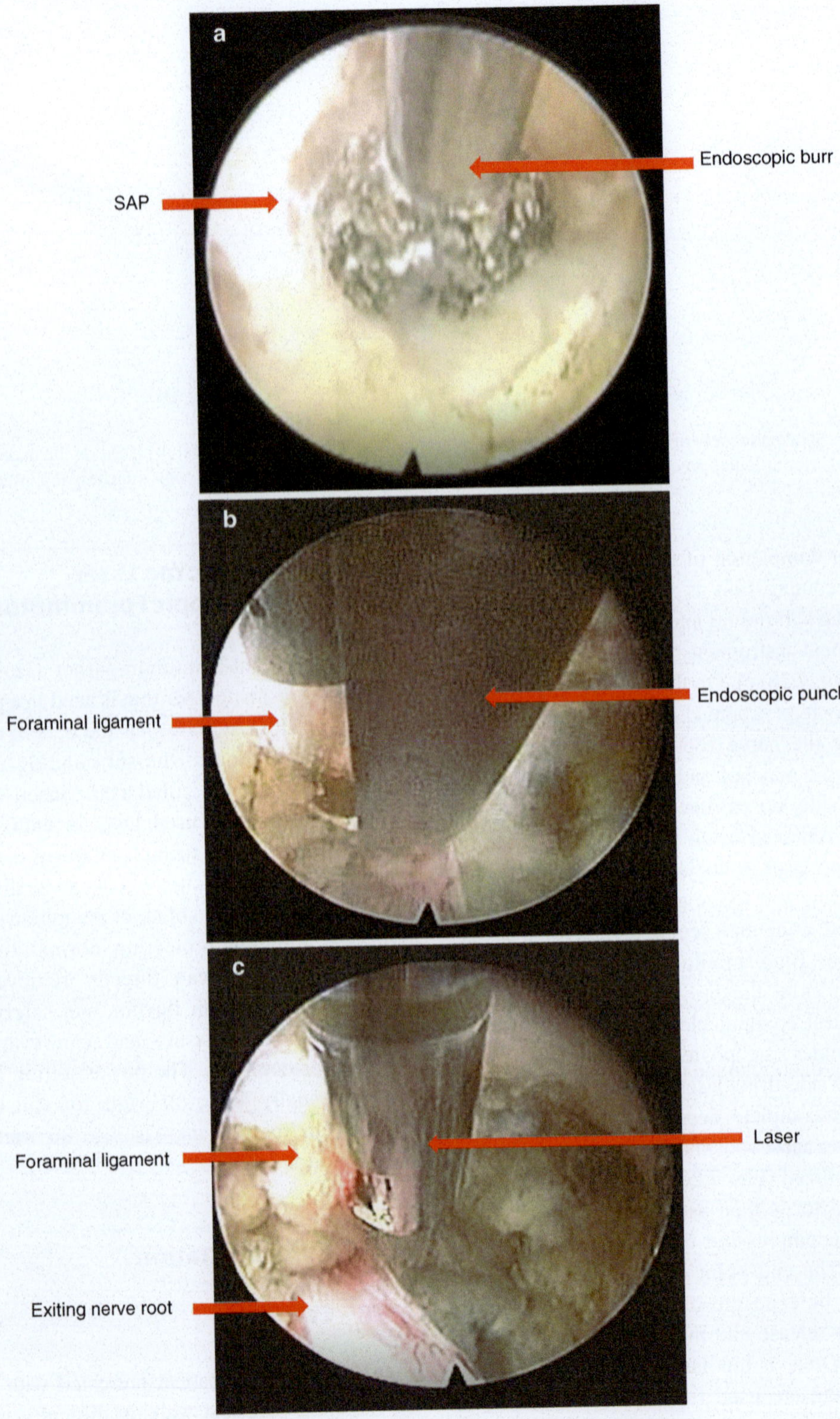

Fig. 7.2 Intraoperative endoscopic view of endoscopic lumbar foraminotomy. (**a**) Foraminal unroofing using endoscopic burr. (**b**) Decompression of the soft tissue is done using punches and forceps. (**c**) Laser is used for more sophisticated decompression. (**d**) Final view of complete foraminal decompression

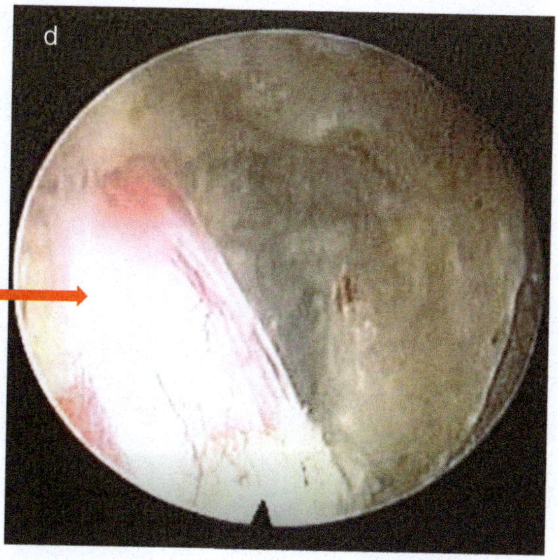

Fig. 7.2 (continued)

on the right L4/5 level caused by disc collapse, ligament hypertrophy, and disc herniation. The patient underwent endoscopic lumbar foraminotomy with removal of herniated disc. Postoperative MR images showed complete decompression of the right L4/5 foraminal stenosis. The patient had complete resolution of his symptoms (Fig. 7.3).

7.5.2 Case 2

A 73-year-old female presented with right leg radiating pain and walking difficulty. She underwent anterior lumbar interbody fusion (ALIF) and percutaneous screw fixation at the L2/3/4/5 levels 2 years earlier. On MR imaging, disc herniation and foraminal stenosis were seen at the L4/5 level which were not visible on the postoperative images taken immediately after her ALIF surgery. Cage subsidence and disc herniation had contributed to the gradual narrowing and stenosis of the L4/5 right foramen. As the L4/5 level was already fused, endoscopic decompression under local anesthesia was selected for this patient. She underwent endoscopic lumbar foraminotomy with removal of herniated disc. Postoperative MR images showed complete decompression of the right L4/5 foraminal area, and the patient showed near-complete resolution of her symptoms (Fig. 7.4, Video 7.1).

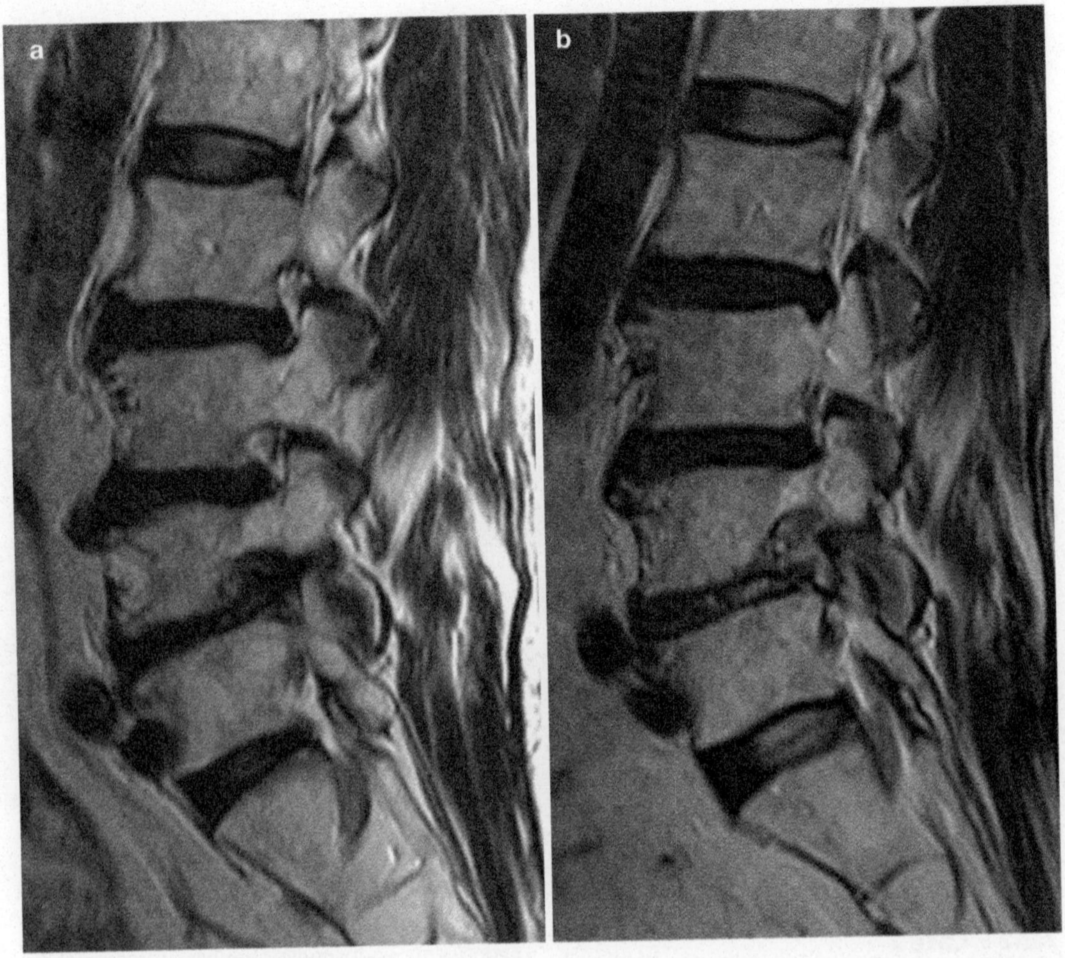

Fig. 7.3 Magnetic resonance (MR) image of right foraminal stenosis at the L4/5 level. (**a**) Preoperative T2-weighted sagittal MR image demonstrating foraminal stenosis. (**b**) Postoperative T2-weighted sagittal MR showing complete decompression

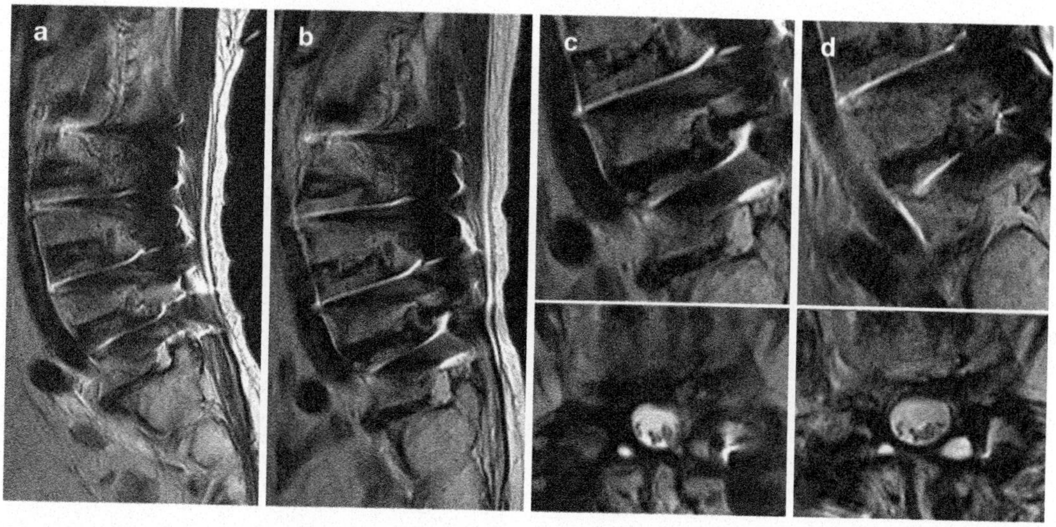

Fig. 7.4 Magnetic resonance (MR) image of right foraminal stenosis at the L4/5 level after fusion surgery. (**a**) MRI after initial fusion surgery showing no sign of foraminal stenosis. (**b**) Gradual decrease in disc height and disc herniation resulting in foraminal stenosis at the L4/5 level on the right side. (**c**) Preoperative T2-weighted sagittal MR image demonstrating foraminal stenosis. (**d**) Postoperative T2-weighted sagittal MR showing complete decompression

7.6 Summary

Endoscopic lumbar foraminotomy is a safe and effective treatment method for lumbar foraminal stenosis. Although there is fairly steep learning, curve, and advances in the surgical technique, the variety and quality of endoscopic equipment and also the use of Ho:YAG laser have helped this procedure become more accessible and practical. Furthermore, endoscopic lumbar foraminotomy under local anesthesia can be considered as a good option for patients who have underlying medical conditions hindering the use of general anesthesia.

References

1. Jenis LG, An HS. Spinal update. Lumbar foraminal stenosis. Neurospine. 2000;25:389–94.
2. Epstein NE. Foraminal and far lateral lumbar disc herniations: surgical alternatives and outcome measures. Spinal Cord. 2002;40:491–500.
3. Reulen HJ, Pfaundler S, Ebeling U. The lateral microsurgical approach to the "extracanalicular" lumbar disc herniation. I: a technical note. Acta Neurochir. 1987;84:64–7.
4. Wiltse LL. The paraspinal sacrospinalis-splitting approach to the lumbar spine. Clin Orthop Relat Res. 1973;91:48–57.
5. Wiltse LL, Spencer CW. New uses and refinements of the paraspinal approach to the lumbar spine. Spine. 1988;13:696–706.
6. Chang HS, Zidan I, Fujisawa N, Matsui T. Microsurgical posterolateral transmuscular approach for lumbar foraminal stenosis. J Spinal Disord Tech. 2011;24:302–7.
7. Donaldson WF, Star MJ, Thorne RP. Surgical treatment for the far lateral herniated lumbar disc. Spine. 1993;18:1263–7.
8. Lejeune JP, Hladky JP, Cotten A, Vinchon M, Christiaens JL. Foraminal lumbar disc herniation. Experience with 83 patients. Spine (Phila Pa 1976). 1994;19:1905–8.
9. Knight M, Goswami A. Management of isthmic spondylolisthesis with posterolateral endoscopic foraminal decompression. Spine. 2003;28:573–81.
10. Schubert M, Hoogland T. Endoscopic transforaminal nucleotomy with foraminoplasty for lumbar disk herniation. Oper Orthop Traumatol. 2005;17:641–61.
11. Jang JS, An SH, Lee SH. Transforaminal percutaneous endoscopic discectomy in the treatment of foraminal and extraforaminal lumbar disc herniations. J Spinal Disord Tech. 2006;19:338–43.
12. Ahn Y, Lee SH, Park WM, Lee HY. Posterolateral percutaneous endoscopic lumbar foraminotomy for L5-S1 foraminal or lateral exit zone stenosis. Technical note. J Neurosurg. 2003;99:320–3.

13. Knight MT, Goswami A, Patko JT, Buxton N. Endoscopic foraminoplasty: a prospective study on 250 consecutive patients with independent evaluation. J Clin Laser Med Surg. 2001;19:73–81.
14. Ahn Y, Oh HK, Kim H, Lee SH, Lee HN. Percutaneous endoscopic lumbar foraminotomy: an advanced surgical technique and clinical outcomes. Neurosurgery. 2014;75:124–33.
15. Ahn Y, Keum HJ, Son S. Percutaneous endoscopic lumbar foraminotomy for foraminal stenosis with postlaminectomy syndrome in geriatric patients. World Neurosurg. 2019;130:E1–7.
16. Ahn Y, Keum HJ, Shin SH, Choi JJ. Laser-assisted endoscopic lumbar foraminotomy for failed back surgery syndrome in elderly patients. Lasers Med Sci. 2020;35:121–9.
17. Ahn Y, Lee U. Use of lasers in minimally invasive spine surgery. Expert Rev Med Devices. 2018;15:423–33.

Microscopic Lumbar Discectomy for Paramedian Disc Herniation with CO_2 Laser

8

Dong Hyun Bae and Junseok Bae

Abstract

Minimally invasive microscopic lumbar discectomy for paramedian disc herniation is the most common surgical technique in the spine field. The herniated disc is treated with the removal of the extruded disc fragment and the removal of the material within the disc space traditionally. On the contrary, fragmentectomy only or laser-assisted small annulotomy has the advantage of effectively removing the disc through a narrow field of view than the conventional scalpel discectomy. According to using laser, normal structures can be preserved as much as possible, and small lesions can be accurately and delicately removed. It has several advantages for lower recurrence rates and postoperative low back pain. It is estimated that laser-induced metaplasia and modulating pro- and anti-inflammatory factors are the mechanisms. As a result, laser-assisted fragmentectomy could be an effective alternative to conventional microdiscectomy techniques.

Supplementary Information The online version of this chapter (https://doi.org/10.1007/978-981-16-2206-9_8) contains supplementary material, which is available to authorized users.

D. H. Bae · J. Bae (✉)
Department of Neurosurgery, Chungdam Wooridul Spine Hospital, Seoul, Republic of Korea

Keywords

Laser discectomy · Laser surgery · Minimally invasive surgery · Open lumbar microdiscectomy · Paracentral disc herniation

8.1 Introduction

Minimally invasive microscopic lumbar discectomy is the most common surgical method in recent years. Traditionally, the annulotomy and discectomy have been performed using a scalpel. However, the annulotomy using a laser can easily do it even in a small space. It is also possible to remove or evaporate small lesions accurately. And it has a mechanism of stabilizing itself by inhibiting tissue regeneration at the laser cauterization site. Therefore, microscopic lumbar discectomy using a laser is a great help in operation much simpler and safer.

8.2 Indications

The indication is almost the same as the conventional microscopic lumbar discectomy for paramedian disc herniation. If there is a disc rupture or protrusion, and there is corresponding low back pain or ipsilateral radiating pain, and there is no improvement to conservative treatment, surgery may be considered. It is also an indication for emergency surgery in case of cauda equina

J. Bae, S.-H. Lee (eds.), *Laser Spine Surgery*, https://doi.org/10.1007/978-981-16-2206-9_8

syndrome or progressive motor weakness. Indications of laser surgery are not different. However, compared to the conventional microscopic discectomy, it can be applied to a smaller and narrower lesion. Therefore, it has the advantage of reducing the area of laminectomy and facet injury.

8.3 Surgical Technique

Most procedures are almost the same as in conventional minimally invasive microdiscectomy with the microscope. A skin incision was made off to the lesion side, which is the most lateral portion of the spinous process at the appropriate disc space after needle localization with x-ray. The typical skin incision was 20-25 mm long. The incision was made to allow the insertion of a 20-mm-wide periosteal elevator laterally to retract the muscle medially once it was subperiosteally dissected from the bone. *Once the lamina was exposed, a lung-shape partial hemilaminectomy with foraminotomy was performed using high-speed drill to expose the ligamentum flavum.* (Fig. 8.1) *Then it was removed by en bloc fashion to expose the epidural space.* (Fig. 8.2) *The affected disc was exposed by cautious retraction of the thecal sac and traversing nerve root.* (Fig. 8.3) Epidural veins around the disc were coagulated with a bipolar coagulator, and the nerve root was gently retracted using a root retractor, exposing the ruptured fragments. Usually, the ruptured disc fragments were removed after they were gently mobilized from beneath the nerve root. But in cases of contained disc herniations, annulotomy was performed with the smallest possible opening using the CO_2 laser (Sharplan 30C, Lumenis, Yokneam, Israel). (Fig. 8.4) By extension of this hole using a CO_2 laser, surgeons can create enough of an annulotomy to remove the fragments under retraction of the traversing nerve root. (Fig. 8.5a, b) At this time, do not shoot the laser too deeply, as it may cause major vessel injury [1] if you shoot the laser far beyond the anterior annulus. *To prevent these complications, it is necessary to fill the disc space with a normal saline when performing*

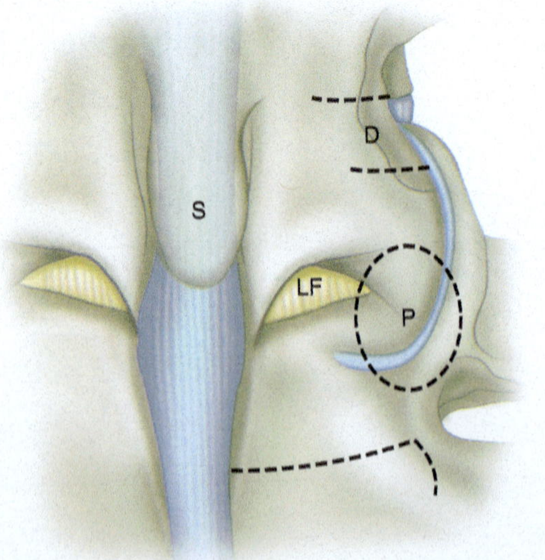

Fig. 8.1 The illustration shows the area of lung-shaped partial hemilaminectomy. The superior border is pars interarticularis or upper endplate, and the lateral border is the virtual extension of the medial border of the inferior level pedicle. The inferior border is the virtual extension of the inferior border of the inferior level pedicle. And the medial border is midline. (S, Spinous process, D, Disc, P, Pedicle, LF, Ligamentum flavum)

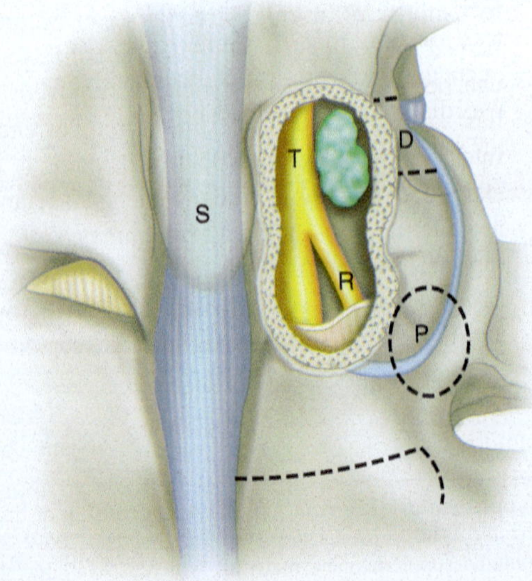

Fig. 8.2 The illustration shows exposure of thecal sac and traversing root after flavectomy as en bloc fashion. (S, Spinous process, D, Disc, P, Pedicle, T, Thecal sac, R, Nerve root)

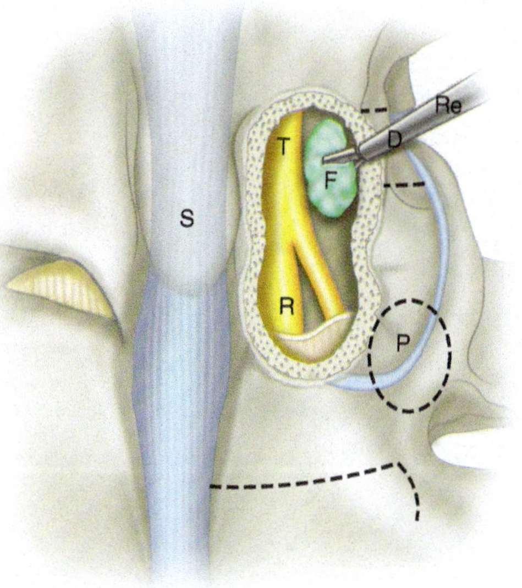

Fig. 8.3 The illustration shows exposure of the ruptured fragment on disc space after gentle retraction of the nerve root. (S, Spinous process, D, Disc, P, Pedicle, T, Thecal sac, R, Nerve root, Re, Retractor, F, Fragment)

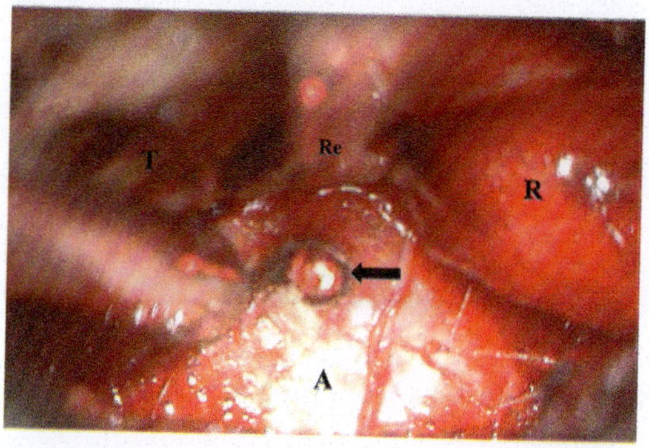

Fig. 8.4 The microscopic view of lumbar microdiscectomy surgery. Small annulotomy (arrow) was performed by laser. (T, Thecal sac, R, Nerve root, Re, Retractor, A, Annulus)

intradiscal laser ablation. (Fig. 8.6) Also, when cauterizing the disc with a laser, there may be nerve root damage caused by the heat of vaporization. Therefore, sufficient normal saline irrigation should be necessary. After confirming the careful inspection for any hidden fragments and release of the nerve root using the microprobe, the wound was closed in a conventional way.

8.4 Postoperative Consideration

Conventional/aggressive discectomy or fragmentectomy/sequestrectomy only are the ways of contemplating surgeon, and it has long been a topic of debate. There are several conflicting literatures. McGirt et al. [2] reported that the incidence of recurrent disc herniation after a fragmentectomy was 7% and for aggressive discectomy was 3.5%. However, Fakouri et al. [3] found that the rate of reherniation in the sequestrectomy group was slightly lower than in the conventional microdiscectomy group. On the other hand, Baek et al. [4] revealed that there was no significant difference in recurrence rates between the fragmentectomy and the conventional microdiscectomy groups. It is difficult to conclude the difference between a conventional discectomy and fragmentectomy in the recurrence rate. Due to laser-induced metaplasia, however, laser-assisted discectomy is believed to decrease recurrence [5, 6].

Postoperative back pain is also a considerable concern of many surgeons. Traditional lumbar discectomy surgery was performed by removal of the extruded disc fragment and removal of the material within the disc space. These surgical methods were known to have a higher incidence of low back pain than fragmentectomy only [7]. However, Baek et al. [4] reported that there were no significant differences in VAS scores after surgery between the fragmentectomy and conventional microdiscectomy groups. Therefore, the method of fragmentectomy only is more favourable to the patient's outcome than the conventional microdiscectomy method. In addition, the laser also acts over the annular nociceptors for its anti-inflammatory and proliferative action [8, 9].

As a result, laser-assisted fragmentectomy could be an effective alternative to conventional microdiscectomy techniques. Because the laser enabled effective removal of disc herniation via a narrow operative corridor without excessive damage of the lamina and the facet joint. And it contributes to preserve normal disc and spinal stability. Therefore, laser-assisted fragmentec-

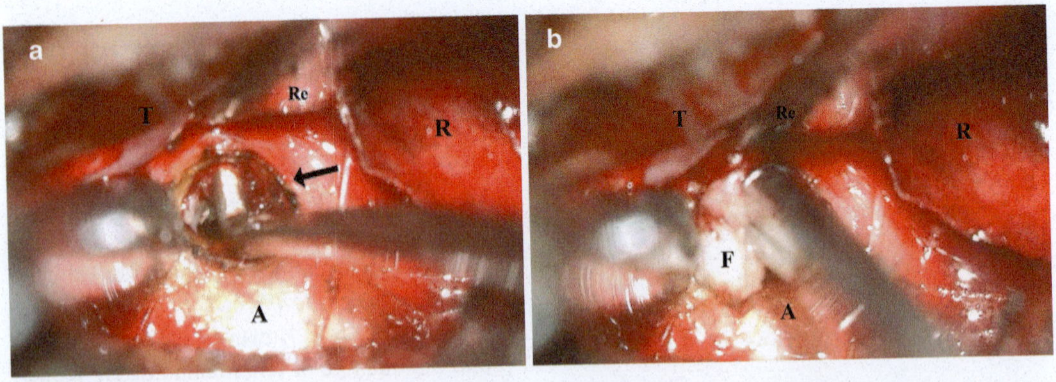

Fig. 8.5 The microscopic view of lumbar microdiscectomy surgery. After the extension of annulotomy (arrow) by laser, (**a**) disc fragment was removed through enough size of annulotomy. (**b**) (T, Thecal sac, R, Nerve root, Re, Retractor, A, Annulus)

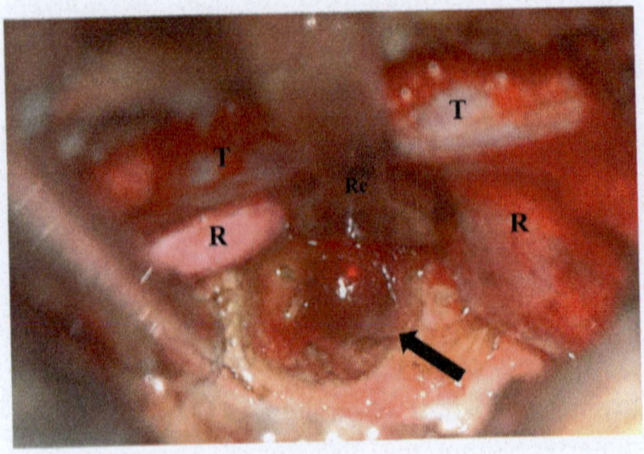

Fig. 8.6 The microscopic view of lumbar microdiscectomy surgery. Fill the disc space with a normal saline. (T, Thecal sac, R, Nerve root, Re, Retractor)

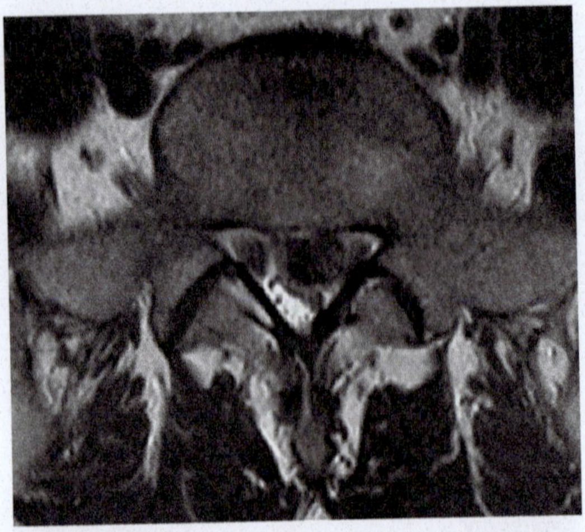

Fig. 8.7 T2-weighted axial magnetic resonance images shows extruded disc particle which is compressing S1 nerve root at the L5-S1 level

tomy is an effective method in the short and long term.

8.5 Case Illustration

A *40*-year-old male patient visited our hospital with lower back pain, left lower leg radiating pain, and numbness lasting a month. He received conservative treatment from other hospitals. Magnetic resonance images (MRI) scans revealed herniated discs at L5-S1, causing left S1 nerve root compromise. (Fig. 8.7) The patient underwent minimally invasive microdiscectomy using laser for herniated disc disease. The operative technique is mentioned above. After gentle retraction of S1 nerve root and thecal sac, ruptured disc fragment was identified through axilla space, and the ruptured particle was removed. Then, the annulotomy was performed by laser. (Fig. 8.8a) the contained disc was removed successfully without nerve root injury. (Fig. 8.8b) *As with this patient, the annular tear was near the midline, and the annulotomy is required through the axilla. In this situation, the use of a scalpel is dangerous, but the use of a laser is safe.* The patient's left lower extremity pain improved after the operation.

In conventional microdiscectomy surgery, most of the surgeon uses scalpel for annulotomy.

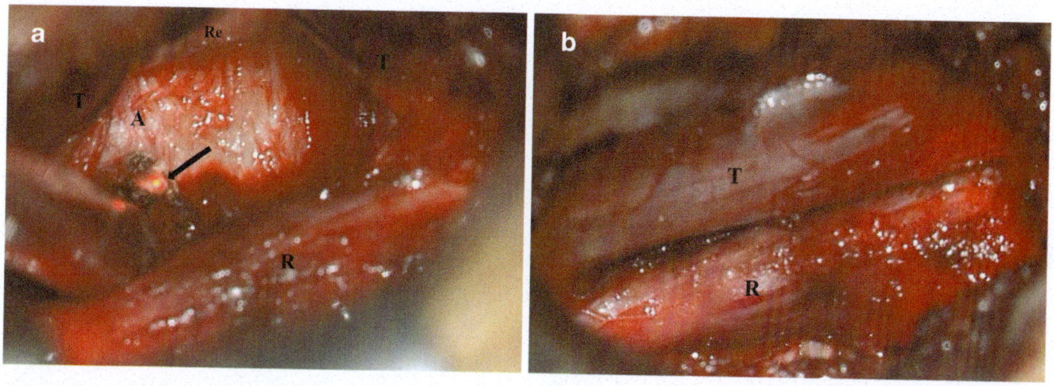

Fig. 8.8 The microscopic view of L5-S1 level. After proper laminectomy and flavectomy, the S1 nerve root and the extruded disc were identified. The ruptured fragment was removed by pituitary rongeur through axilla space. Then, the annulotomy was performed with laser.(arrow) (**a**) Complete decompression of the left S1 nerve root and the thecal sac is achieved.(**b**)

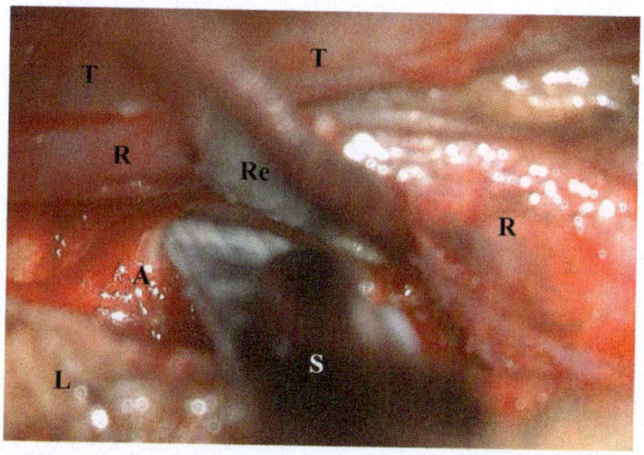

Fig. 8.9 The microscopic view of conventional annulotomy with No. 15 scalpel. (T, Thecal sac, R, Nerve root, Re, Retractor, A, Annulus, L, Lamina, S, No.15 scalpel)

(Fig. 8.9) It occupies most of the surgical corridor and can make riskiness of nerve root injury. On the other hand, in the case of this patient, the laser can focus exactly on and evaporate the targeted annulus through small corridor.

8.6 Summary

Microscopic lumbar discectomy for paramedian disc herniation is one of the most commonly performed surgeries in the spine area, and the minimally invasive technique is becoming universal. Fragmentectomy only or laser-assisted small annulotomy has the advantage of effectively removing the disc in a narrow field of view than the conventional scalpel discectomy and preserving normal structures. And the laser has advantages over scalpel use in terms of preciseness. These are the ability to be used on delicate tissues, minimal tissue manipulation, less bleeding, swelling, and trauma. Therefore, it is useful in the small spaces involved in paramedian herniated discs.

References

1. Jeon S-H, Lee S-H, Choi W-C. Iliac artery perforation following lumbar discectomy with microsurgical carbon dioxide laser: a report of a rare case and discussion on the treatment. Spine. 2007;32(3):E124–E5.
2. McGirt MJ, Ambrossi GLG, Datoo G, Sciubba DM, Witham TF, Wolinsky J-P, et al. Recurrent disc herniation and long-term back pain after primary lumbar discectomy: review of outcomes reported for limited versus aggressive disc removal. Neurosurgery. 2009;64(2):338–45.
3. Fakouri B, Patel V, Bayley E, Srinivas S. Lumbar microdiscectomy versus sequestrectomy/free fragmentectomy: a long-term (> 2 y) retrospective study of the clinical outcome. Clin Spine Surg. 2011;24(1):6–10.
4. Baek G-S, Kim Y-S, Lee M-C, Song J-W, Kim S-K, Kim I-H. Fragmentectomy versus conventional microdiscectomy in single-level lumbar disc herniations: comparison of clinical results and recurrence rates. J Korean Neurosurg Soc. 2012;52(3):210.
5. Kim J-S, Choi G, Jin S-R, Lee S-H. Removal of a discal cyst using a percutaneous endoscopic interlaminar approach: a case report. Photomed Laser Surg. 2009;27(2):365–9.

6. Oh H-S, Kim J-S. Clinical Application of CO_2 Laser. CO_2 Laser: Optimisation and Application. 2012:357.
7. Soliman J, Harvey A, Howes G, Seibly J, Dossey J, Nardone E. Limited microdiscectomy for lumbar disk herniation: a retrospective long-term outcome analysis. Clin Spine Surg. 2014;27(1):E8–E13.
8. Fukuda TY, Tanji MM, Silva SR, Sato MN, Plapler H. Infrared low-level diode laser on inflammatory process modulation in mice: pro-and anti-inflammatory cytokines. Lasers Med Sci. 2013;28(5):1305–13.
9. Plapler H, Mancini MW, Sella VR, Bomfim FR. Evaluation of different laser wavelengths on ablation lesion and residual thermal injury in intervertebral discs of the lumbar spine. Lasers Med Sci. 2016;31(3):421–8.

Discectomy of Calcified Disc Herniation Using CO_2 Laser

9

Yong Soo Choi

Abstract

Lumbar disc herniation is a relatively common disease among spinal diseases. With the development of invasive and non-invasive treatments, treatment methods are very diverse, and the prognosis is improving day by day. However, the treatment for calcified disc herniation during such lumbar disc herniation has a slightly different treatment method compared to the soft disc herniation. Hard disc herniation is because there are quite a few cases where it is not easy to remove. Calcified intervertebral disc herniation is often not easily separated from the surrounding tissues and tends to be difficult to remove with mechanical tools. Lasers offer a very effective and safe way to treat such hard disc herniation. By using a laser, calcified intervertebral disc herniation can be removed more easily and safely, thereby increasing the success rate of surgery.

Keyword

Hard disc · Calcified disc · Disc herniation · Discectomy · CO_2 laser

Y. S. Choi (✉)
Department of Neurosurgery, Chungdam Wooridul Spine Hospital, Seoul, Republic of Korea
e-mail: yong@wooridul.co.kr

9.1 Introduction

Surgical removal of a calcified disc herniation is more complex than removing a soft disc herniation [1]. The hard intervertebral disc is firmly attached to the surrounding tissues and is not easily removed, and there is a high possibility of adhesion with the nerve tissues, and it is often difficult to be held by mechanical devices. When removing a hard disc rupture, open microdiscectomy is preferred due to adhesion of surrounding tissues and hard disc herniation fragments [2]. Rarely has been described for effective and safe removal of calcified intervertebral discs [3]. When removing the calcified prolapsed intervertebral disc, complications such as nerve damage or insufficient disc resection are likely to occur [4]. Therefore, it should be devised to effectively and safely remove the calcified prolapsed intervertebral disc. Microdiscectomy is currently the standard method for removing a prolapsed intervertebral disc [5, 6]. In the surgical field of view, the nerve tissue and the prolapsed intervertebral disc are identified, the nerve tissue can be safely retracted, and tools for disc resection are effectively used. In particular, lasers are more useful than other mechanical tools when removing calcified intervertebral discs. By using a laser, nerve damage is minimized, and the calcified intervertebral disc is well separated from the surrounding tissue. It also allows to remove remaining hard parts. The laser, which is used in various ways

J. Bae, S.-H. Lee (eds.), *Laser Spine Surgery*, https://doi.org/10.1007/978-981-16-2206-9_9

during surgery, is also an excellent tool when removing calcified intervertebral discs.

9.2 Surgical Technique

The incidence of calcified disc herniation is not statistically known, but it is not uncommonly found. If the disc herniation is not absorbed or removed effectively, it can harden over time. In addition, the calcified disc fragment may prolapse with the soft disc material surrounding it. When these calcified intervertebral discs compress the neural tissue, pain and neurological symptoms may be presented. In these cases, effective decompression may be required if symptoms are not relieved, and symptoms persist or worsen. Calcified intervertebral discs can be removed using open spinal surgery or endoscopic discectomy. When the calcified intervertebral disc is removed by open surgery, the hard prolapsed disc is often difficult to incise with a surgical knife and may sometimes need to be removed with an electric drill or large-sized instruments. When these tools are used, the defect of the intervertebral disc becomes large, resulting in a sudden degenerative change of the intervertebral disc, a decrease in the height of the intervertebral disc, or damage to the neural structure. The CO_2 laser provides a safe and effective surgical procedure without its drawbacks in removing calcified prolapsed intervertebral discs using a large tool. If a surgical approach such as laminectomy is performed with a microscope field of view, neural structures such as the dura and nerve root are identified. When these nerve structures are towed with a retractor, the intervertebral disc would be seen. The calcified prolapsed intervertebral disc is visible in the microscope field. Discectomy is performed by determining the extent of the prolapsed intervertebral disc. If the calcified intervertebral disc is small, it can be burned out with a CO_2 laser. If the size of the calcified prolapsed intervertebral disc is large, a plan should be made for discectomy for effective and safe complete removal. The CO_2 laser is a positive and ideal tool when a large calcified prolapsed intervertebral disc is surgically removed. If the hard intervertebral disc is surrounded by soft intervertebral discs and extruded, the boundary line is secured by burning around the hard part using a laser. (Fig. 9.1) Afterwards, the hard part is separated from the periphery and floated, and these parts are easily removed with physical tools. The prolapsed intervertebral disc that has not been removed can be removed cleanly using a laser. (Fig. 9.2) If a hard intervertebral disc is attempted to be removed with tools such as a surgical knife without a laser, the boundaries of the hard tissue cannot be accurately known, and the soft normal disc may be excessively damaged. Also, the connected soft tissue may interfere with the removal of the hard disc. Lasers that can be used during spinal surgery, especially CO_2 lasers, can be used

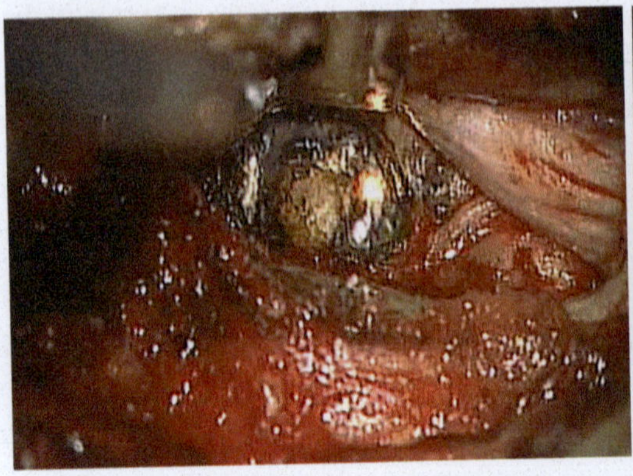

Fig. 9.1 The calcified prolapsed intervertebral disc on left L5 ~ S1 level was confirmed after laminectomy and flavectomy, and the boundary was burned with CO2 laser.

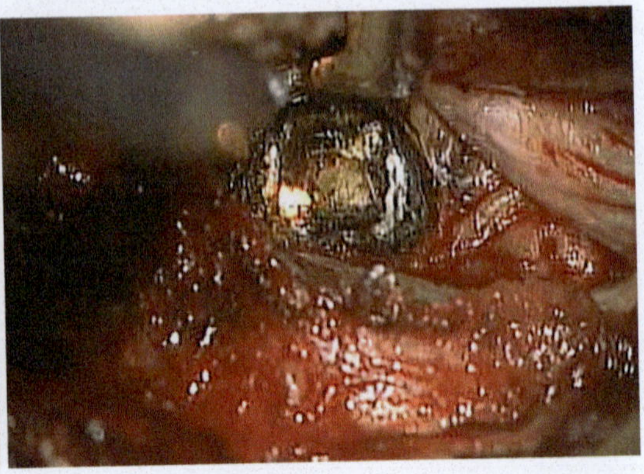

The hard part is separated from the surrounding tissues using a laser and becomes easy to remove

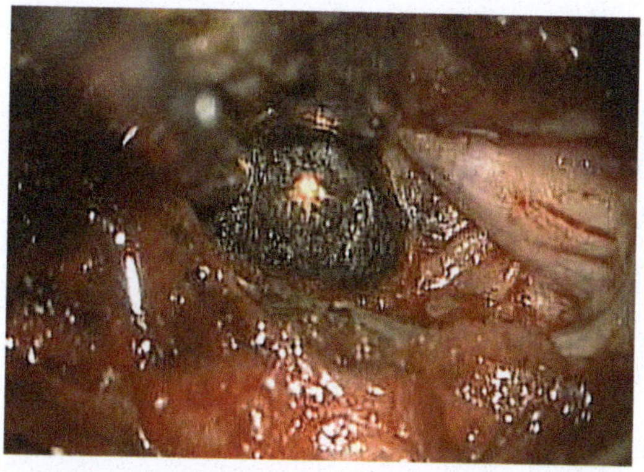

Fig. 9.2 The hard intervertebral disc separated from the surrounding tissue may be removed using mechanical tools but may be selectively removed while maintaining normal intervertebral disc tissue by removing it using a laser

in a variety of ways. One of them can be easily used to remove the hard disc, that is, the calcified prolapsed disc. Laser discectomy is more accurate and easier to perform than using a mechanical tool.

9.3 Conclusion

It is rare that calcified intervertebral disc herniation is described. If symptoms occur due to the hard prolapsed intervertebral disc compressing the nerve, it is necessary to remove it. The hard disc is often adhered to the surrounding tissues, and it tends to be difficult to remove with mechanical tools, so it is more difficult than removing a soft disc prolapse. Lasers are useful in overcoming these difficulties and effectively and safely removing calcified prolapsed intervertebral discs.

References

1. Shao J, Yu M, Jiang L, et al. Differences in calcification and osteogenic potential of herniated discs according to the severity of degeneration based on Pfirrmann grade: a cross-sectional study. BMC Musculoskelet Disord. 2016;17:191.
2. Katayama Y, Matsuyama Y, Yoshihara H, et al. Comparison of surgical outcomes between macro discectomy and micro discectomy for lumbar disc herniation: a prospective randomized study with surgery performed by the same spine surgeon. J Spinal Disord Tech. 2006;19:344–7.
3. Kim HS, Adsul N, Ju YS, et al. Full endoscopic lumbar discectomy using the calcification floating technique for symptomatic partially calcified lumbar herniated nucleus pulposus. World Neurosurg. 2018;119:500–5.
4. Dabo X, Ziqiang C, Yinchuan Z, et al. The clinical results of percutaneous endoscopic interlaminar discectomy (PEID) in the treatment of calcified lumbar disc herniation: a case-control study. Pain Physician. 2016;19:69–76.
5. Postacchini F, Postacchini R. Operative management of lumbar disc herniation: the evolution of knowledge and surgical techniques in the last century. Acta Neurochir Suppl. 2011;108:17–21.
6. Maroon JC. Current concepts in minimally invasive discectomy. Neurosurgery. 2002;51:S137–45.

10 Microscopic Lumbar Discectomy for Foraminal and Extraforaminal Disc Herniation Using CO_2 Laser

Dong-Ju Yun

Abstract

Disc herniation that is confined to the neural foramen area is called foraminal lumbar disc herniation (FLDH). Herniated discs arising outwardly of the neural foramen constitute extraforaminal lumbar disc herniation (EFLDH). Microscopic lumbar discectomy via the paraspinal approach is considered the gold standard for surgical treatment of FLDH and EFLDH. However, there is a possibility of postoperative complications due to the complex anatomical structures, narrow surgical field, excessive neural retraction, and incomplete decompression. Lumbar microdiscectomy via the paraspinal approach for FLDH and EFLDH using a carbon dioxide (CO_2) laser can minimize spinal nerve traction and tissue damage. In this chapter, we describe the surgical method of lumbar microdiscectomy via the paraspinal approach for FLDH and EFLDH using a CO_2 laser and discuss the usefulness of CO_2 use.

Keywords

Foraminal · Extraforaminal · Intervertebral disc · Laser · Microscopic

10.1 Introduction

Foraminal, intraforaminal, far-lateral, extreme-lateral, and extracanalicular disc herniation are terms used to define disc herniation into the intervertebral foramen or lateral area of the intervertebral foramen. Herniated discs that are confined to the neural foramen area are called foraminal lumbar disc herniation (FLDH). Herniated discs arising outwardly of the neural foramen are called extraforaminal lumbar disc herniation (EFLDH). FLDH and EFLDH are reported to constitute 7%–12% of disc herniations [1–4]. They most often at the L3–L4 or L4–L5 level, followed by L5–S1 [4]. FLDH and EFLDH compress the exiting spinal nerve and dorsal root ganglion (DRG), thus, causing extreme radiating pain in the leg.

There are several reports of surgical management for this condition. In 1968, Wiltse et al. first reported the paraspinal approach for lumbar arthrodesis [5]. In 1985, Recoules-Arche reported a surgical method with the transmuscular approach in the treatment of FLDH and EFLDH [6]. In 1987, Reulen et al. and Fankhauser et al. reported a microsurgical approach via the paramuscular and transmuscular techniques for surgical treat-

Supplementary Information The online version of this chapter (https://doi.org/10.1007/978-981-16-2206-9_10) contains supplementary material, which is available to authorized users.

D.-J. Yun (✉)
Department of Neurosurgery, Busan Wooridul Spine Hospital, Busan, South Korea
e-mail: djyunns@wooridul.co.kr

J. Bae, S.-H. Lee (eds.), *Laser Spine Surgery*, https://doi.org/10.1007/978-981-16-2206-9_10

ments for FLDH and EFLDH [7, 8]. In 1996, Reulen et al. reported the microsurgical anatomy required to treat EFLDH at the L5–S1 level through a lateral approach [9, 10]. Since then, many studies have been reported on the paraspinal approach in FLDH and EFLDH [10–14]. Microscopic lumbar discectomy via the paraspinal approach has been used as an effective surgical treatment for FLDH and EFLDH. This technique minimizes the damage to the surrounding tissues and preserves the facet joint to avoid postoperative instability, which may require fusion surgery [15]. However, there have been reports of postoperative leg pain and dysesthesia after the paraspinal approach for FLDH and EFLDH due to excessive neural manipulation or incomplete decompression [3, 11, 14, 15]. In the paraspinal approach, the space between the facet joint and spinal nerve is usually narrow; therefore, in order to remove the disc material, the spinal nerve needs to be manipulated to access the disc space. However, the spinal nerve should not be manipulated excessively, and the facet joint should not be removed excessively to obtain the proper surgical view.

Microscopic lumbar discectomy via the paraspinal approach for FLDH and EFLDH using a carbon dioxide (CO_2) laser can minimize spinal nerve traction and tissue damage. It has been reported to provide good clinical outcomes [3, 15, 16]. In this chapter, we describe the surgical method of microscopic lumbar discectomy via the paraspinal approach for FLDH and EFLDH using a CO_2 laser and discuss the usefulness of CO_2 use.

10.2 Indications

- When the herniated lumbar disc is located below the pedicle or outside the pedicle, compressing the spinal nerve is identified through neuroimaging, such as magnetic resonance imaging (MRI).
- Neuroimaging findings correspond with the clinical manifestation.
- When back and radicular pain do not improve or symptoms worsen even with conservative treatment.
- If the patient has neurologic deficiencies, such as severe motor weakness.

10.3 Surgical Technique

The bony structures that constitute the intervertebral foramen of the lumbar spine include the upper and lower pedicles, dorsal aspect of the vertebral body, ventral aspect of the facet joints, and pars intercularis. The operative window for the paraspinal approach is created by the lateral surface of pars intercularis and the ventral and lateral surfaces of the facet joint on the medial side; the lower edge of the pedicle and cranial transverse process or prominent accessory process, if present, on the cranial side; and the upper edge of the caudal transverse process on the caudal side. The operative window gradually narrows as it descends from the L1–L2 level to the L5–S1 level.

Going down to the lower lumbar level, the distance from the spinous process to the lateral margin of pars intercularis increases gradually, and the lamina gradually covers the waist of the vertebral body. The transverse process moves downward, and there are many prominent accessory processes at the lower lumbar level. The course of the nerve changes at different levels and is altered by disc herniation.

The facet joint becomes larger, and the facet articulation changes gradually from the sagittal direction to the coronal direction. When performing the paraspinal approach, at the upper lumbar level, a sufficient operative window can be obtained by removing a small bony structure; however, at the lower lumbar level, more bony structures must be removed [3] (Fig. 10.1).

Following the removal of these bony structures, the intertransverse ligaments must be removed to access the foraminal or extraforaminal area. In the intertransverse space, these ligaments act as septa that divide the anterior and posterior musculature of the lumbar spine. In shape and composition, the intertransverse ligaments are more like membranes than true ligaments. The intertransverse ligaments are attached to the cranial and caudal transverse processes. Medially, the ligaments are connected to the pars intercularis and the capsule of the facet joint. Laterally, they are attached to the thoracolumbar fascia [17] (Fig. 10.1).

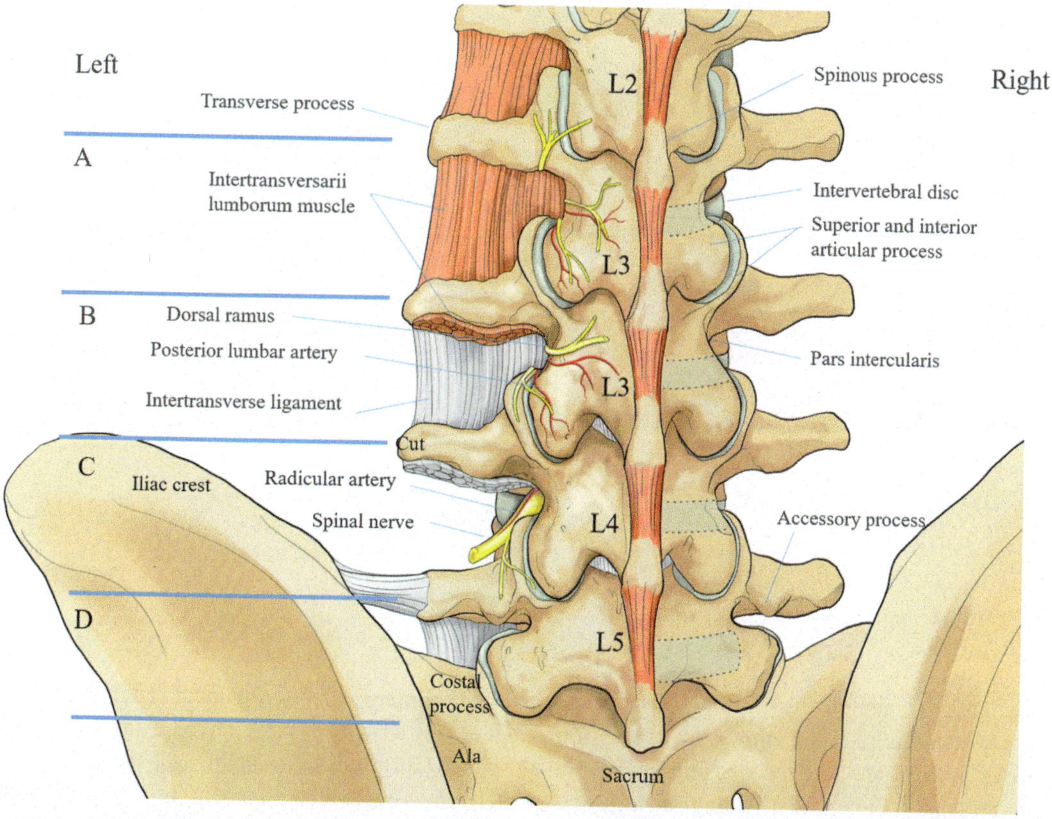

Fig. 10.1 The surgical anatomic features of the paraspinal approach. Left: L2–5 vertebrae that include muscular, osseous, ligamentous, vascular, and neural structures. Area **a**: After the dissection between the multifidus and longissimus muscle, the intertransversarii lumborum muscle can be identified. Area **b**: After removal of the intertransversarii lumborum muscle, the intertransverse ligament can be identified. The dorsal ramus and posterior lumbar artery break through the intertransverse ligament. Area **c**: After removal of the intertransverse ligament, the spinal nerve can be identified. Area **d**: intertransverse ligament between the L5 transverse process and the costal process of the sacrum. A prominent accessory process below the L5 transverse process can be identified. Right: From L2–L3 down to L5–S1, the disc space is obscured by the pars intercularis and facet joints. The distance from the spinous process to the lateral margin of the pars intercularis also increases

10.3.1 L1–L2, L2–L3, L3–L4, and L4–L5

The patient lies in the prone knee chest position on the table. Lateral radiographs are taken to check the surgical level. Usually, 2.5–3.5 cm lateral to the midline, a 3–4-cm vertical skin incision is placed, and the subcutaneous tissue and thoracolumbar fascia are dissected. The fibrous septum is identified between the multifidus and longissimus muscle. Using preoperative MRI or computed tomography (CT), it is helpful to check the position of the fibrous septum between the multifidus muscle and the longissimus muscle at the index level. Dissection is performed between the multifidus and longissimus muscles using the fingertip and a pair of scissors. If a fibrous septum is not identified, a fingertip dissection is performed between the muscles. The facet joint, pars intercularis, and cranial and caudal transverse processes are checked with a fingertip (Fig. 10.2). A self-retractor (Papavero–Caspar speculum, B Braun, Germany) is inserted after pulling or removing the intertransversarii lumborum muscle that crosses between the transverse processes. Lateral radiographs are obtained to verify the surgical level again. The operative table is tilted to the other side by approximately 10°–30°. The

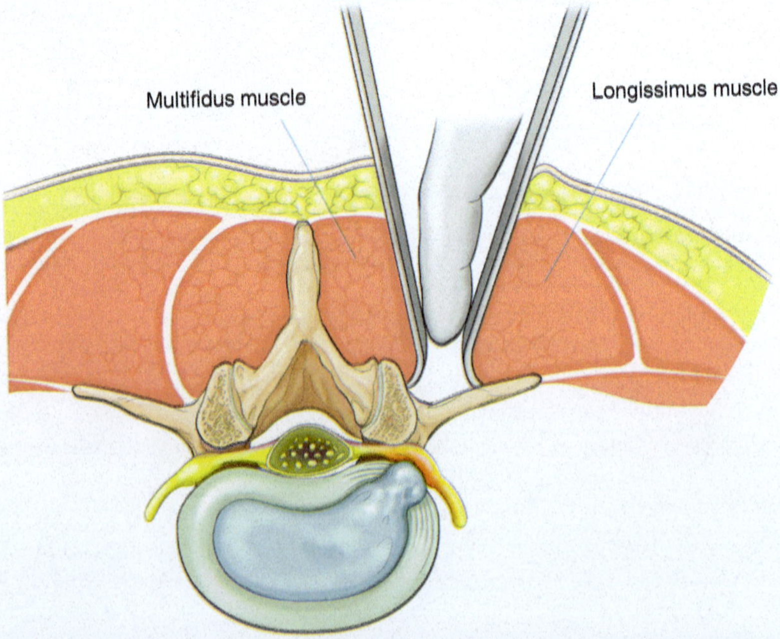

Fig. 10.2 Splitting between the multifidus and longissimus muscles using the fingertip

cranial transverse process, mammillary process, pars intercularis, facet joint, and caudal transverse process are rechecked using an operative microscope (Fig. 10.3). Using a high-speed diamond-tipped burr, the outer part of pars intercularis is drilled along with the lower part of the cranial transverse process and the outer part of the superior articular process (Fig. 10.4).

Drilling the lateral part of the pars intercularis is an important step in the surgery. As it descends from L1 to L5, the lamina gradually widens outward. DRGs are mostly located below or outside the pedicle at the L1–L2, L2–L3, and L3–L4 levels. In contrast, at the L4–L5 and L5–S1 levels, they are mostly located below or inside the pedicle. The distance from the pars intercularis to the outer boundary of the spinal cord is relatively short at L1–L2, L2–L3, and L3–L4 levels and is relatively long at L4–L5 and L5–S1 levels [18]. Therefore, the size of drilling the pars intercularis should be relatively small at L1–L2, L2–L3, and L3–L4 levels and relatively large at L4–L5 and L5–S1 levels [13]. When drilling the outer surface of the superior articular process, the operative table must be tilted to the contralateral side and undercut as much as possible to preserve the facet joint.

The intertransverse ligament is detached from the bony structure and removed using a Kerrison punch (B Braun, Germany) (Figs. 10.5 and 10.6). The intertransverse ligament is removed carefully to avoid damaging the neurovascular bundle and fat tissue around the spinal nerve and ganglion. When the intertransverse ligament is removed, the fibroadipose tissue, radicular arteries and veins, and primary dorsal ramus are located above the spinal nerve and ganglion. Radicular arteries and veins and the primary dorsal ramus should be preserved, if possible. However, if necessary, the radicular arteries and veins are coagulated using bipolar cautery to prevent bleeding. The primary dorsal ramus may also be cut for retraction of the spinal nerve. The herniated disc material is checked, and the spinal nerve and ganglion are retracted. Excessive manipulation of the spinal nerve and ganglion should be avoided. The herniated disc material is removed using a CO_2 laser attached to a microscope (Sharplan 30C, Lumenis, Yokneam, Israel). By using a pinpoint-sized laser beam, the herniated disc material can be precisely removed while minimizing the retraction of the spinal nerve and ganglion (Fig. 10.7). The remaining disc material is checked using a probe, and subtotal discec-

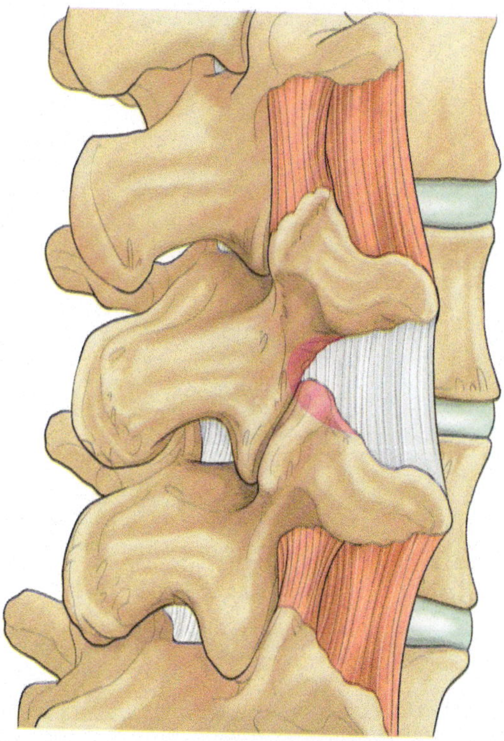

Fig. 10.3 After dissection of the intertransversarii lumborum muscle. Zone of resection: Parts of pars intercuralis and the superior articular process are marked to be removed with a drill

tomy is performed using pituitary forceps. In the case of foraminal stenosis, foraminal widening is performed using a curved foraminal punch and currets. After confirming free mobilization and release of the spinal nerve, sophisticated haemostasis is performed. The drain is then inserted, and the conventional wound closure technique is performed.

10.3.2 L5–S1

Because of the large coronal facet joint, oblique pedicle, the proximity of the iliac crest or prominent sacral ala, and higher frequency of prominent accessory process, the paraspinal approach at the L5–S1 level provides limited surgical field compared with that at L1–L5 level [19]. These changes require more bone removal to expose the DRG, spinal nerve, and disc space at the L5–S1 level. The surgical procedure before dissection of the fibrous septum between the multifidus and longissimus muscles is the same as that in the paraspinal approach at the L1–L5 level—using a fingertip and a pair of scissors. Fingertip dissection is performed to confirm the triangular space

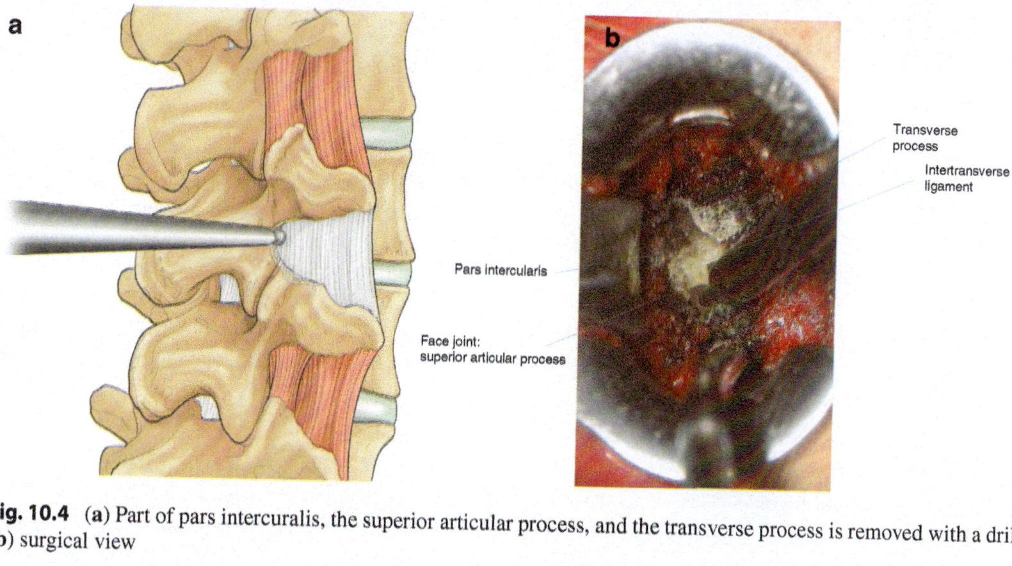

Fig. 10.4 (**a**) Part of pars intercuralis, the superior articular process, and the transverse process is removed with a drill. (**b**) surgical view

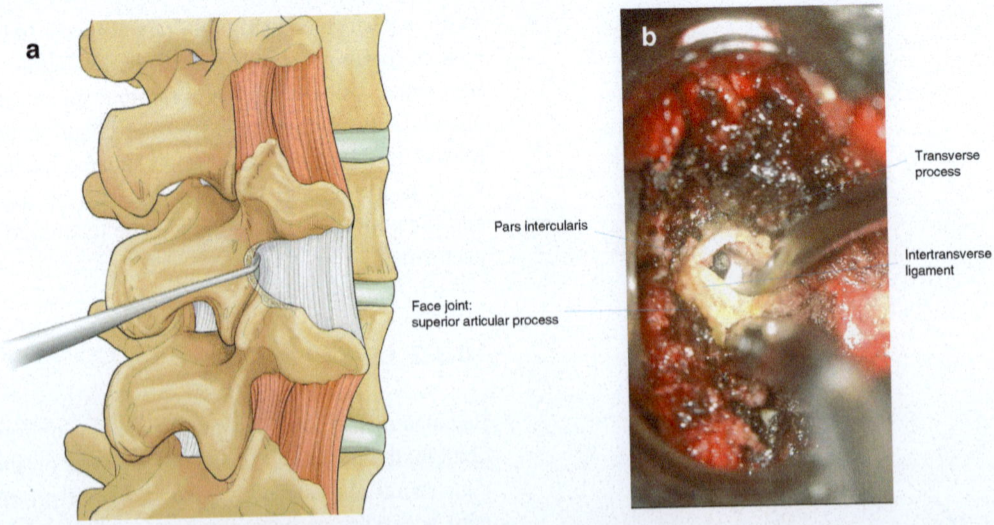

Fig. 10.5 (**a**) After removing a part of the bone, use a curret to detach the intertransverse ligament from the bone. (**b**) surgical view

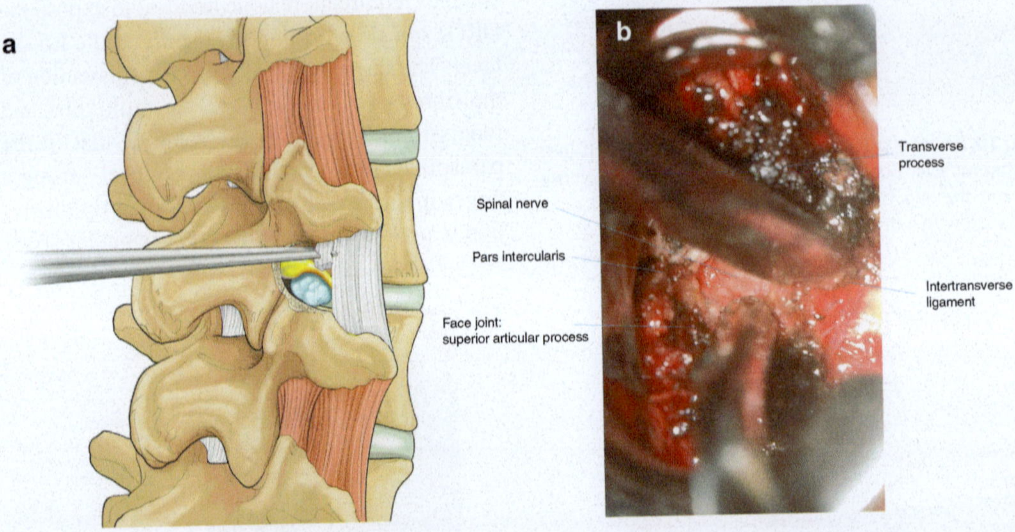

Fig. 10.6 (**a**) The intertransverse ligament is removed using a Kerrison punch. (**b**) surgical view

bordered by the L5 transverse process, lateral margin of L5–S1 facet joint, and the upper rim of the sacrum with the costal process. A self-retractor (Papavero–Caspar speculum, B Braun) is inserted, and lateral radiography is obtained to re-check the surgical level.

The operative table is tilted to the opposite side by 30°–40°. Using an operative microscope, the L5 transverse process, mammillary process, pars intercularis, facet joint, and the upper rim of the sacrum with the costal process are checked. The facet joint, pars intercularis, and costal process of the sacrum can obscure the disc space and the course of the L5 spinal nerve. The outer part of the pars intercularis, the lower edge of L5 transverse process, and the outer part of the superior articular process are drilled using a high-speed diamond-tipped burr. A part of the alar and costal processes is also removed, if necessary. Care must be taken to avoid damage to the spinal nerve during drilling. The intertransverse ligament above the L5 spinal nerve and ganglion is

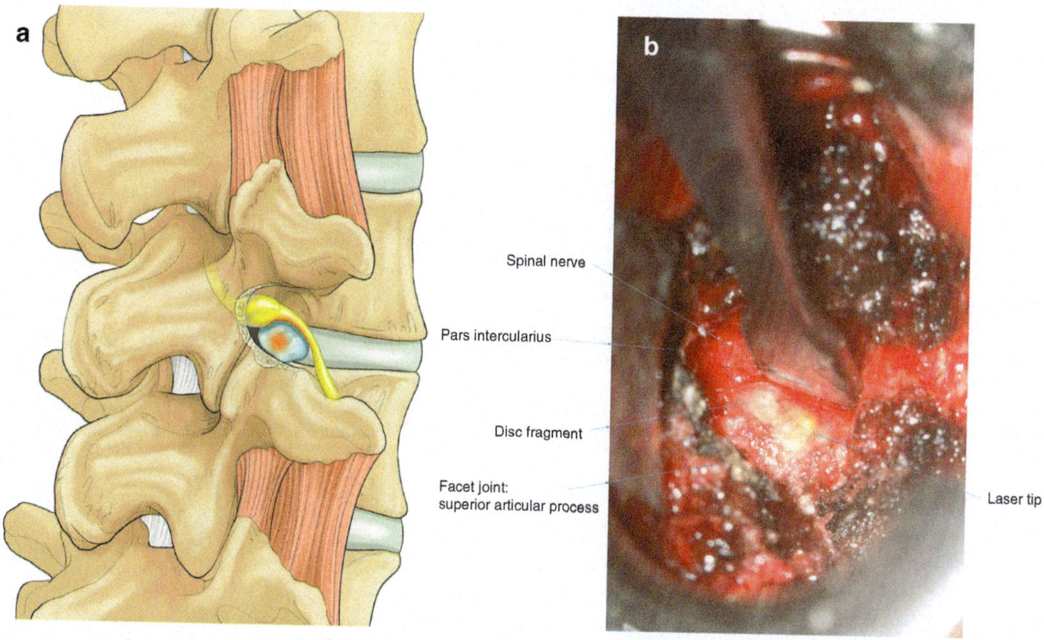

Fig. 10.7 (**a**) After removing the intertransverse ligament, check the herniated disc compressing the spinal nerve. The spinal nerve is retracted, and the herniated disc material is removed using a CO_2 laser. (**b**) surgical view

identified. The intertransverse ligament is removed using a Kerrison punch. The intertransverse ligament is carefully removed to avoid damaging the neurovascular bundle and fat tissue around the L5 spinal nerve and ganglion [12]. When the intertransverse ligament is removed, the fibroadipose tissue, radicular arteries and veins, and primary dorsal ramus are located above the spinal nerve and ganglion. Radicular arteries and veins and the primary dorsal ramus should be preserved, if possible. However, if necessary, the radicular arteries and veins are coagulated using bipolar cautery to prevent bleeding. The primary dorsal ramus may be cut for retraction of the spinal nerve. The herniated disc material is checked, and the spinal nerve and ganglion are retracted. Excessive manipulation of the spinal nerve and ganglion should be avoided. The herniated disc material is removed using a CO_2 laser attached to a microscope (Sharplan 30C, Lumenis). Using a pinpoint-sized laser beam, the herniated disc material can be precisely removed while minimizing the retraction of the spinal nerve and ganglion. The subsequent surgical procedure is the same as previously described (Fig. 10.8).

10.4 Case Illustration

***Case 1*:** Microscopic lumbar discectomy via paraspinal approach at L4–L5

A 59-year-old man was admitted to the hospital due to severe pain in the right leg. The visual analogue scale (VAS) score was 10, and the motor grade in the right ankle was III. An up-migrated herniated lumbar disc was observed in the right foraminal area on MRI. Microscopic lumbar discectomy using a CO_2 laser was performed through the paraspinal approach. Postoperative MRI confirmed that the herniated disc material was completely removed. Immediately after the surgery, the VAS score decreased to 2. The ankle motor grade also improved to grade V (Fig. 10.9).

***Case 2*:** Microscopic lumbar discectomy via the paraspinal approach at L5–S1

A 63-year-old female patient was admitted to the hospital with severe pain in the right leg and back. The VAS score was 10. An up-migrated herniated lumbar disc was observed in the right

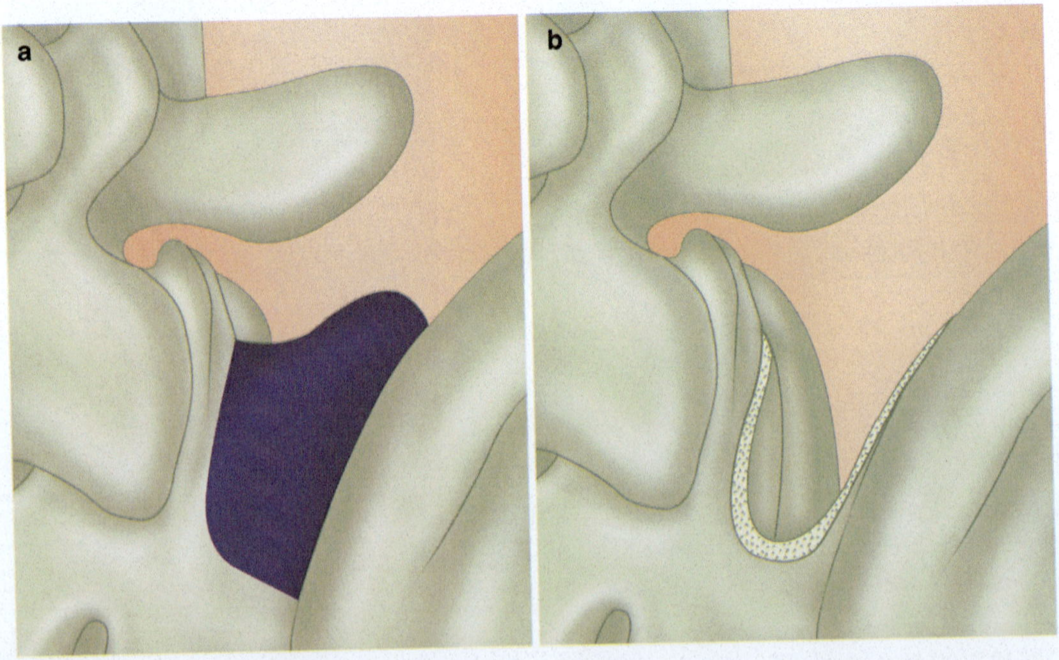

Fig. 10.8 (**a**) The anatomic relationships of osseous boundaries and the area of bone resection at L5–S1. A: Resection of an osseous triangle (lateral margin of the facet joint, the upper rim of the sacrum with the costal process [dotted line]) should be done to access the foraminal and extraforaminal area. (**b**) after resection of the osseous triangle

foraminal area on MRI. Microscopic lumbar discectomy using a CO_2 laser was performed through the paraspinal approach. Postoperative MRI confirmed that the herniated disc material was completely removed. Immediately after the surgery, the VAS decreased to 1 (Fig. 10.10).

10.5 Summary

Microscopic lumbar discectomy via the paraspinal approach is reported as the gold standard for the surgical treatment of FLDH or EFLDH [3]. The success rate of microscopic lumbar discectomy via the paraspinal approach is reported to be 72%–83% [20, 21]. However, there have been reports of postoperative leg pain and dysesthesia with the paraspinal approach for FLDH and EFLDH due to excessive neural manipulation or incomplete decompression [3, 11, 14, 15].

DRG located in the foraminal or extraforaminal zone is susceptible to mechanical or dermal irritation damage. Due to the narrow surgical field, excessive surgical manipulation of DRG can cause postoperative leg pain and dysesthesia [3]. When using a laser during microscopic lumbar discectomy via the paraspinal approach, manipulation of the neural structures should be minimized. In 1986, there was the first report of the use of neodymium: yttrium-aluminium-garnet (Nd: YAG) laser in lumbar disc surgery. Since then, there have been many reports of spine surgery using lasers [3, 15, 16, 22–24]. The laser removes the disc material by vaporization [25]. The diameter of the focused laser beam is less than 0.5 mm, while the width of surgical instruments, such as pituitary forceps, is greater than 5 mm [3]. Therefore, using a laser during microscopic lumbar discectomy via the paraspinal approach can remove lesions more precisely. When using a laser in microscopic lumbar discectomy via the paraspinal approach, an advantage is that disc material can be precisely removed while minimizing damage to the surrounding tissues and neural retraction even in a narrow surgical field of view. However, thermal injury of the neural structure caused by uncon-

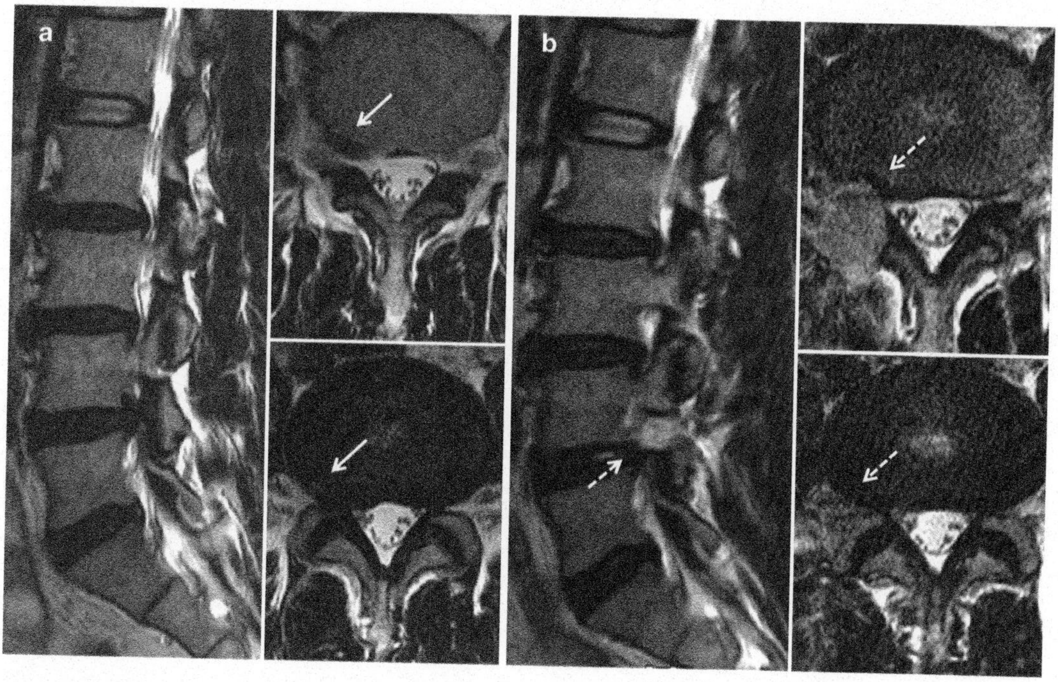

Fig. 10.9 **Case 1:** Microscopic lumbar discectomy via paraspinal approach at L4–L5. (**a**) Preoperative MRI L spine images: white arrow indicates up-migrated herniated lumbar disc at the foraminal area at L4–L5. (**b**) Postoperative MRI L spine images. The white dotted arrow shows that the herniated disc was removed completely. MRI: magnetic resonance imaging

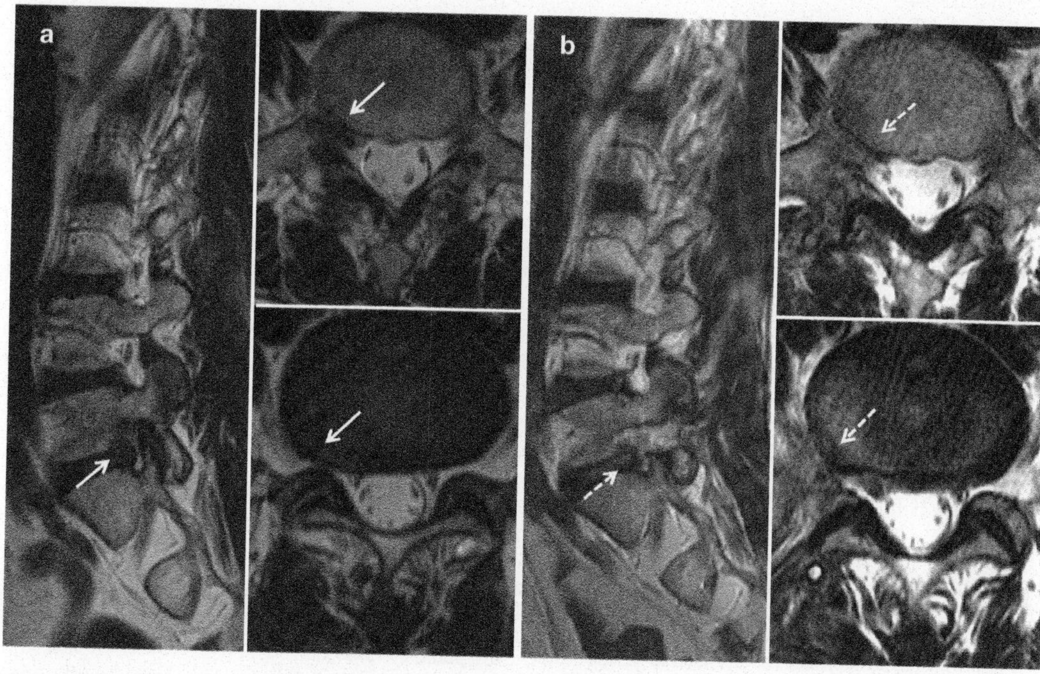

Fig. 10.10 **Case 2:** Microscopic lumbar discectomy via the paraspinal approach at L5–S1. (**a**) Preoperative MRI L spine images. The white arrow indicates up-migrated herniated lumbar disc at the foraminal area at L5–S1. (**b**) Postoperative MRI L spine images. The white dotted arrow shows that the herniated disc was removed completely. MRI: magnetic resonance imaging

trolled laser irradiation is a serious and irreversible neurologic sequela; therefore, it must be used with great care.

If spine surgeons accurately understand the anatomical structure and surgical method required for the paraspinal approach for FLDH and EFLDH and perform surgery with minimizing neural retraction using a CO_2 laser, postoperative clinical results can be improved, and complications can be reduced.

References

1. Siebner HR, Faulhauer K. Frequency and specific surgical management of far lateral lumbar disc herniations. Acta Neurochir. 1990;105:124–31. https://doi.org/10.1007/BF01669995.
2. Epstein NE. Evaluation of varied surgical approaches used in the management of 170 far-lateral lumbar disc herniations: indications and results. J Neurosurg. 1995;83:648–56. https://doi.org/10.3171/jns.1995.83.4.0648.
3. Ahn Y, Lee U, Lee YJ, Keum HJ. Laser-assisted microdiscectomy for far lateral lumbar disc herniation at the L5-S1 level. Photomed Laser Surg. 2018;36:555–61. https://doi.org/10.1089/pho.2018.4497.
4. Epstein NE. Foraminal and far lateral lumbar disc herniations: surgical alternatives and outcome measures. Spinal Cord. 2002;40:491–500. https://doi.org/10.1038/sj.sc.3101319.
5. Wiltse LL, Bateman JG, Hutchinson RH, Nelson WE. The paraspinal sacrospinalis-splitting approach to the lumbar spine. J Bone Joint Surg Am. 1968;50:919–26. https://doi.org/10.2106/00004623-196850050-00004.
6. Recoules-Arche D. Surgery of disk hernia of the lumbar vertebral canal. Neurochirurgie. 1985;31:61–4.
7. Reulen HJ, Pfaundler S, Ebeling U. The lateral microsurgical approach to the "extracanalicular" lumbar disc herniation. I: A technical note. Acta Neurochir. 1987;84:64–7. https://doi.org/10.1007/BF01456353.
8. Fankhauser H, de Tribolet N. Extreme lateral lumbar disc herniation. Br J Neurosurg. 1987;1:111–29. https://doi.org/10.3109/02688698709034347.
9. Reulen H-J, Müller A, Ebeling U. Microsurgical anatomy of the lateral approach to extraforaminal lumbar disc herniations. Neurosurgery. 1996;39:345–51.; Discussion 350-1. https://doi.org/10.1097/00006123-199608000-00022.
10. Kotil K, Akcetin M, Bilge T. A minimally invasive transmuscular approach to far-lateral L5-S1 level disc herniations: a prospective study. J Spinal Disord Tech. 2007;20:132–8. https://doi.org/10.1097/01.bsd.0000211268.43744.2a.
11. Lee DY, Lee SH. Microdecompression for extraforaminal L5-S1 disc herniation; the significance of concomitant foraminal disc herniation for postoperative leg pain. J Korean Neurosurg Soc. 2008;44:19–25. https://doi.org/10.3340/jkns.2008.44.1.19.
12. Jang JS, An SH, Lee SH. Clinical analysis of extraforaminal entrapment of L5 in the lumbosacral spine. J Korean Neurosurg Soc. 2004;36:383–7.
13. Tessitore E, de Tribolet N. Far-lateral lumbar disc herniation: the microsurgical transmuscular approach. Neurosurgery. 2004;54:939–42.; Discussion 942. https://doi.org/10.1227/01.neu.0000115154.62636.77.
14. Viswanathan R, Swamy NK, Tobler WD, Greiner AL, Keller JT, Dunsker SB. Extraforaminal lumbar disc herniations: microsurgical anatomy and surgical approach. J Neurosurg. 2002;96:206–11. https://doi.org/10.3171/spi.2002.96.2.0206.
15. Lee DY, Lee SH. Carbon dioxide (CO_2) laser-assisted microdiscectomy for extraforaminal lumbar disc herniation at the L5-S1 level. Photomed Laser Surg. 2011;29:531–5. https://doi.org/10.1089/pho.2010.2954.
16. Kim JS, Oh HS, Lee SH. Usefulness of carbon dioxide laser for recurrent lumbar disc herniation. Photomed Laser Surg. 2012;30:568–72. https://doi.org/10.1089/pho.2012.3288.
17. Bogduk N. Clinical and radiological anatomy of the lumbar spine. Elsevier Health Sciences. 2012:45–6.
18. Hasegawa T, Mikawa Y, Watanabe R, An HS. Morphometric analysis of the lumbosacral nerve roots and dorsal root ganglia by magnetic resonance imaging. Spine (Phila Pa 1976). 1996;21:1005–9. https://doi.org/10.1097/00007632-199605010-00001.
19. Zhang HJKSNS. Koonja. Surgical atlas of spine. 2010:373–6.
20. Kunogi J, Hasue M. Diagnosis and operative treatment of intraforaminal and extraforaminal nerve root compression. Spine (Phil Pa 1976). 1991;16:1312–20. https://doi.org/10.1097/00007632-199111000-00012.
21. Chang SB, Lee SH, Ahn Y, Kim JM. Risk factor for unsatisfactory outcome after lumbar foraminal and far lateral microdecompression. Spine (Phil Pa 1976). 2006;31:1163–7. https://doi.org/10.1097/01.brs.0000216431.69359.91.
22. Choy D, Case R, Zickel R, Kaplan M, Ascher P, Eron LJTLrae, Orthopedic Research Society. Percutaneous laser ablation of lumbar disc: a preliminary report of in-vitro and in-vivo experience in animals and four human patients. 1987;12:323.
23. Houck PM. Comparison of operating room lasers: uses, hazards, guidelines. Nurs Clin North Am. 2006;41:193–218, vi. https://doi.org/10.1016/j.cnur.2006.01.004.
24. Kim JS, Lee SH. Carbon dioxide (CO_2) laser-assisted ablation of lumbar discal cyst. Photomed Laser Surg. 2009;27:837–42. https://doi.org/10.1089/pho.2008.2397.
25. Stein E, Sedlacek T, Fabian RL, Nishioka NS. Acute and chronic effects of bone ablation with a pulsed holmium laser. Lasers Surg Med. 1990;10:384–8. https://doi.org/10.1002/lsm.1900100412.

Transforaminal Endoscopic Thoracic Discectomy with Ho:Yag Laser

11

Junseok Bae

Abstract

Symptomatic thoracic disc herniation (TDH) is rare and surgical intervention is even more uncommon. Several surgical approaches have been developed to address adequate surgical decompression with minimal approach-related morbidity. Transforaminal endoscopic thoracic discectomy (TETD) has brought in a paradigm shift in the management of thoracic disc herniation in its least approach-related complications and wider application for various levels of herniation. Ho:Yag laser is an essential surgical instrument for endoscopic discectomy for safe and effective surgery. In this chapter, authors describe tips and trick of thoracic endoscopic discectomy using laser.

Keywords

Thoracic disc herniation · Spinal endoscopy
Ho:YAG laser · Foraminoplasty
Transforaminal endoscopic thoracic discectomy

Supplementary Information The online version of this chapter (https://doi.org/10.1007/978-981-16-2206-9_11) contains supplementary material, which is available to authorized users.

J. Bae (✉)
Department of Neurosurgery, Chungdam Wooridul Spine Hospital, Seoul, Republic of Korea

11.1 Introduction

Thoracic disc herniation is an important but rare degenerative pathology that may cause significant disability including back pain and neural symptoms including radicular pain and myelopathy [1–3]. The incidence of symptomatic thoracic disc herniation (TDH) has been reported to be 0.25% to 0.75% of all the spinal disc diseases. However, diagnosis of TDH is increasing with the development of magnetic resonance image (MRI). Studies have reported that the prevalence of TDH ranges from 11.1% to 14.5%. In 75% of patients with TDH, the affected level is below T8 and is mostly at T11–T12 [1–5]. Given the unique surgical challenges presented by thoracic discectomy, despite several surgical techniques being described, they have not been accepted universally. No consensus has been reached regarding the indications for disc removal except for severe myelopathy. Symptomatic relief after selective epidural block was evaluated to confirm the diagnosis. Transforaminal endoscopic thoracic discectomy (TETD) can minimize the approach-related complications. However, compared to open surgery, endoscopic decompression is difficult to apply for all forms of disc herniation due to its small operating field, limited equipment availability, and limited working mobility.

J. Bae, S.-H. Lee (eds.), *Laser Spine Surgery*, https://doi.org/10.1007/978-981-16-2206-9_11

11.2 Indications

Thoracic disc herniation can be classified as central, centrolateral, or lateral depending on the location of the herniated disc [4, 6–8]. Because TETD is characterized by the foramen approach at the posterior lateral side, it can be applied to all soft thoracic disc herniations, regardless of location, from lateral to central herniation. In general, indications are soft central or centrolateral disc herniations at any levels radiologically concordant with symptoms [4]. Surgery needs to be considered when patients' symptoms are not responding to conservative treatments. For experienced surgeons, the indication can be carefully extended to migrated or calcified herniations [6, 7, 9–11]. However, TETD is not practically applicable in case of hard disc herniation combined with ossification of the posterior longitudinal ligament. These are often adherent to the surrounding dural sac causing dural calcification. It is difficult to dissect the layer between the hernia and ventral dura or to remove the hernia without dural leak. Significant or progressive myelopathy is not an absolute contraindication [12–14]. The surgeon should be cautious in addressing endoscopy for these patients.

11.3 Surgical Technique

Surgery was performed in a prone position under local anesthesia and conscious sedation. Midazolam or fentanyl may be given intravenously to relieve pain and sedation during the procedure. The degree of sedation is controlled to respond to the physician's verbal command during the procedure. Skin entry point was determined by drawing a line from the posterior annulus at the midpedicular level to the lateral margin of the facet joint on axial computed tomography scan or magnetic resonance imaging, usually located approximately 6–7 cm from the midline (Fig. 11.1). An access angle of about 45–60 degrees is recommended for removal of the disc in the subarticular zone. After infiltration of the local anesthesia, a 6-inch-long 18-G needle was inserted aimed at the midpedicular line on anteroposterior (AP) fluoroscopic view and the posterior vertebral body line on lateral fluoroscopic view. Also in oblique view, the needle tip should be placed between the pedicle and the rib head (Fig. 11.2a). Epidurography was performed, followed by epidural anesthetic infiltration (Fig. 11.2b). The needle was advanced into the disc space following discography using a mixture of radiopaque dye (Telebrix; Guerbet, France), indigo carmine, and normal saline in a 2:1:2 ratio. A guide wire was inserted through the needle. Serial dilation and sequential reaming of ventral and lateral aspect of superior articular facet was performed over the wire, to expand the neural foraminal window. Then, the 4.7-mm spinal endoscope (TESSYS; joimax GmbH, Karlsruhe, Germany) was introduced (Fig. 11.3). After approaching the disc space, internal discal decompression is performed using laser or forceps. After finding the annular tear point, the herniated disc can be easily removed. Under direct visualization, a blue-stained herniated fragment could be identified. The posterior longitudinal ligament (PLL) was resected to expose the ventral epidural space. Holmium:yttrium-aluminum-garnet (Ho:YAG) laser (VersaPulse; Lumenis, Yokneam, Israel) was used to ablate the posterior annulus and the PLL with minimal thermal

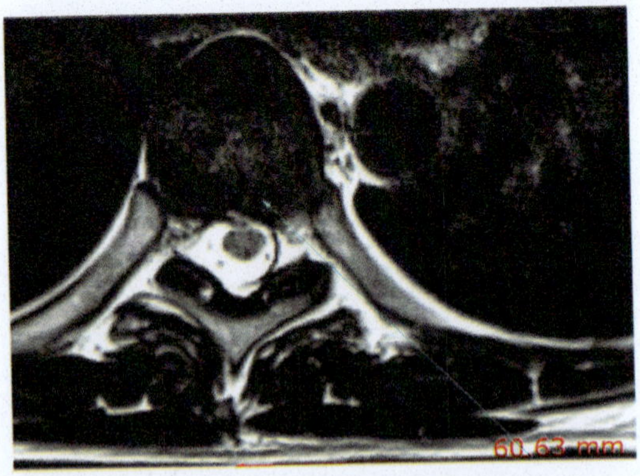

Fig. 11.1 Skin entry point was determined by drawing a line from the posterior annulus at the midpedicular level to the lateral margin of the facet joint on axial computed tomography scan or magnetic resonance imaging, usually located approximately 6–7 cm from the midline

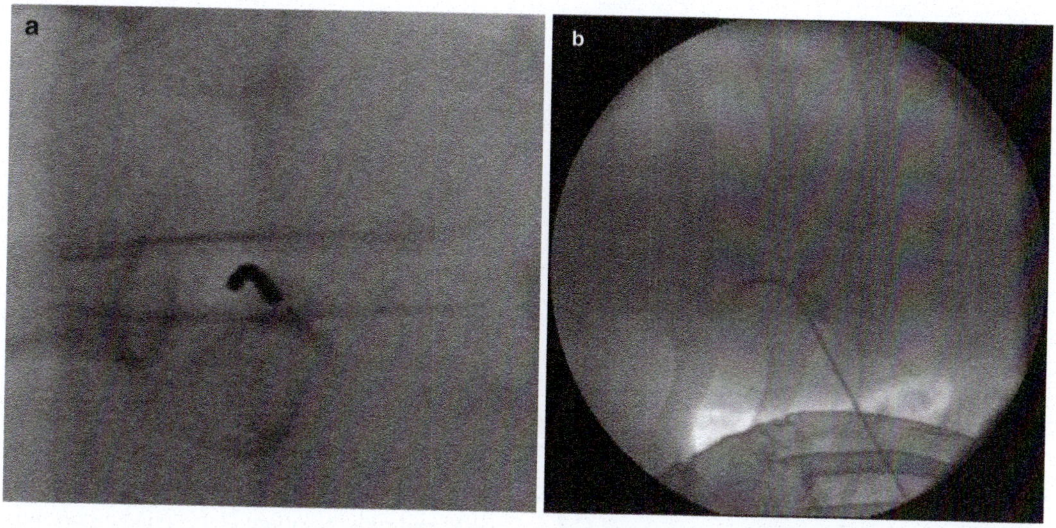

Fig. 11.2 In oblique view, the needle tip should be placed between the pedicle and the rib head (**a**). Epidurography was performed followed by epidural anesthetic infiltration (**b**)

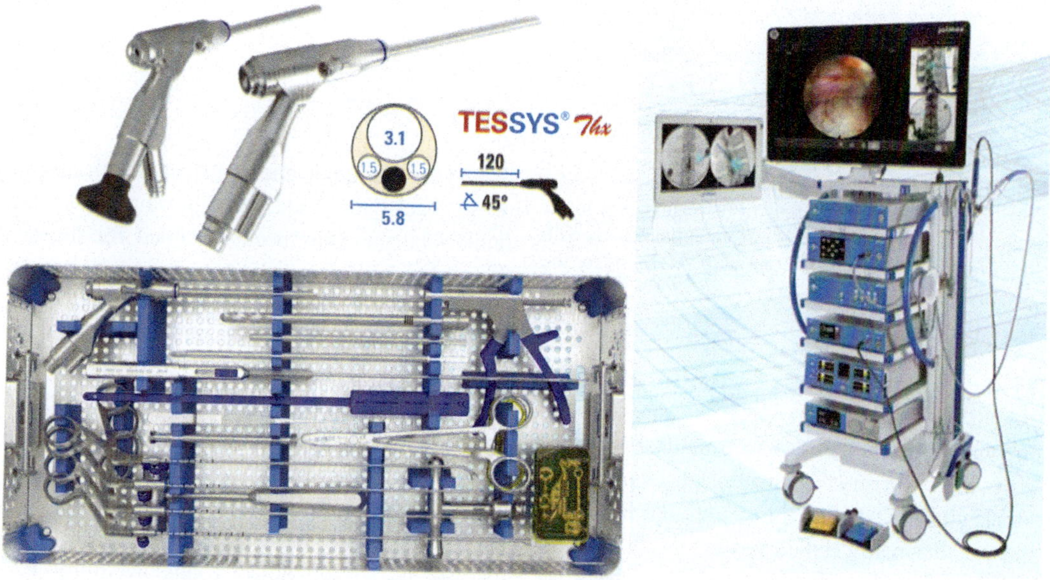

Fig. 11.3 4.7-mm with 45-degree optic angle spinal endoscope (TESSYS thx; joimax GmbH, Karlsruhe, Germany), endoscopic instruments, and endoscopic trolley

necrosis (Fig. 11.4). Ho:YAG laser is effective for (1) internal decompression within the posterior annulus at initial stage, (2) shrinkage and resecting the thickened posterior annulus around the annulus tear, (3) resection of the PLL for exposing the ventral epidural space for removal of transligamentous extrusion, and (4) resection of osteophyte or traction spur. The herniated fragment was removed with endoscopic forceps. After adequate decompression, the skin was closed with subcuticular suture and sterile dressing.

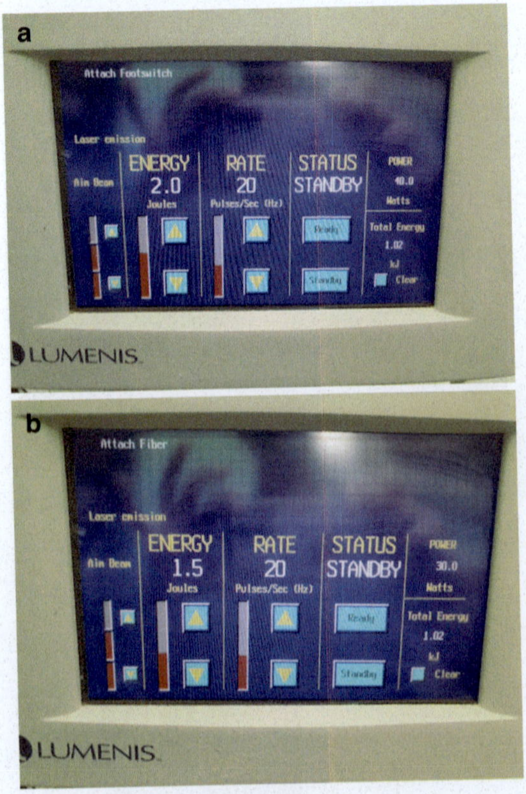

Fig. 11.4 Ho:YAG laser setting for thoracic endoscopic discectomy. Laser energy needs to be regulated to lower as closer to the neural tissue. Note that initial 2 Joule with 20 Hz rate (**a**) is adjusted to 1.5 J with 20 Hz (**b**) for the late stage of decompression

11.4 Postoperative Consideration

Patients were encouraged to ambulate immediately after surgery. Neurological examination should confirm whether the symptom is improved and whether motor deficit has occurred. In addition, postoperative MR can be used to check for complete decompression of the lesion. The patient may be discharged after several hours of observation. At discharge, oral antibiotics are considered to prevent procedure-related infection.

11.5 Case Illustration

Bae et al. reported 92 consecutive patients (mean age was 48.9 years, 57 males) who underwent TETD from 2001 to 2018 met the inclusion criteria. Patients underwent surgery at different levels: 16 patients for T2–3 to T5–6, 41 cases for T6–7 to T8–9, and 35 patients for T9–10 to T12–L1. After mean 38.4 ± 32.3 months of follow-up, all patients showed a significant improvement in pain (7.6 to 1.6 for VAS and 68.2% to 13.2% for ODI, $p < 0.05$ for both). According to the modified Macnab's criteria, 44 patients reported an excellent outcome (47.8%), 39 (42.4%) showed good outcomes, 8 (8.7%) of them had a fair outcome, and only 1 patient (1.1%) had a poor outcome. Two patients had symptomatic recurrent herniation. Of these, one patient underwent TETD and the other patient improved with conservative treatment.

11.5.1 Case 1

A 50-year-old male patient presented with chronic dorsal back pain with radiating pain on the left flank. The pain has been sustained for the last 5 years without responding to conservative treatments including epidural block, physical therapy, and pain medications. Preoperative pain visual analogue score of pain was 7 and Oswestry disability index was 32%. MRI and CT scan showed centrolateral soft disc herniation at the T7–8 level (Fig. 11.5). Transforaminal endoscopic thoracic discectomy was performed under the awakened anesthesia (Figs. 11.6 and 11.7). Under the direct endoscopic visualization, fragmentectomy was done with endoscopic forceps and Ho:YAG laser (Fig. 11.8, 11.9, 11.10, 11.11, 11.12, and 11.13). Full decompression was achieved after operation (Fig. 11.14). His chronic pain was alleviated and was discharged on the same day.

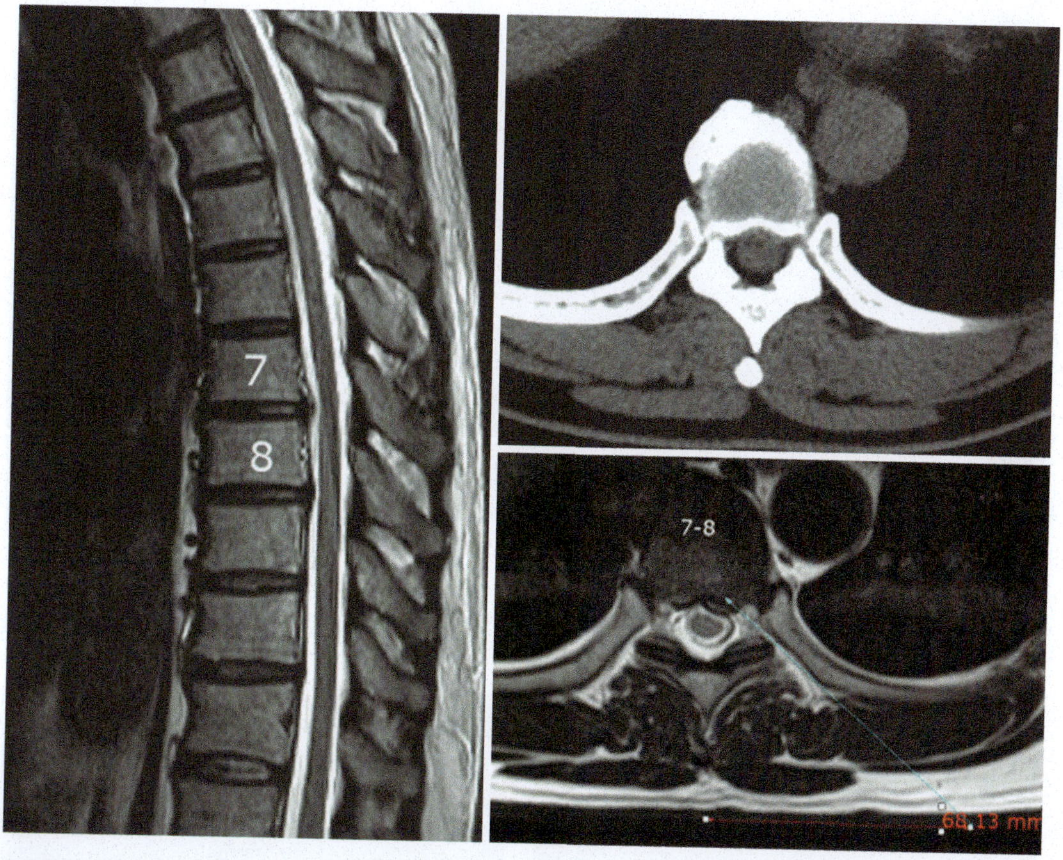

Fig. 11.5 Preoperative MRI and CT scan shows left centrolateral soft disc herniation at the T7–8 level

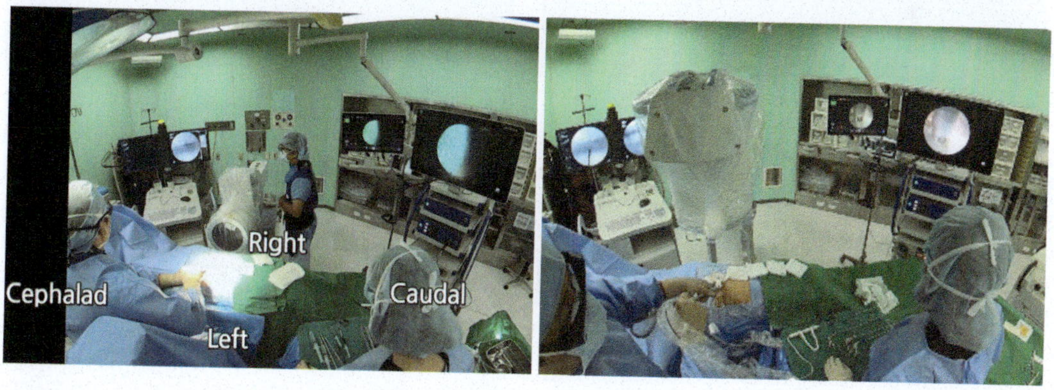

Fig. 11.6 Intraoperative photo of operation theater. The surgeon and scrub nurse are standing on the left side C-arm machine and endoscopic monitor on its tower placed on the other side. Note that the surgeon is holding a laser tip and its line covered with sterilized plastic drape on the right photo

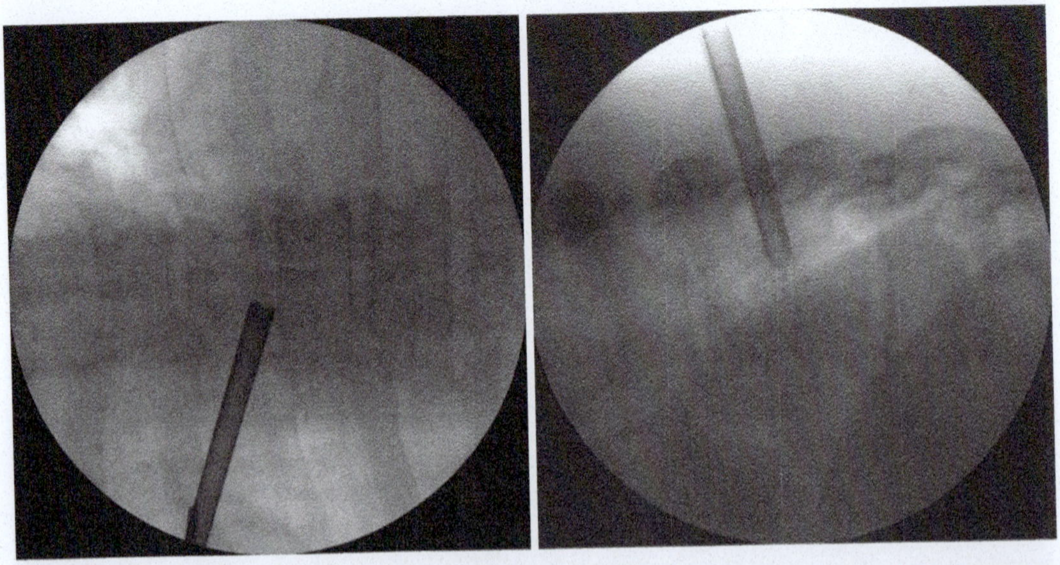

Fig. 11.7 Fluoroscopic view of transforaminal working channel placement. Note that it is located on the medial pedicle line on the AP view and posterior vertebral line on the lateral view

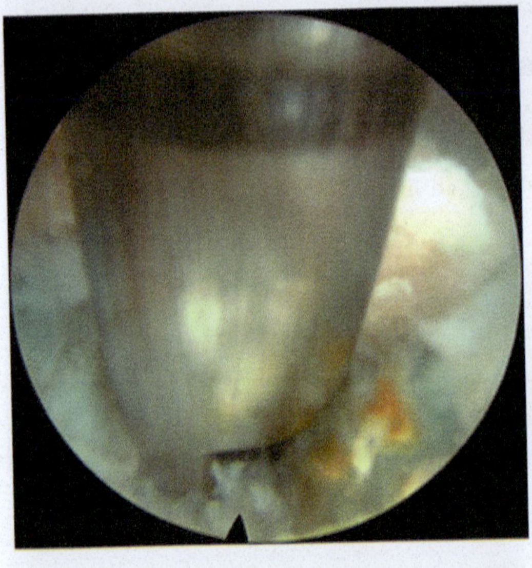

Fig. 11.8 Intraoperative photo of transforaminal endoscopic thoracic discectomy. Laser is performed for internal decompression of subligamentous intraannular herniated disc that is stained in blue color with indigo carmine. Laser is effective than forceps for decompression within narrow thoracic intervertebral disc space

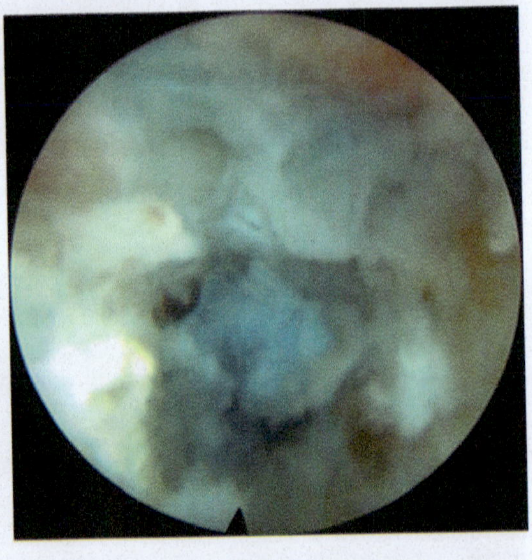

Fig. 11.9 Intraoperative photo showing loose fragment is coming out after initial decompression

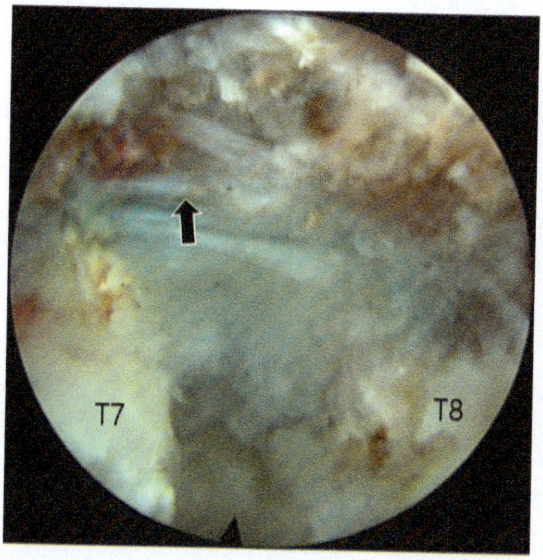

Fig. 11.10 Intraoperative photo showing the posterior longitudinal ligament (arrow) and thickened posterior annulus

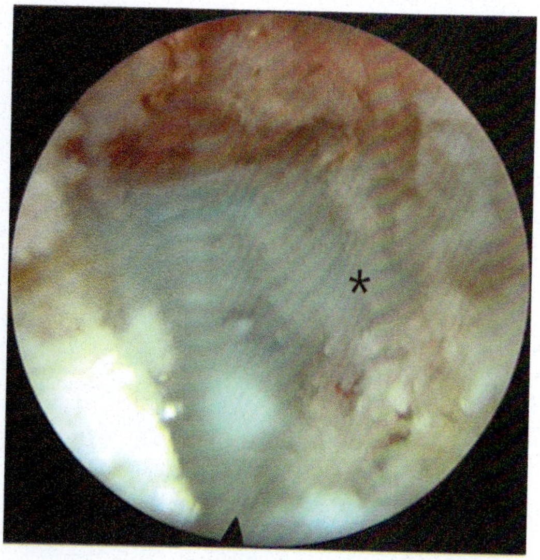

Fig. 11.12 Intraoperative photo showing the ventral epidural space and transligamentous hernia (*)

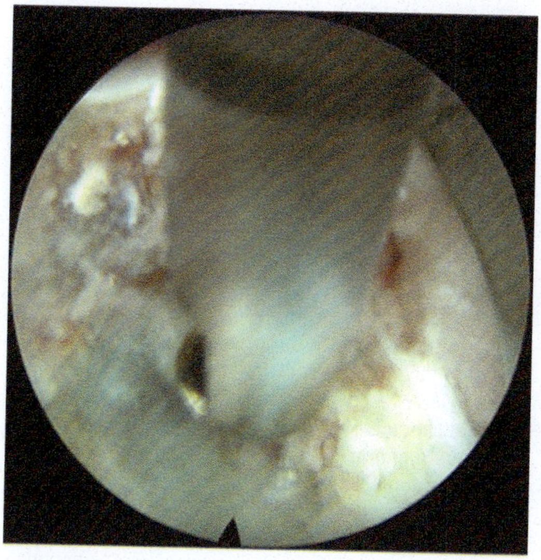

Fig. 11.11 Intraoperative photo showing laser is resecting the PLL to expose the ventral dural and transligamentous hernia

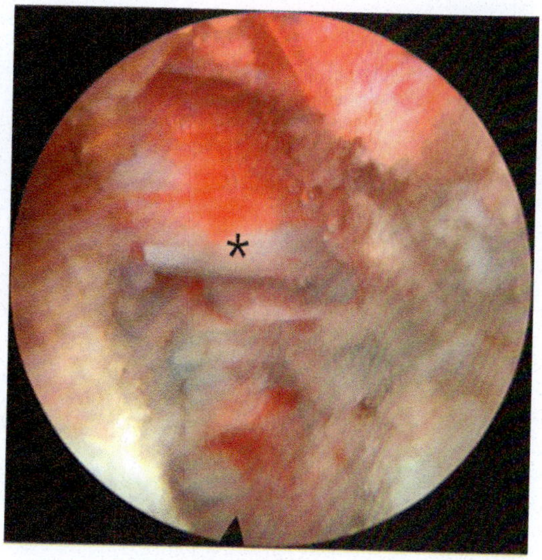

Fig. 11.13 Intraoperative photo showing full decompression of the dural sac (*)

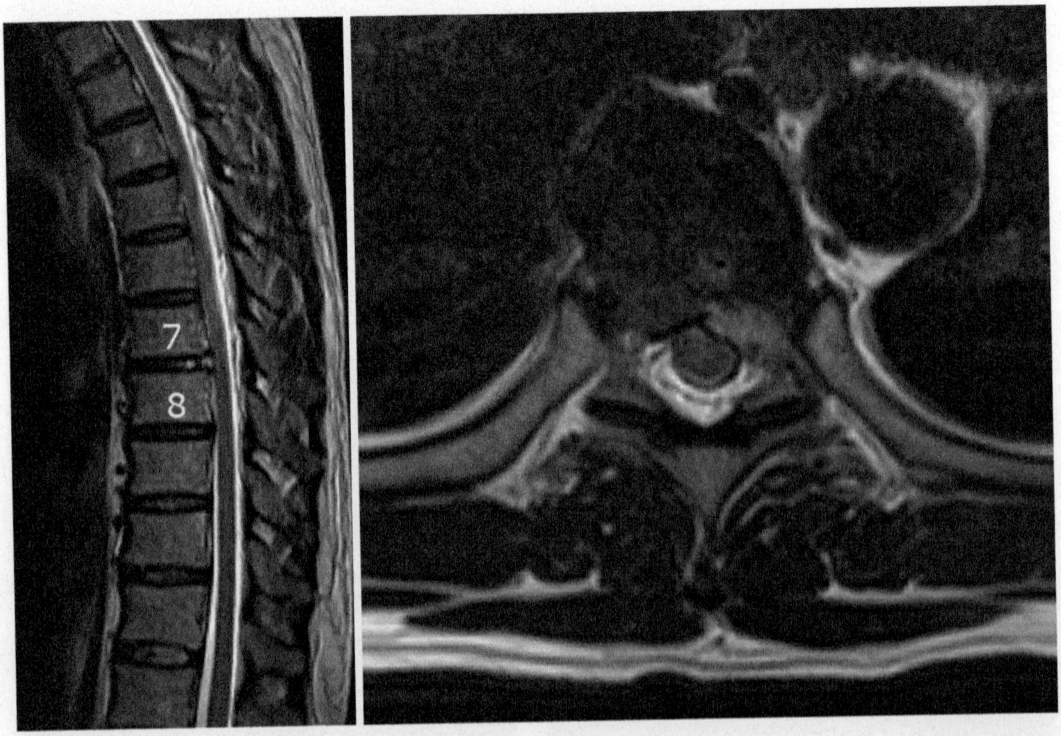

Fig. 11.14 Postoperative MRI showing decompressed state at the T7–8 level. There's a small amount of irrigation fluid left in the disc space which is absorbed in a few days

11.6 Summary

There are increasing evidence showing the possible utilization of spinal endoscopy with Ho:YAG laser in the management of thoracic disc herniations. Transforaminal endoscopic thoracic discectomy is a feasible, effective, minimally invasive treatment option with favorable clinical results in carefully selected (soft, paramedian to lateral disc herniations) patients, when performed by well-experienced surgeons.

References

1. Shimada S, Tamaki N. Assessment of safety and feasibility of spinal endoscope in the thoracic and lumbar region: a cadaveric study. Kobe J Med Sci. 2001;47(6):263–72.
2. Wilke A, Wolf U, Lageard P, Griss P. Thoracic disc herniation: a diagnostic challenge. Man Ther. 2000;5(3):181–4.
3. Brown CW, Deffer PA Jr, Akmakjian J, Donaldson DH, Brugman JL. The natural history of thoracic disc herniation. Spine (Phila Pa 1976). 1992;17(6 Suppl):S97–102.
4. Bae J, Chachan S, Shin SH, Lee SH. Transforaminal endoscopic thoracic discectomy with foraminoplasty for the treatment of thoracic disc herniation. J Spine Surg. 2020;6(2):397–404.
5. Gloyer MA, Cadosch D, Galldiks N, Gautschi OP. Thoracic disc herniation with affection of the anterior spinothalamic tract: a case report and review of literature. Neurol India. 2011;59(4):627–8.
6. Bae J, Chachan S, Shin SH, Lee SH. Percutaneous endoscopic thoracic discectomy in the upper and midthoracic spine: a technical note. Neurospine. 2019;16(1):148–53.
7. Wagner R, Telfeian AE, Iprenburg M, Krzok G, Gokaslan Z, Choi DB, et al. Transforaminal endoscopic foraminoplasty and discectomy for the treatment of a thoracic disc herniation. World Neurosurg. 2016;90:194–8.
8. Choi KY, Eun SS, Lee SH, Lee HY. Percutaneous endoscopic thoracic discectomy; transforaminal approach. Minim Invasive Neurosurg. 2010;53(1):25–8.
9. Yue B, Chen B, Zou YW, Xi YM, Ren XF, Xiang HF, et al. Thoracic intervertebral disc calcification and

herniation in adults: a report of two cases. Eur Spine J. 2016;25(Suppl 1):118–23.
10. Paolini S, Tola S, Missori P, Esposito V, Cantore G. Endoscope-assisted resection of calcified thoracic disc herniations. Eur Spine J. 2016;25(1):200–6.
11. Nie HF, Liu KX. Endoscopic transforaminal thoracic foraminotomy and discectomy for the treatment of thoracic disc herniation. Minim Invasive Surg. 2013;2013:264105.
12. Song KJ, Kim KB, Lee KB. Sequestrated thoracic disc herniation mimicking a tumoral lesion in the spinal canal: a case report. Clin Imaging. 2012;36(4):416–9.
13. Quint U, Bordon G, Preissl I, Sanner C, Rosenthal D. Thoracoscopic treatment for single level symptomatic thoracic disc herniation: a prospective followed cohort study in a group of 167 consecutive cases. Eur Spine J. 2012;21(4):637–45.
14. Deviren V, Kuelling FA, Poulter G, Pekmezci M. Minimal invasive anterolateral transthoracic transpleural approach: a novel technique for thoracic disc herniation. A review of the literature, description of a new surgical technique and experience with first 12 consecutive patients. J Spinal Disord Tech. 2011;24(5):E40–8.

Microscopic Thoracic Discectomy for Paramedian Disc Herniation with CO_2 Laser

12

Han Joong Keum

Abstract

Thoracic disc herniation is a potentially disabling condition that is technically difficult to manage, is associated with various complications, and is unfamiliar to many surgeons. The ideal surgical approach for thoracic disc herniations is still not available. Microscopic thoracic discectomy using posterolateral trajectories has been typically favored for smaller, noncalcified, and/or laterally displaced herniations, but modifications have enabled easier access and less manipulation of the neural structures. Furthermore, the introduction of CO_2 laser into the operative field has enabled removal of thoracic disc herniations which were previously inaccessible, further broadening the indication for microscopic thoracic discectomy while reducing the operation field and nerve manipulation necessary for successful surgery.

Keywords

Thoracic disc herniations · Discectomy · Laminotomy · Laser · Minimally invasive spine surgery

H. J. Keum (✉)
Department of Neurosurgery, Chungdam Wooridul Spine Hospital, Seoul, Republic of Korea
e-mail: hanj@wooridul.co.kr

12.1 Introduction

Thoracic disc herniation is a potentially disabling condition that is technically difficult to manage, is associated with various complications, and is unfamiliar to many surgeons. The choice of surgical approach for symptomatic thoracic disc herniation has been determined by several factors including the size of the herniation, its relationship to the midline sagittal plane, and the degree of calcification. The variety of available techniques indicates that a single method may not be practical for every case, and the surgeon may need to tailor the technique based on the morphology of the herniation as well as the symptom presentation of the patient.

The ideal surgical approach should provide proper visibility of the cord, enable complete access to the herniation, cause minimal morbidity to the patient, and have easily reproducible results. A number of operative techniques including transthoracic, lateral extracavitary, and posterolateral approaches have been introduced to allow the surgeons to safely remove herniated discs [1–3]. Transthoracic and extracavity approaches provide good access to the herniation, a lack of surgical and anatomic familiarity and also potential complication risks including cerebrospinal fluid leak control, post-thoracotomy pain, and cardiopulmonary complications may influence selection of this

J. Bae, S.-H. Lee (eds.), *Laser Spine Surgery*, https://doi.org/10.1007/978-981-16-2206-9_12

approach [4–6]. Posterolateral approaches have the least risk of complications, but have not provided sufficient access to the central areas of discs [7].

Microscopic thoracic discectomy using posterolateral trajectories has been typically favored for smaller, noncalcified, and/or laterally displaced herniations. These surgical techniques include laminotomy and medical facetectomy, transfacet pedicle-sparing, and transpedicular approaches [8–10]. Laminectomy alone has been largely abandoned because of poor clinical outcomes [11, 12]. Modifications of these techniques have enabled easier access and less manipulation of the neural structures when undergoing a posterolateral approach (Fig. 12.1). An oblique paraspinal approach using a tubular retractor has also been proven to be a good alternate posterolateral method to treat thoracic disc herniations and can be used for more centralized disc herniations (Fig. 12.1) [13, 14]. Furthermore, the introduction of CO_2 laser into the operative field has enabled removal of thoracic disc herniations which were previously inaccessible or difficult to remove with less compromise to the normal structure.

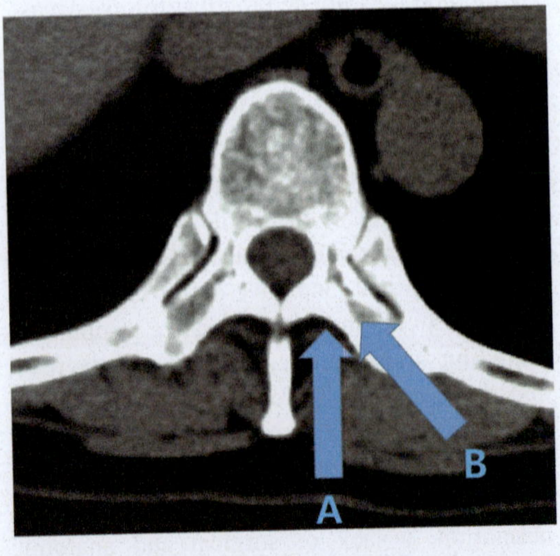

Fig. 12.1 Direction and trajectories of the posterolateral (**A**) and oblique paraspinal approach (**B**)

12.2 Indications

Soft or calcified, paramedian to laterally displaced disc herniations can be removed through the posterolateral approach. More centrally placed herniations can be removed more efficiently using oblique paraspinal approach. Although soft disc herniations have been treated more frequently with an endoscopic approach, open discectomy is still considered a better option in calcified discs or larger disc herniations causing neurological deficits or myelopathic symptoms.

12.3 Surgical Technique

12.3.1 Posterolateral Approach

The patient is placed in a prone position on the operating table under general anesthesia. After identifying and marking the target level, skin preparation and draping is done. A longitudinal incision of approximately 3 cm long is made, centered over the disc space. Subperiosteal dissection is done to expose the posterior elements on the affected side. After identification of the correct facet joint, the operating microscope is introduced into the operative field. An interlaminar laminotomy is conducted using a high-speed drill which includes partial removal of the superior and inferior arches, as well as 2–3 mm of the medial aspect of the facet joint (Fig. 12.2). Kerrison punches are used to enlarge the hemilaminotomy medially to the lateral edge of the dural sac. The superior and medial borders of the pedicle associated with lower vertebral body area are palpated with a probe. This provides exposure of approximately 5 mm of the lateral portion of the disc, which is sufficient to undertake the discectomy. Partial removal of the caudal pedicle may be done to further expose the disc space. Epidural bleeding is controlled with bipolar cauterization after identification of the

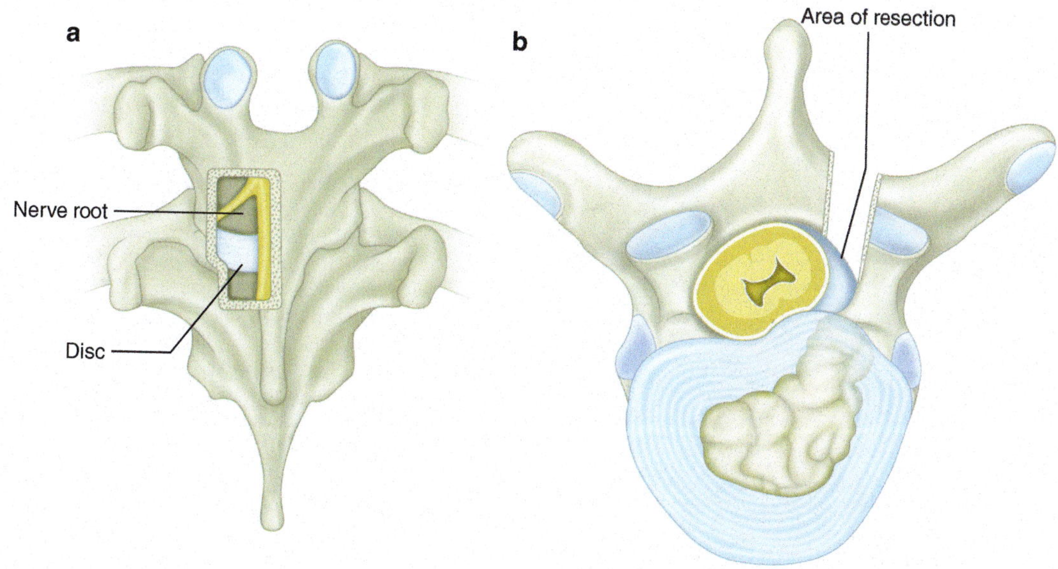

Fig. 12.2 Drawing of the area of bone resection required to expose the disc and the lateral edge of the thecal sac. (**a**) Unilateral intralaminar laminotomy is done, including the superior and inferior laminar arches, as well as of the medial 2–3 mm of the facet joint. (**a**) Posterior view. (**b**) Axial view

dural edge and exiting nerve root. Any free fragments of disc material can be removed, and the disc space is entered lateral to the thecal sac below the exiting root. The disc is further removed using angled curettes and disc forceps. The more medially located disc herniations, down-biting curettes may be used to push down the herniated fragments before removal to avoid cord manipulation.

12.3.2 Oblique Paraspinal Approach

The patient is placed in a prone position on the operating table under general anesthesia. After identifying and marking the target level, skin preparation and draping is done. A longitudinal skin incision is made approximately 5–6 cm lateral to the posterior midline, and an initial dilator is placed over the superior aspect of the base of the caudal transverse process. Then, sequential dilators are inserted, and an 18- or 20-mm tubular retractor is docked and attached to the table mount. The docking area of transverse process is drilled out to create a more oblique angle of the tubular retractor. The table can be rotated away from the surgeon to give better visualization of the midline structures. The lateral facet and proximal transverse process is exposed using monopolar cauterization. A high-speed drill is used to remove the rostral portion of the caudal transverse process and the lateral portion of the facet joint. After drilling the superior aspect of the pedicle, the foraminal bleeding is controlled with bipolar cautery. Careful dissection is performed to identify the exiting root. The exposed field should include the lateral margin of the thecal sac and the exiting nerve root. Through oblique inclination of the microscope and the operation table, discectomy can be done with minimal cord retraction and manipulation.

12.4 Application of CO_2 Laser During Microscopic Thoracic Discectomy

The usefulness of CO_2 laser as a surgical tool for removal of soft and calcified disc herniations has been reported in various situations [15–18]. The most significant benefit is the ability of the pinpoint laser to ablate and remove disc herniations

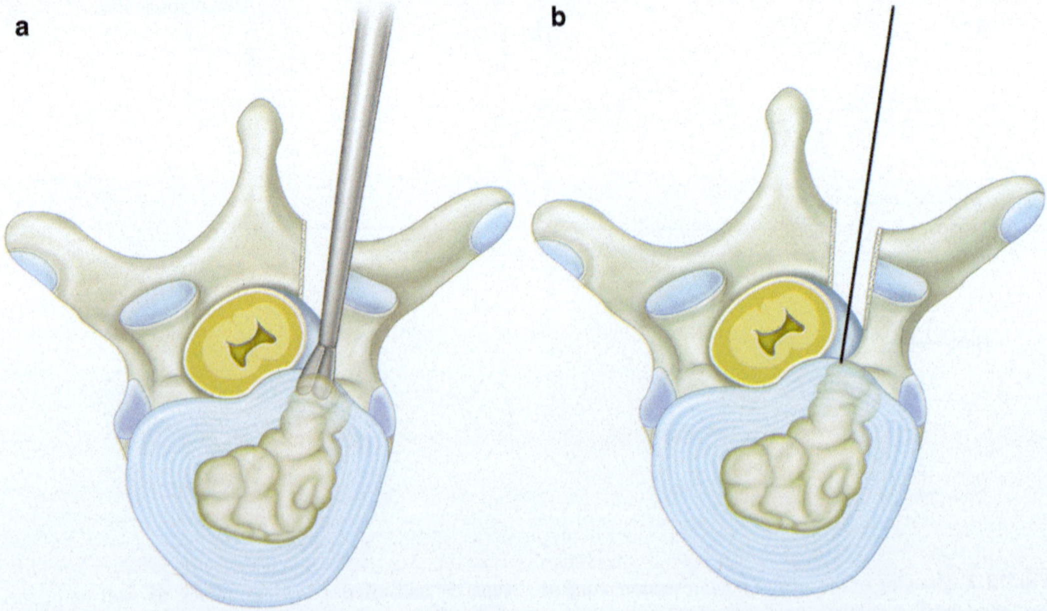

Fig. 12.3 Comparison of the discectomy using laser and pituitary rongeurs. (**a**) Conventional discectomy using mechanical instruments may require considerable neural manipulation and extensive bone resection. (**b**) The pin-point laser of less than 0.5 mm diameter enables discectomy in small operation field with minimal nerve retraction

in a tight and narrow surgical field with minimal retraction of adjacent neural tissue (Fig. 12.3). Compared to a pituitary forceps which has a width of at least 5 mm, the diameter of the laser beam is less than 0.5 mm, which enables precise cutting and evaporation of the herniated disc within a very small operation field. This enables the surgeon to minimize the amount of bone removal necessary to create an adequate surgical field and may help in reducing complications such as total facetectomy and instability. Also, the CO_2 laser can effectively remove calcified discs or osteophytes with no risk of inserting any bulky instruments and causing any iatrogenic injuries. Another advantage of the laser is that sophisticated tissue dissection is possible without damage to neural elements. Inflammatory fibrous adhesion or even scarring from a previous operation can be delicately dissected using CO_2 laser and can reduce the risk of dural tear, intraoperative bleeding, and trauma to normal tissue. The most important disadvantage of laser surgery is the risk of thermal injury to neural tissues. Excessive laser application to the dural sac or nerve root may cause some profound or even irreversible neurologic damages. Also, thermal injury to other normal tissues by uncontrolled laser irradiation may cause unexpected tissue necrosis and degeneration in the skin, muscle, ligaments, bone, and disc. Therefore, laser irradiation should be strictly controlled by an expert surgeon during the entire procedure.

12.5 Case Illustration

12.5.1 Case 1

A 43-year-old male patient presented with a sudden onset of excruciating back pain and left side dominant leg pain, especially at the anterior aspect of the thigh, and walking difficulty which

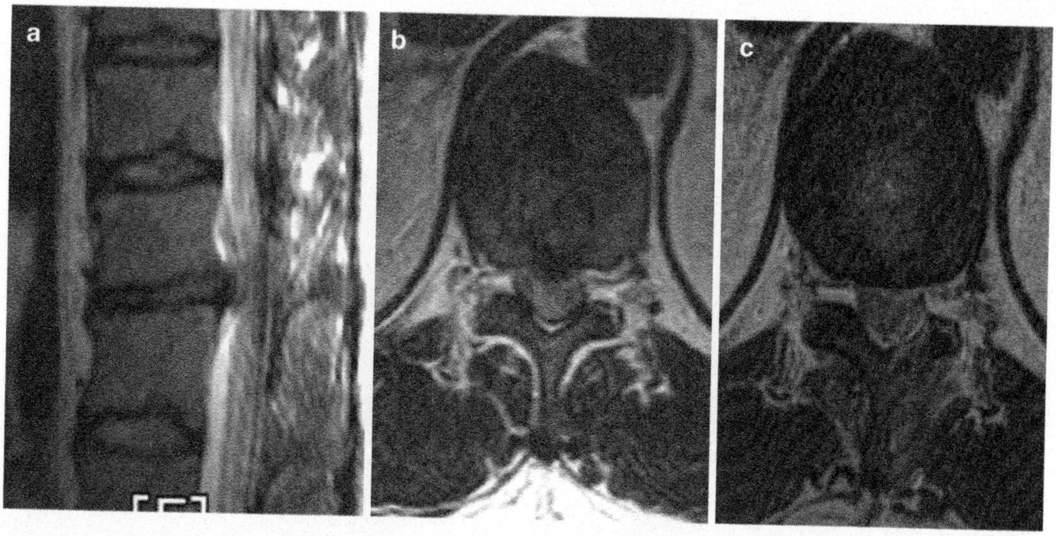

Fig. 12.4 Magnetic resonance (MR) image of a soft disc herniation at the T11/12 level. (**a**) Preoperative T2-weighted sagittal MR image demonstrating soft disc herniation. (**b**) A T2-weighted axial image showing centrolateral disc herniation. (**c**) Postoperative T2-weighted sagittal MR showing complete decompression

began 2 weeks prior to admission. On magnetic resonance (MR) imaging, a left centrolateral soft disc herniation with spinal cord compression at the T11/12 level was identified. The patient underwent posterolateral approach for removal of the thoracic disc herniation using CO_2 laser. Postoperative MR images showed decompression of the spinal cord. The patient had complete resolution of his symptoms (Fig. 12.4).

12.5.2 Case 2

A 33-year-old female presented with long-standing thoracic back pain and walking difficulty, along with numbness and weakness in both lower extremities. On MR imaging, a calcified right paracentral disc herniation with spinal cord compression at the T11/12 level was identified. The patient underwent posterolateral approach for removal of the thoracic disc herniation using CO_2 laser along with down-bite curettes. Partial pediculectomy was done to widen the operation field. Postoperative MR imaging showed decompression of the spinal cord, and gradual resolution of all her symptoms was seen (Fig. 12.5).

12.5.3 Case 3

A 43-year-old female presented with long-standing thoracic back pain and walking difficulty, as well as weakness in the lower extremities and urinary incontinence. On MR imaging, a large left paracentral disc herniation with spinal cord compression was seen at the T8/9 level. The patient underwent paraspinal oblique approach for removal of the thoracic disc herniation using CO_2 laser. Postoperative MR imaging showed complete decompression of the spinal cord and complete resolution of all her symptoms (Fig. 12.6).

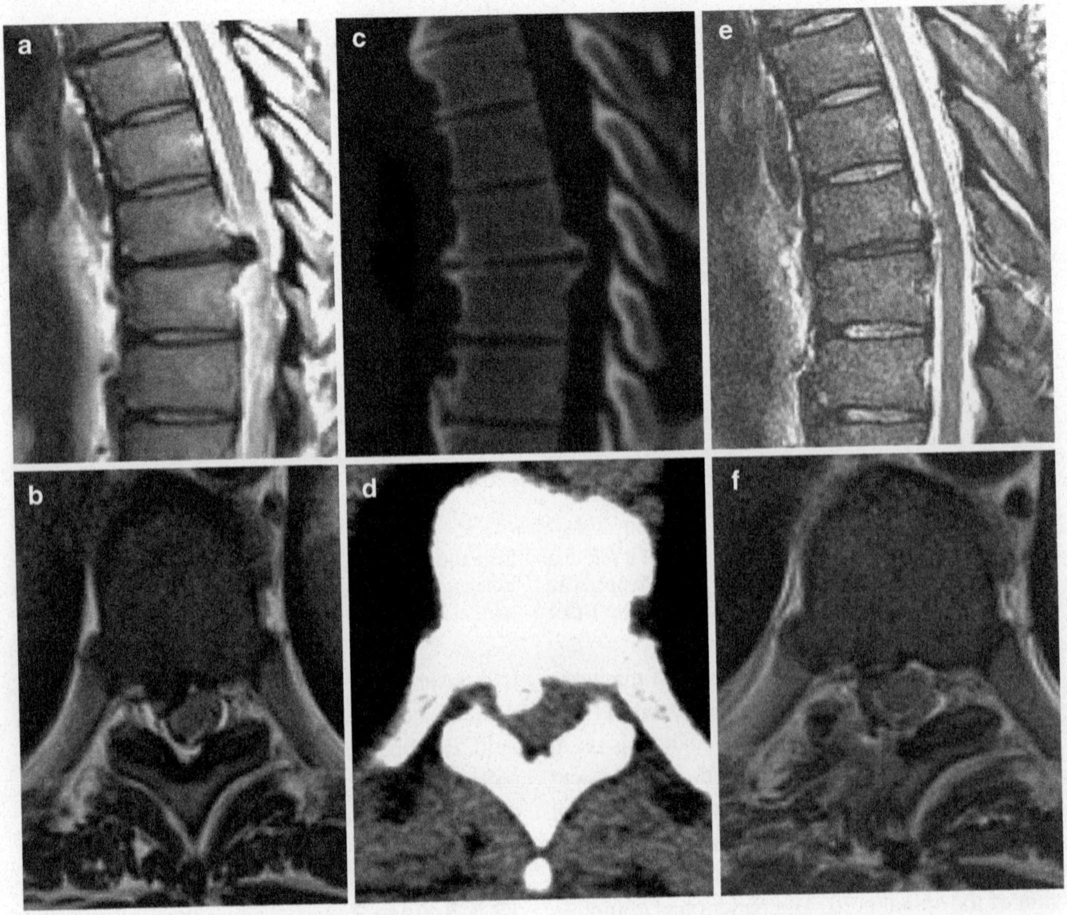

Fig. 12.5 Magnetic resonance (MR) image of a calcified disc herniation at the T11/12 level. (**a**, **b**) Preoperative T2-weighted sagittal and axial MR image showing disc herniation. (**c**, **d**) Computed tomography (CT) sagittal reconstruction image showing calcified disc. (**e**, **f**) Postoperative T2-weighted sagittal MR showing complete decompression

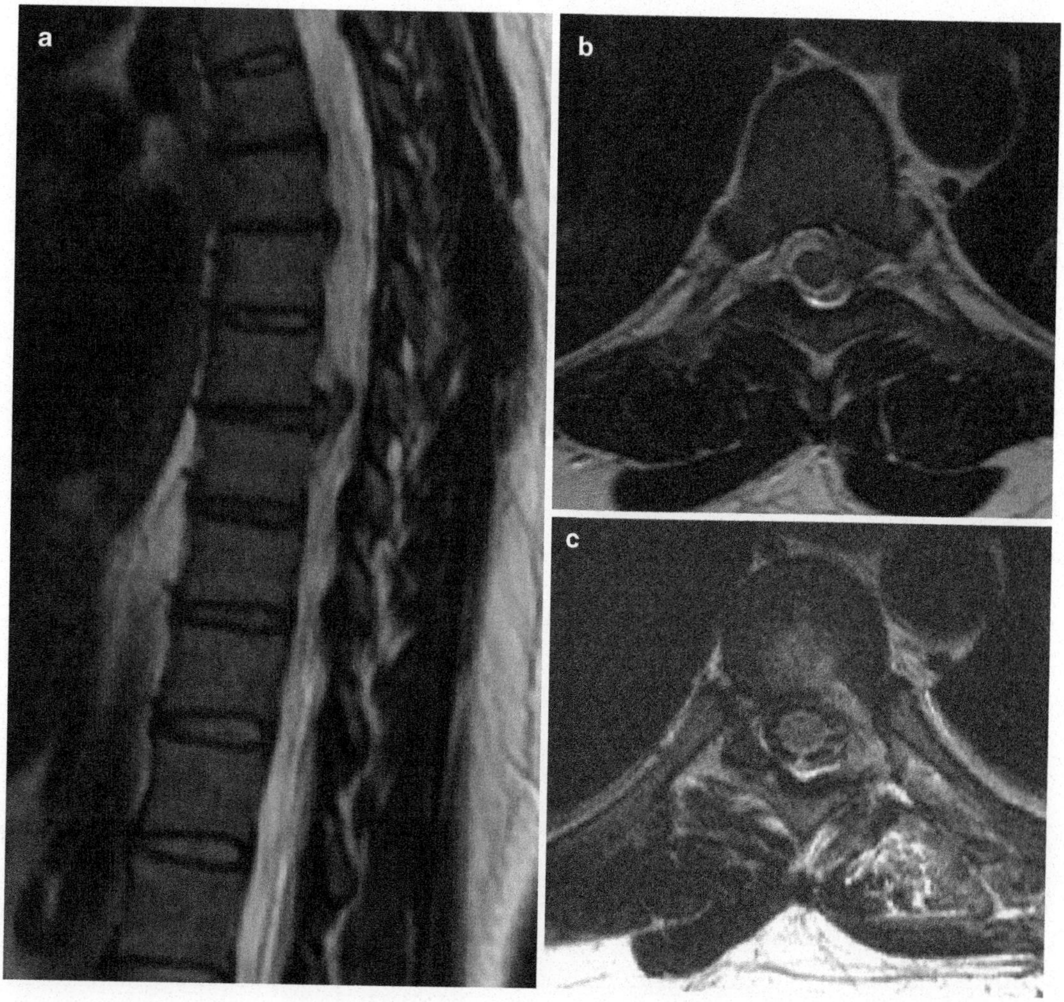

Fig. 12.6 Magnetic resonance (MR) image of a soft disc herniation at the T8/9 level. (**a**) Preoperative T2-weighted sagittal MR image demonstrating soft disc herniation. (**b**) A T2-weighted axial image showing a large paracentral disc herniation. (**c**) Postoperative T2-weighted sagittal MR showing paraspinal oblique trajectory and complete decompression

12.6 Summary

Microscopic thoracic discectomy can be successfully used for a broad range of thoracic disc herniations, including more central, calcified, and large disc herniations. The advantages of this approach include anatomic familiarity, lower morbidity, and infrequent requirement for instrumental stabilization. The use of CO_2 laser for discectomy has further broaden the indication for posterolateral discectomy while reducing the operation field and nerve manipulation necessary for successful surgery.

References

1. Sharma SB, Kim JS. A review of minimally invasive surgical techniques for the management of thoracic disc herniations. Neurospine. 2019;16:24–33.
2. Bouthors C, Benzakour A, Court C. Surgical treatment of thoracic disc herniation: an overview. Int Orthop. 2019;43:807–16.
3. Sivakumaran R, Uschold TD, Brown MT, Patel NR. Transfacet and transpedicular posterior approaches to thoracic disc herniations: consecutive case series of 24 patients. World Neurosurg. 2018;120:e921–31.
4. Foreman PM, Naftel RP, Moore TA, Hadley MN. The lateral extracavitary approach to the thoracolumbar spine: a case series and systematic review. J Neurosurg Spine. 2016;24:570–9.
5. Mayer HM. The microsurgical anterior approach to T5-T10 (mini-TTA). In: Mayer HM, editor. Minimally invasive spine surgery: a surgical manual. Berlin: Springer; 2000. p. 59–66.
6. Kasliwal MK, Deutsch H. Minimally invasive retropleural approach for central thoracic disc herniation. Minim Invasive Neurosurg. 2011;54:167–71.
7. Börm W, Bäzner U, König RW, et al. Surgical treatment of thoracic disc herniations via tailored posterior approaches. Eur Spine J. 2011;20:1684–90.
8. Stillerman CB, Chen TC, Day JD, Couldwell WT, Weiss MH. The transfacet pedicle-sparing approach for thoracic disc removal: cadaveric morphometric analysis and preliminary clinical experience. J Neurosurg. 1995;83:971–6.
9. Patterson RH Jr, Arbit E. A surgical approach through the pedicle to protruded thoracic discs. J Neurosurg. 1978;48:768–72.
10. Black P. Laminotomy/medial facet approach in the excision of thoracic disc herniation. Neurosurg Focus. 2000;9:E6.
11. McCormick WE, Will SF, Benzel EC. Surgery for thoracic disc disease. Complication avoidance: overview and management. Neurosurg Focus. 2000;9:E13.
12. Fessler RG, Sturgill M. Review: complications of surgery for thoracic disc disease. Surg Neurol. 1998;49:609–18.
13. Cho JY, Lee SH, Jang SH, Lee HY. Oblique paraspinal approach for thoracic disc herniations using tubular retractor with robotic holder: a technical note. Eur Spine J. 2012;21:2620–5.
14. Kim JS, Lee SH, Moon KH, Lee HY. Surgical results of the oblique paraspinal approach in upper lumbar disc herniation and thoracolumbar junction. Neurosurgery. 2009;65:95–9.
15. Sherk HH, Rhodes A. Laser discectomy. In: Sherk HH, editor. Lasers in orthopedics. Philadelphia: J. B. Lippincott; 1990. p. 185–9.
16. Kim JS, Lee SH. Carbon dioxide (CO_2) laser-assisted ablation of lumbar discal cyst. Photomed Laser Surg. 2009;27:837–42.
17. Lee DY, Lee SH. Carbon dioxide (CO_2) laser-assisted microdiscectomy for extraforaminal lumbar disc herniation at the L5-S1 level. Photomed Laser Surg. 2011;29:531–5.
18. Ahn Y, Moon KS, Kang BU, Hur SM, Kim JD. Laser assisted posterior cervical foraminotomy and discectomy for lateral and foraminal cervical disc herniation. Photomed Laser Surg. 2012;30:510–5.

Posterior Microscopic Cervical Discectomy with CO_2 Laser

13

Ju-Wan Seuk and Junseok Bae

Abstract

Posterior microscopic cervical discectomy is an effective surgical option for the treatment of cervical radiculopathy. CO_2 laser is an effective tool for minimally invasive spinal surgery in both percutaneous and open spinal procedures. Posterior microscopic cervical discectomy with CO_2 laser procedure can be used as a sharp cutting tool in a limited surgical field rather than conventional discectomy using micro-forceps and may also improve efficiency by reducing intraoperative bleeding, operation time, and risk of tissue damage.

Keywords

Posterior microscopic cervical discectomy · Cervical foraminal disc rupture · Posterior cervical foraminotomy · CO_2 laser · Limited surgical field

Supplementary Information The online version of this chapter (https://doi.org/10.1007/978-981-16-2206-9_13) contains supplementary material, which is available to authorized users.

J.-W. Seuk · J. Bae (✉)
Department of Neurosurgery, Chungdam Wooridul Spine Hospital, Seoul, Republic of Korea

13.1 Introduction

Posterior cervical foraminotomy (PCF) and discectomy is an effective surgical treatment for symptomatic cervical degenerative disease [1, 2]. Although anterior cervical decompression surgery has shown good results, posterior cervical decompression still provides symptom relief for radiculopathy patients [3]. The value of the posterior approach is avoidance of the complication attendant to anterior approaches, such as esophageal injury, vascular injury, recurrent laryngeal nerve paralysis, dysphagia, and accelerated degeneration of adjacent motion segments after fusion [4].

The minimally invasive PCF minimizes the side effects of the posterior approach such as postoperative neck pain and muscle spasm [1, 4, 5]. However, in PCF, limited exposure of the disc space due to the anatomical characteristics of the cervical spine is one of its major disadvantages [6]. The foraminal dimension in the cervical spine is relatively small, so the working space is also limited. To remove a herniated disc fragment in the cervical foramen by using mechanical forceps, wide foraminal exposure and excessive nerve retraction are required. Occasionally, it is very difficult to effectively remove the herniated fragment due to the following reasons:

1. Use of a carbon dioxide (CO_2) laser for PCF and discectomy ensures less bone resection

J. Bae, S.-H. Lee (eds.), *Laser Spine Surgery*, https://doi.org/10.1007/978-981-16-2206-9_13

and less epidural bleeding during a micro-discectomy.
2. The sharp photo-ablation effect of the laser scalpel enables sophisticated decompression in a small surgical field within a limited surgical field.

13.2 Indications and Contraindications

13.2.1 Indications

Radiculopathy from lateral disc herniation at the cervical spine.

Persistent or recurrent root symptoms following anterior cervical discectomy and fusion.

Anterior cervical approaches are relatively contraindicated (e.g., tracheostomy, prior irradiation).

13.2.2 Contraindications

Primary axial neck pain without neurological symptoms

Gross cervical instability at the involved level

Excessive burden of ventral disease (e.g., OPLL)

Cervical myelopathy

Severe cervical kyphotic deformity

Symptomatic cervical central disc herniation or stenosis

13.3 Surgical Technique

The skin incision is made approximately 1 cm lateral to the midline.

If a retractor system is used, very small incisions are necessary (1.5 to 2 cm).

With the use of a retractor, blunt dissection is performed down to the level of the lamina.

If a tubular retractor system is used, serial dilators are used to bluntly widen the approach through the muscles, and finally the tubular retractors are placed.

The retractor should be placed on the interlaminar space (two-thirds) and on the facet joint (one-third).

Expose and mark the interlaminar space of the appropriate level and check again with fluoroscopy.

Expose the medial parts of the capsule of the facet joint and perform a foraminotomy with a high-speed drill with a small Kerrison rongeur.

Extend the foraminotomy and undercut the facet joint laterally until the entire foramen is patent but preserve at least 50% of the facet, because significant postoperative neck pain and instability will be possible.

Resect the ligamentum flavum and expose the lateral edge of the dura and the exiting nerve root.

The collection of veins overlying the nerve root was coagulated and removed for better visualization of the nerve (Fig. 13.1).

After removing sequestered free fragments using micro-forceps, the nerve root was gently retracted to reveal the compressive disc fragment.

Compressive disc fragment was evaporated using a CO_2 laser attached to a microscope (Figs. 13.2 and 13.3).

When retracting the nerve root, be sure to check and protect the anterior nerve root because

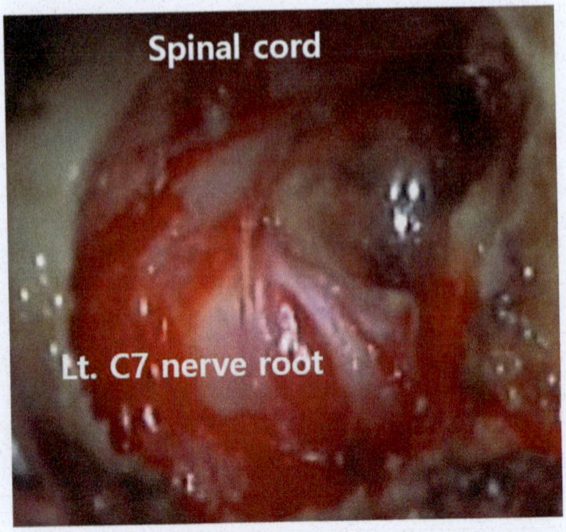

Fig. 13.1 Intraoperative microscopic image. Note the compressed exiting nerve root and spinal cord

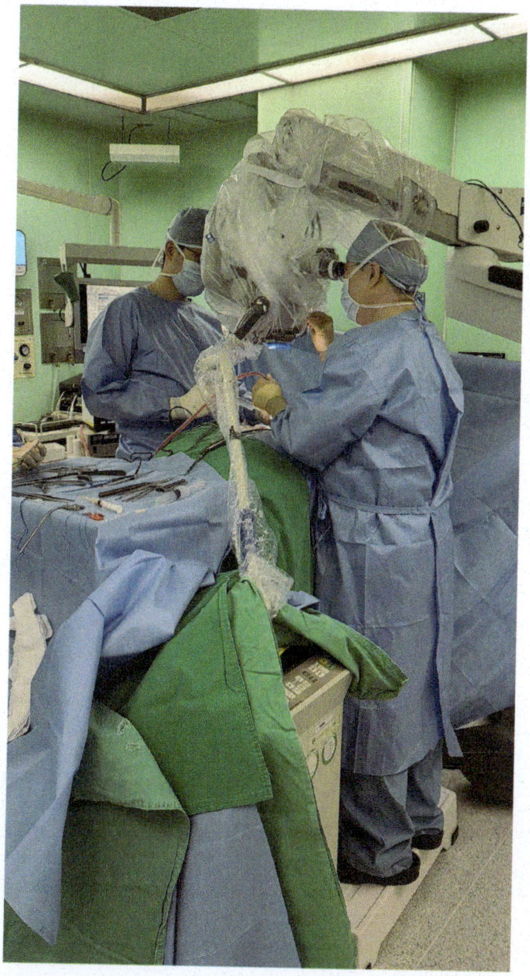

Fig. 13.2 Operative field image. Using the CO_2 laser-equipped surgical microscope

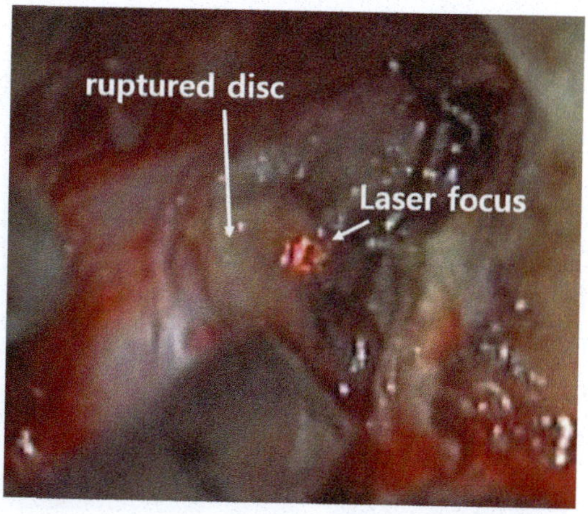

Fig. 13.3 Intraoperative microscopic image. Note the gently retracted exiting nerve root, ruptured disc, and pointed CO_2 laser beam

it is located further caudal than the dorsal nerve root.

The pinpoint size laser was used at a power level of 10 W, which allows safe and precise evaporation.

And it has to be more delicate than the lumbar spine surgery, so intermittent laser use is safer than continuous laser use.

It is recommended to make a small hole at the annulus or disc hernia site, and perform fragmentectomy, to reduce the possibility of recurrence.

After sufficient decompression, hemostasis was achieved and the wound was closed with insertion of hamovac.

13.4 Case Illustration

The patient is a 56-year-old man who presented with left upper extremity radiating pain. Conservative treatment was maintained for 1 month, but symptoms did not improve. An MRI of the cervical spine (Fig. 13.4) was notable for a ruptured disc at the left foraminal area at C67 level. Finally, CO_2 laser-assisted PCF and discectomy was performed. On the postoperative MRI (Fig. 13.5), the ruptured disc was well removed, and it was confirmed that the left C7 nerve root was well decompressed. The patient had an uneventful postoperative recovery.

13.5 Summary

Posterior microscopic cervical discectomy with CO_2 laser is an effective surgical option for the treatment of cervical radiculopathy. In spinal surgery, laser systems have advantages over using a scalpel in terms of precision. The diameter of the focused beam of a CO_2 laser is <0.5 mm, whereas the width of small disc forceps is *5 mm. This small spot size enables selective tissue ablation in a narrow surgical bed [6]. It can be used precisely and delicately, so there is less bleeding, less swelling, and less trauma, thanks to minimal tis-

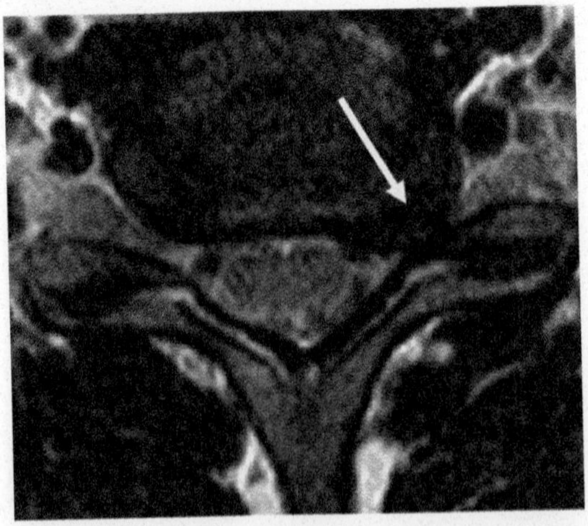

Fig. 13.4 Preoperative MRI axial image. Ruptured disc at left C67 foramen was identified

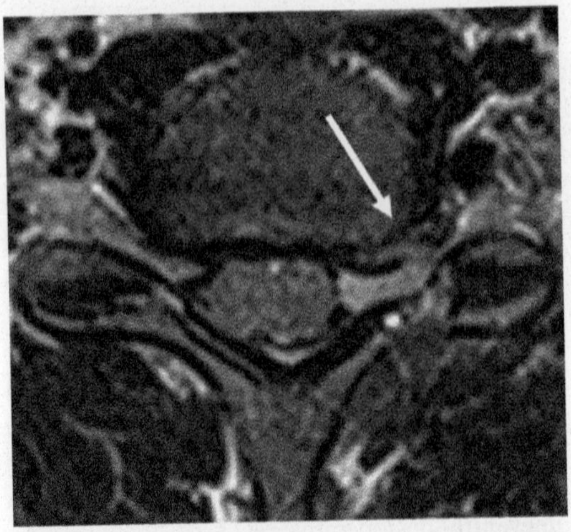

Fig. 13.5 Postoperative MRI axial image. Facet was preserved and ruptured foraminal disc was well removed

sue manipulation [6–8]. Therefore, laser is an effective tool for minimally invasive spinal surgery in both percutaneous and open spinal procedures [8–15]. CO_2 laser-assisted PCF procedure can be used as a sharp cutting tool in a limited surgical field and may improve efficiency by reducing intraoperative bleeding, operation time, and risk of tissue damage.

A laser can be used to remove herniated disc material or osteophytes and reduce intradiscal pressure by vaporization [16]. And CO_2 laser is also believed to decrease reherniation after discectomy caused by laser-induced metaplasia.

References

1. Ratliff JK, Cooper PR. Cervical laminoplasty: a critical review. J Neurosurg. 2003 April;98(3 Suppl):230–8.
2. Ducker TB, Zeidman SM. The posterior operative approach for cervical radiculopathy. Neurosurg Clin N Am. 1993;4:61–74.
3. Khoo LT, Perez-Cruet MJ, Laich DT, Fessler RG. Posterior cervical microendoscopic foraminotomy. In: Perez-Cruet MJ, Fessler RG, editors. Outpatient spinal surgery. St. Louis: Quality Medical Publishing, Inc.; 2006. p. 71–93.
4. Fessler RG, Khoo LT. Minimally invasive cervical microendoscopic foraminotomy: an initial clinical experience. Neurosurgery. 2002 November;51(5 Suppl):S37–45.
5. Siddiqui A, Yonemura KS. Posterior cervical mircoendoscopic diskectomy and laminoforaminotomy. In: Kim DH, Fessler RG, Regan JJ, editors. Endoscopic spine surgery and instrumentation: percutaneous procedures. New York: Thieme; 2005. p. 66–73.
6. Ahn Y, Moon KS, Kang B-U, Hur SM, Kim JD. Laser-assisted posterior cervical foraminotomy and discectomy for lateral and foraminal cervical disc herniation. Photomed Laser Surg. 2012;30(9):510–5.
7. Lee DY, Lee SH. Carbon dioxide (CO_2) laser-assisted microdiscectomy for extraforaminal lumbar disc herniation at the L5-S1 level. Photomed Laser Surg. 2011;29:531–5.
8. Jeon SH, Lee SH, Choi WC. Iliac artery perforation following lumbar discectomy with microsurgical carbon dioxide laser: a report of a rare case and discussion on the treatment. Spine (Phila Pa 1976). 2007;32:E124–5.
9. Kim JS, Lee SH. Carbon dioxide (CO_2) laser-assisted ablation of lumbar discal cyst. Photomed Laser Surg. 2009;27:837–42.
10. Kim JS, Choi G, Jin SR, Lee SH. Removal of a discal cyst using percutaneous endoscopic interlaminar approach: a case report. Photomed Laser Surg. 2009;27:365–9.
11. Ahn Y, Lee SH, Shin SW. Percutaneous endoscopic cervical discectomy: clinical outcome and radiographic changes. Photomed Laser Surg. 2005;23:362–8.
12. Choy DS, Hellinger J, Hellinger S, Tassi GP, Lee SH. 23rd anniversary of percutaneous laser disc decompression (PLDD). Photomed Laser Surg. 2009;27:535–8.

13. Lee DY, Ahn Y, Lee SH. Percutaneous endoscopic lumbar discectomy for adolescent lumbar disc herniation: surgical outcomes in 46 consecutive patients. Mt Sinai J Med. 2006;73:864–70.
14. Lee SH, Ahn Y, Choi WC, Bhanot A, Shin SW. Immediate pain improvement is a useful predictor of long-term favorable outcome after percutaneous laser disc decompression for cervical disc herniation. Photomed Laser Surg. 2006;24:508–13.
15. Lee SH, Ahn Y, Lee JH. Laser-assisted anterior cervical corpectomy versus posterior laminoplasty for cervical myelopathic patients with multilevel ossification of the posterior longitudinal ligament. Photomed Laser Surg. 2008;26:119–27.
16. Ivanov AA, Faizan A, Ebraheim NA, Yeasting R, Goel VK. The effect of removing the lateral part of the pars interarticularis on stress distribution at the neural arch in lumbar foraminal microdecompression at L3-L4 and L4-L5. Anatomic and finite element investigations. Spine. 2007;32:2462–6.

Posterior Endoscopic Cervical Foraminotomy and Discectomy with Ho:Yag Laser

14

Yong Soo Choi

Abstract

Posterior endoscopic cervical foraminotomy (PECF) is one of the minimally invasive procedures that solve the lateral pathology of cervical spine that can cause radiating pain. In the past, it was performed as an operation to enlarge the incision, but due to the recent development of the endoscope, effective treatment with minimal incision has become possible. At the same time, with the development of lasers along with endoscopy, these treatment techniques are creating a better prognosis through more sophisticated and effective methods. It is important to understand in which cases these techniques are performed properly and how to safely and effectively perform these techniques.

Keywords

Posterior endoscopic cervical foraminotomy (PECF) · Cervical nerve root decompression Posterior cervical laser discectomy · Posterior cervical foraminotomy · Posterior cervical laminoforaminotomy

Y. S. Choi (✉)
Department of Neurosurgery, Chungdam Wooridul Spine Hospital, Seoul, Republic of Korea
e-mail: yong@wooridul.co.kr

14.1 Introduction

In 1944, Spurling and Scoville performed posterior cervical foraminotomy to treat osteophytes or lateral disc herniation and proved that it was effective and safe [1]. The cervical anterior approach can show very good postoperative progress by performing neural decompression by discectomy, foraminotomy, or increasing the disc height. However, there is a high frequency of fusion surgery after discectomy, and there is a risk of injury to the trachea, esophagus, carotid artery, or jugular vein. On the other hand, posterior cervical foraminotomy or laminoforaminotomy can decompress the nerve roots without risk of damage to the organs located in front of the neck, and the frequency of interbody fusion is less. However, it can cause muscle pain, muscle spasm, or cervical kyphosis after surgery by dissection of the posterior cervical muscle structures [2]. In 2001, Adamson reported that performing posterior cervical foraminotomy using a microendoscopy showed excellent results similar to open posterior cervical foraminotomy while significantly reducing muscle damage [3]. In 2007, Ruetten performed a full endoscopic posterior cervical foraminotomy and reported an excellent course of effective nerve decompression with minimal muscle damage [4]. Since then, endoscopic technology has been further developed, leading to safe and effective discectomy using laser.

J. Bae, S.-H. Lee (eds.), *Laser Spine Surgery*, https://doi.org/10.1007/978-981-16-2206-9_14

14.2 Indications

The indications of posterior endoscopic cervical foraminotomy and discectomy are as follows:

- Foraminal disc herniation
- Lateralized disc extrusion
- Foramina stenosis
- Osteophyte compressing nerve root
- Facet cyst compressing nerve root
- Residual foraminal pathology following anterior approach

Posterior endoscopic cervical foraminotomy (PECF) is an indication for lateralized disc herniation, foraminal stenosis, and nerve root compression due to osteophytes. Furthermore, it can be performed in cases that a nerve root is compressed due to a facet cyst and to effectively expand the remaining foraminal stenosis after anterior approach surgery. Since endoscopic foraminal decompression is a technique that resolves a lesion caused by compression of a nerve root, radiating pain associated with compressed nerve root can be significantly reduced. Axial neck pain without radiating pain is not appropriate for PECF. Ventral lesions such as OPLL, central disc extrusion and broad hard disc extrusion, and severe spinal cord compression are contraindicated in endoscopic cervical foraminotomy. In addition, in cases of deformity or instability of the cervical spine, it should be performed carefully or replaced with fusion surgery.

14.3 Surgical Technique

For posterior endoscopic cervical procedures, endotracheal general anesthesia is preferred over local anesthesia. The reason is that for the posterior cervical approach, the patient should be in a prone position and not move while the procedure is performed with the neck flexed. It is difficult for most patients to maintain this posture, and severe pain and unintentional movement may occur when a nerve root is retracted, which can cause fatal damage to the spinal cord and nerve roots. Electromyography (EMG) and somatosensory evoked potentials (SSEPs) monitoring can be performed to effectively protect nerves and decompress nerves during the procedure, which can be very helpful in some cases.

The patient's position can be either prone or sitting, but Mayfield head fixation must be performed in the seated position, and may not be used in the prone position. Mayfield head fixation is an invasive fixation device on the head, so prone position without head fixation is advantageous to avoid headaches and scalp wounds after the procedure. Therefore, it is preferred to perform the posterior cervical spine approach in the prone position (Fig. 14.1a). The patient's eyes, forehead, chest, and abdomen should be padded so as not to be pressed, and the neck should be flexed to the extent that the airway does not narrow. The operating table is placed in the center of the operating room, and the anesthesia machine is located above the patient's head, and the C-arm and its monitor, the machine tower including the endoscope monitor, the laser machine, and the surgical instrument table are located in an appropriate position around the operating table. The surgeon and assistant perform the procedure without interference (Fig. 14.1b).

After sterilizing the procedural site and covering the surgical drape, fluoroscopic images confirm the surgical site and the initial entry point. An 18G needle is inserted from the skin to the foraminotomy or laminoforaminotomy point under the fluoroscopic guide, and the target point is the V-point, which is the lamino-facetal junction at the level of the lesion (Fig. 14.2). After the correct trajectory for access to the endoscope is confirmed, the wire is inserted into the 18G needle, and the needle is removed after skin incision (Fig. 14.3). Serial dilators split the paraspinal muscles to provide space for the working sleeve of endoscope. After the working sleeve has a space for entry, push it in until it comes into close contact with the lamina and facet of the cervical spine and the wire and dilators are removed. There are two types of working sleeves with and without screw grooves, and there are types with rounded ends and types with oblique cuts

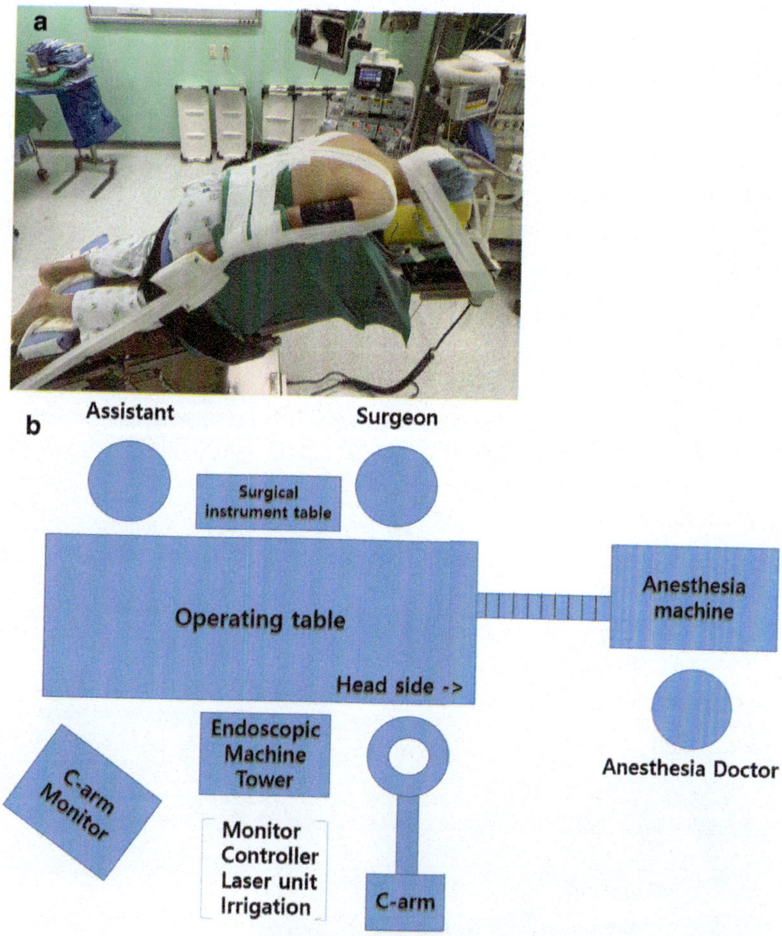

Fig. 14.1 (**a**) Prone position without head fixation. The patient's neck was flexed and fixed softly, the airways should be firmly maintained, and the face, chest, and limbs should be supported with pads to prevent pressure. During the procedure, the hips should be pulled up so that the patient's body does not slide down. (**b**) The operating bed is placed in the center of the operating room, the anesthesia device is located above the patient's head, and the surgeon and assistant nurse are on the left side of the prone patient. If the surgeon is left-handed, it is convenient for the surgeon to be on the patient's right side. An endoscopic monitor, instruments, and C-arm are placed opposite the surgeon

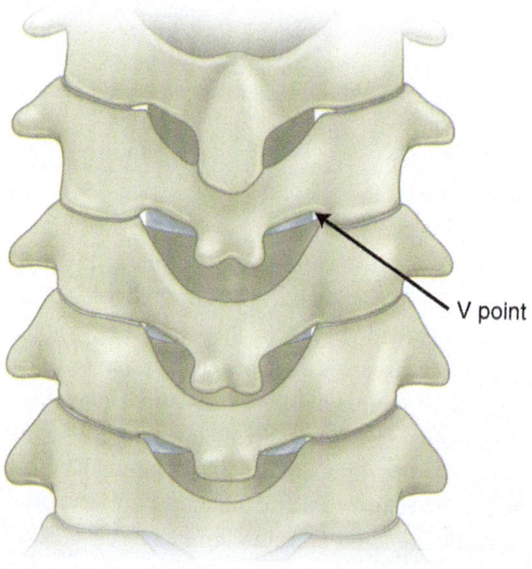

Fig. 14.2 Target point is the lamino-facetal junction (V-point)

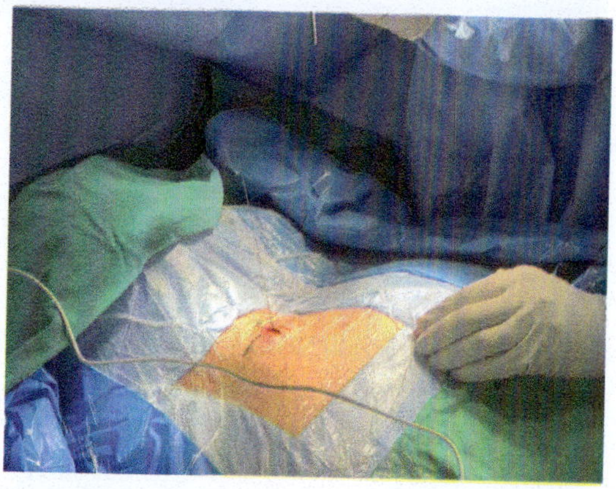

Fig. 14.3 The guide wire inserted from the skin to the target point is an important step during the early stage of the procedure because it makes the way for the dilators and the working sleeve

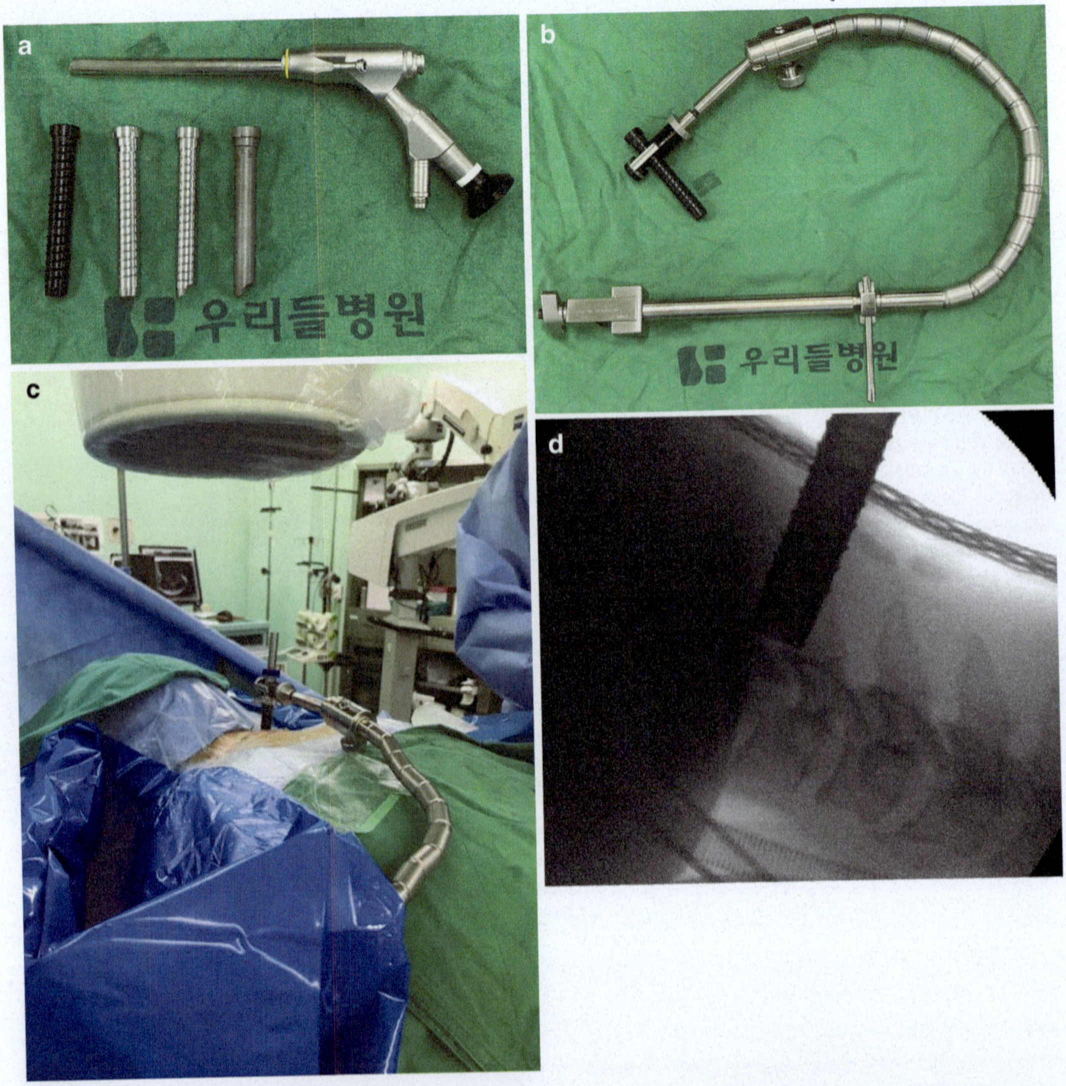

Fig. 14.4 (**a**) Working sleeves are made of metal and plastic and are available with and without screw grooves with rounded ends and types with oblique cuts. (**b**, **c**) The metal arm connects and fixes the working sleeve and the surgical table so that the working sleeve does not move when performing endoscopic procedures. (**d**) In the C-arm view, the working sleeve is fixed to the target point as shown in the radiograph

(Fig. 14.4a). The appropriate kind of working sleeve is selected according to different situations. The working sleeve is fixed by means of a metal arm that is connected to the surgical table (Fig. 14.4b–d). When the endoscope enters the working sleeve described above, a V-point consisting of the cervical lamina and facet is observed. After arranging the muscle tissue that obstructs the visual field, foraminotomy is performed from the lamino-facetal junction using endoscopic drills (Fig. 14.5). After foraminotomy is performed from the lower margin of the pedicle at the upper level to the upper margin of the pedicle at the lower level, the nerve root wrapped with soft tissue is shown. If decompression is needed in the medial part, the lamina can be further drilled out to expose the ligamentum flavum covering the dura. If this ligamentum flavum is carefully removed using an endoscopic punch or forceps, the dura surrounding the cervical spinal cord can be exposed. When exposed to this dura, the pressure in the endoscopic irrigation fluid should be reduced to prevent iatrogenic cord compression. Bipolar cauterization controls bleeding around the nerve root and dura. After organizing the soft tissue and performing hemostasis to secure the field of view of the endoscope, expand the range of nerve decompression. In general, in the vertical direction, the nerve root decompression is performed by securing a space from the lower margin of the upper pedicle to the upper margin of the lower pedicle (Fig. 14.6a, b). In some cases, a pediculotomy that drills a part of the pedicle may be performed in case neural decompression is not sufficient, and the space is narrow for retraction of neural structures to remove the herniated intervertebral disc. To the lateral boundary, the nerve root is decompressed by drilling to the lateral margin of the pedicle. The facet joint should be drilled by half to avoid spinal instability. After the lateral margin and nerve root of the dura are identified, a herniated intervertebral disc would be found (Fig. 14.6a, b). Most herniated discs are located in the axillary portion of the nerve root. The ruptured disc is removed using a holmium:yttrium-aluminum-garnet laser after retraction of the nerve root superiorly. At the end of this procedure, it is confirmed by palpating the nerve root using an endoscopic probe and visualizing the free nerve root if the nerve root is well decompressed.

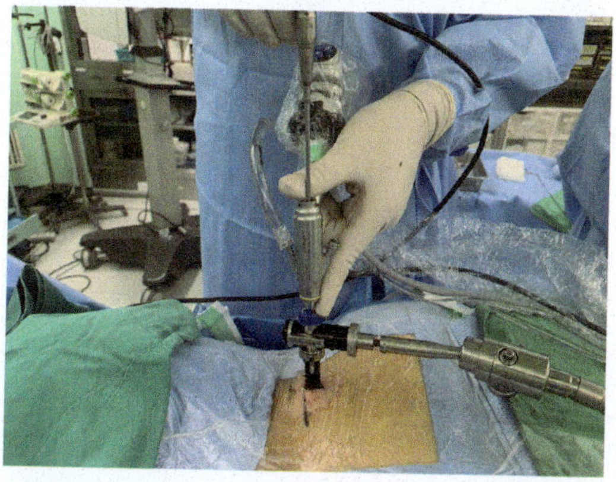

Fig. 14.5 The endoscope enters into the working sleeve and the surgical site is checked through the monitor, and a foraminotomy or laminoforaminotomy is performed using an endoscope drill. The endoscope is fixed with one hand and another hand holds the drill and moves it

14.4 Complications

There are several possible complications in performing posterior endoscopic cervical foraminotomy. There may be dura or neural injury while performing this procedure, which is statistically unlikely, but should be performed carefully as it may be caused by careless or incompetent techniques. Hemostasis should be actively performed because neurological symptoms may occur due to nerve compression due to bleeding after the

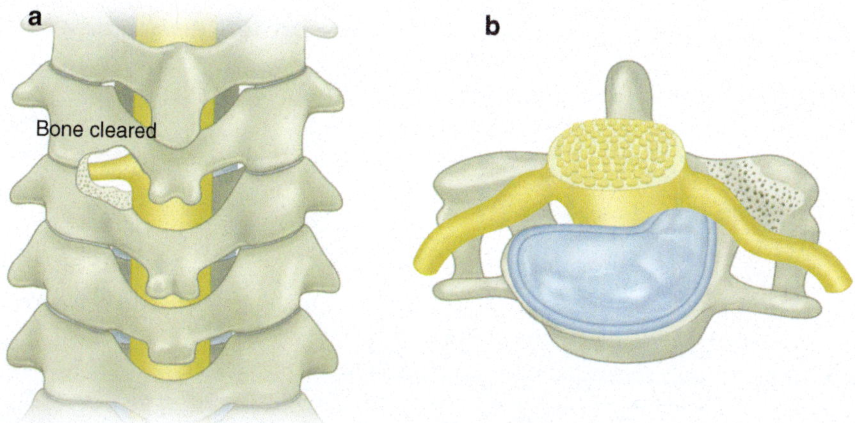

Fig. 14.6 (**a**, **b**) After foraminotomy or laminoforaminotomy was performed, the lateral margin of the nerve root and dura was identified after the soft tissue was cleaned. Typically, the herniated intervertebral disc is observed on the axillar area of the nerve root

procedure. If the pressure of the endoscopic irrigation water increases, nerve compression may occur, so the flow of irrigation water must be continuously monitored during the procedure. Since the treatment site skin may not be healed, wound management should be well done after the procedure, and appropriate disinfection and antibiotic administration should be performed to prevent wound infection.

14.5 Case Illustration

- Case 1

A 42-year-old female office worker presented with symptoms of right scapular pain, right arm lateral pain, tingling sensation, and numbness in the right thumb and index finger, which developed 2 months ago. Not only could she sit still; she couldn't turn her neck, and the pain prevented her from lying down and sleeping. The pain was getting worse for 2 months. The pain did not improve despite taking painkillers. Her muscle strength was normal, but the Spurling sign was positive on the right. Cervical MRI suggested a lateral disc herniation on the right side between the fifth and sixth cervical vertebrae, which was compressing the nerve root of the sixth cervical vertebra (Fig. 14.7). The patient underwent PECF, and a prolapsed intervertebral disc holding it in the axillar portion of the nerve root in the endoscopic field of view was found and removed with a Ho:Yag laser (Fig. 14.8a, b). The procedural time was about 40 minutes, and all of the patient's symptoms immediately disappeared

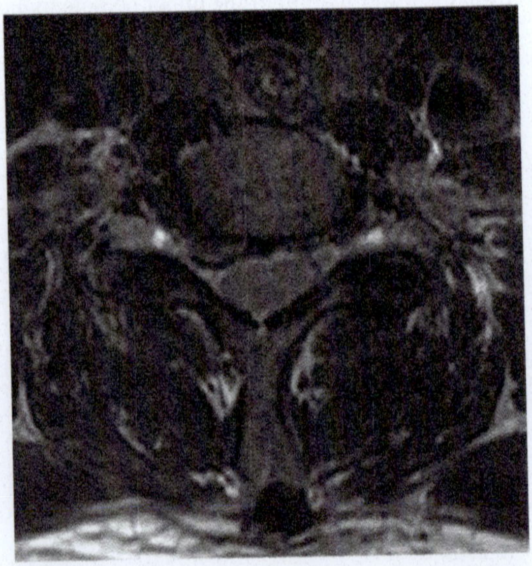

Fig. 14.7 A lateral disc herniation on the right side between the fifth and sixth cervical vertebrae was compressing the nerve root of the sixth cervical vertebra on the axial view of magnetic resolution image

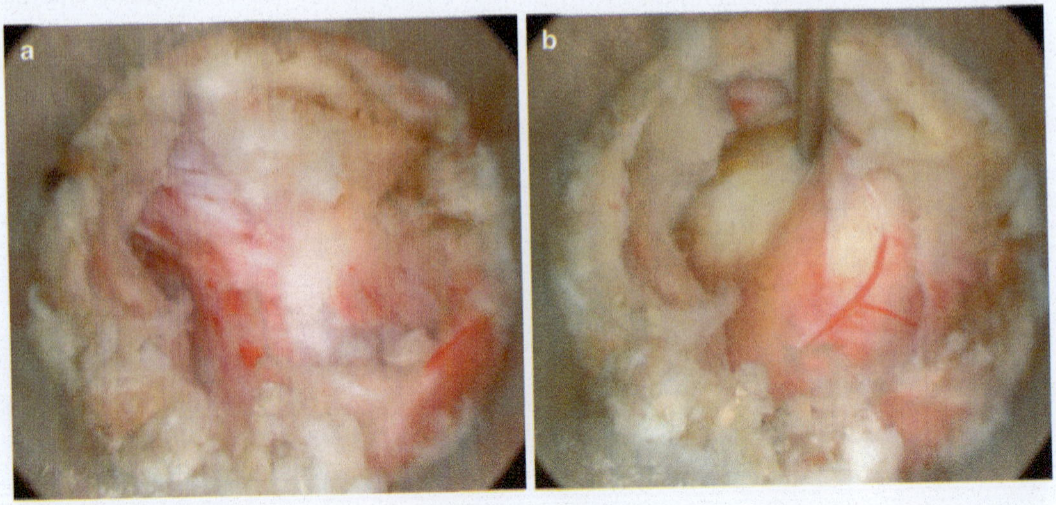

Fig. 14.8 (**a**) After foraminotomy, the lateral margin of the sixth nerve root and dura was identified in the endoscopic field of view. (**b**) When the sixth nerve root is retracted upward, the intervertebral disc that was compressing the nerve root is identified on the axillar area of the nerve root

after the procedure. She returned home 2 days later and did not feel any pain, so she could now move and live freely and sleep comfortably.

- Case 2

A 60-year-old woman presented with pain in the back of her right arm. She underwent an artificial intervertebral disc implantation between cervical spine 6–7 at another hospital 8 months ago (Fig. 14.9), and the above symptoms gradually developed. When she turned her head to the right, she complained of pain in the right arm. So, even though there were no problems with the intervertebral disc, she had been unable to turn her neck. In cervical MRI, the protrued intervertebral disc at the right C6-7, where the artificial disc was inserted, compressed the seventh cervical nerve root (Fig. 14.10). She underwent PECF, and the prolapsed intervertebral disc compressing the nerve root in the endoscopic field of view was removed using a laser (Fig. 14.11). Her symptoms were alleviated, and after that, the movement of her neck became normal, and the

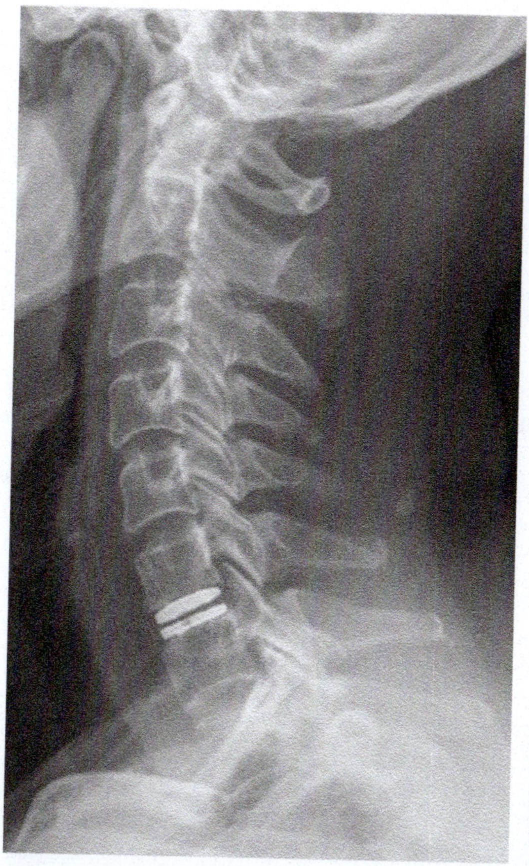

Fig. 14.9 The patient underwent an artificial intervertebral disc implantation between cervical spines 6 and 7 at another hospital 8 months ago

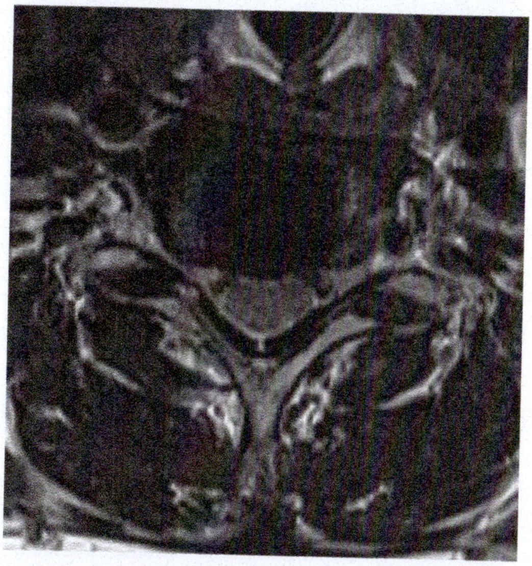

Fig. 14.10 The remaining intervertebral disc located on the right side between cervical vertebrae 6 and 7, where the artificial disc was inserted, protruded, and pressed the seventh cervical nerve root on the axial view of magnetic resolution image

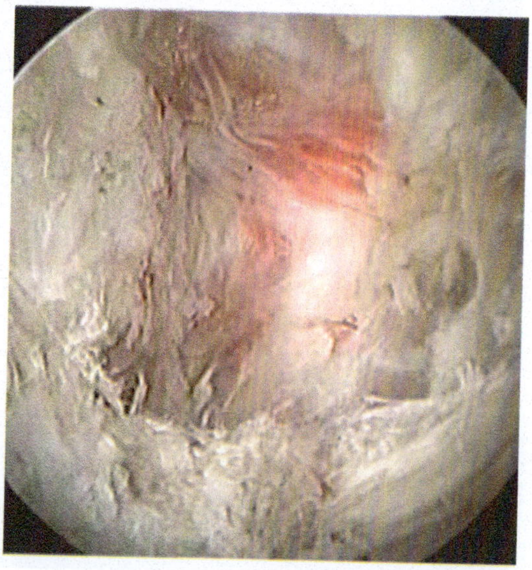

Fig. 14.11 The prolapsed intervertebral disc was compressing the seventh nerve root in the endoscopic field of view

artificial intervertebral disc also moved normally. After surgery, MRI suggests that the nerve root is decompressed (Fig. 14.12).

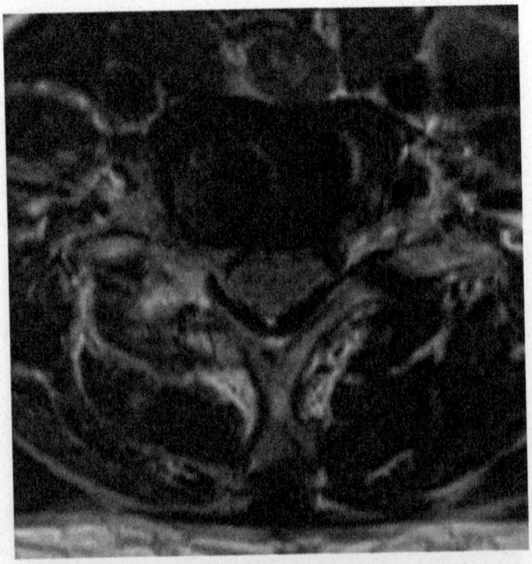

Fig. 14.12 Postoperative MRI confirmed that the seventh nerve root was decompressed anteroposteriorly

References

1. Spurling RG, Scoville WB. Lateral rupture of the cervical intervertebral disc: a common cause of shoulder and arm pain. Sug Gynecol Obstet. 1944;78:350–8.
2. Won S, Kim CH, Chung CK, et al. Clinical outcomes of single-level posterior percutaneous endoscopic cervical foraminotomy for patients with less cervical lordosis. J Minim Invasive Spine Surg Tech. 2016;1(1):11–7.
3. Adamson TE. Microendoscopic posterior cervical laminoforaminotomy for unilateral radiculopathy: results of a new technique in 100 cases. J Neurosurg. 2001;95:51–7.
4. Ruetten S, Komp M, Merk H, Godolias G. A new full-endoscopic technique for cervical posterior foraminotomy in the treatment of lateral disc herniations using 6.9-mm endoscopes: prospective 2-year results of 87 patients. Minim Invasive Neurosurg. 2007;50:219–26.

15 Anterior Endoscopic Cervical Discectomy with Ho:YAG Laser

Junseok Bae

Abstract

Anterior endoscopic cervical discectomy is an effective treatment for soft disc herniation causing cervical radiculopathy and myelopathy. In particular, Ho:YAG laser is the most important surgical tool for efficient and accurate surgery under the endoscopic visualization in a narrow space. In this chapter, we will describe tips and pearls for the use of endoscopic laser in anterior cervical endoscopic discectomy.

Keywords

Anterior endoscopic cervical discectomy
Cervical disc herniation · Ho:YAG laser
Foraminal disc herniation · Central disc herniation

15.1 Introduction

Anterior endoscopic cervical discectomy is an effective treatment for soft disc herniation causing cervical radiculopathy and myelopathy [1–6]. Tajima et al. reported the first percutaneous anterior cervical discectomy procedure [7]. Techniques such as percutaneous cervical automated nucleotomy, percutaneous cervical laser decompression, and percutaneous cervical endoscopic laser discectomy have been developed with advancement of endoscopic instrument and side-firing laser. In particular, Ho:YAG laser is the most important surgical tool for efficient and accurate surgery under the endoscopic visualization in a narrow space [8]. In this chapter, we will describe tips and pearls for the use of endoscopic laser in anterior cervical endoscopic discectomy.

15.2 Indications

The indication is soft cervical disc herniation located at the central, paramedian, and foraminal area that causes radiculopathy or myelopathy concordant with the radiological finding with unsuccessful improvement of symptom after appropriate conservative treatment [2, 3, 7–11]. Contraindications are calcified disc herniation, sequestrated disc herniation, severe spondylosis with disc space narrowing (disc space <3 mm), cervical myelopathy, spondylolisthesis, instability, fracture, tumor, or infection.

Supplementary Information The online version of this chapter (https://doi.org/10.1007/978-981-16-2206-9_15) contains supplementary material, which is available to authorized users.

J. Bae (✉)
Department of Neurosurgery, Chungdam Wooridul Spine Hospital, Seoul, Republic of Korea

J. Bae, S.-H. Lee (eds.), *Laser Spine Surgery*, https://doi.org/10.1007/978-981-16-2206-9_15

15.3 Surgical Technique

The operation is performed under local or general anesthesia. For a comfortable surgery during local anesthesia, evaluation of the patient's neck by palpation of the vertebral body before surgery is essential. Patients who are too sensitive and prone to gag or who have agoraphobia are recommended for general anesthesia. Midazolam and fentanyl are given intravenously for conscious sedation. The amount of sedative is carefully adjusted by an anesthesiologist during local procedures. At all stages of surgery, the patient should ensure that there is no discomfort to ensure a safe operation. It is advantageous to monitor changes in symptoms, and it helps the surgeon to perform a safe procedure to recognize the nerve structure. Immediate pain relief after decompression of the hernia can be confirmed by the aroused patient. In general anesthesia, nerve monitoring should be applied during surgery.

The patient is in a supine position with the neck slightly extended on a radiolucent operating table (Fig. 15.1). Then, check the index level by taking anteroposterior and lateral perspective images. In case of paramedian or foraminal disc herniation, the contralateral approach is recommended. The midline, disc space, and medial edge of the SCM muscle are indicated by surface landmarks. After facilitating the pulsation of the carotid artery, gently move the visceral compartment, including the trachea and esophagus, with the index and third fingers to the opposite side (Fig. 15.2a, b). The access needle is inserted into the disc space between the tips of your fingers (Fig. 15.2c). Care should be taken when inserting into the midline of the anterior collar to prevent damage to the longus colli muscle. Under the lateral perspective, the needle advances into the posterior disc space. Discography is performed to show the contrast agent leaks into the epidural space (Fig. 15.3). Acid degenerate nuclei can be stained blue when using indigo carmine. A guide wire is inserted through the needle. With a sequential dilator (Fig. 15.4), the working tube is introduced to reach the posterior vertebral body (Figs. 15.5 and 15.6). This is important to avoid unnecessary resection of the normal nucleus during decompression and to perform selective fragment resection. A 3.9 mm endoscope (CESSYS ventral, joimax GmbH, Germany) is introduced into the working tube (Fig. 15.7). After removing the subligamentous herniated debris, defects in the posterior longitudinal ligament (PLL) can be identified. Side-firing holmium:YAG laser is used to release fibrotic anchoring posterior annulus and herniated fragment (Fig. 15.8). Herniated fragments of the epidural space can be seen through the torn PLL layer. Further opening of the PLL with side-firing laser exposes and mobilizes the epidural hernia. Herniated fragment can be removed with grabbing forceps (Fig. 15.9). For foraminal herniation, opening of the posterior uncinated process is necessary for adequate foraminal approach with endoscopy. An endoscopic reamer, diamond drill, or laser is used to remove the posterior part of the uncinated process (Fig. 15.10). In summary, the side-firing Ho:YAG laser (Fig. 15.11) is useful in (1) shrinking of the thickened posterior annulus and resecting posterior bone spur to open proper visualization into the posterior surface of intervertebral disc space, (2) thinning the degenerated PLL, (3) opening of the defects in

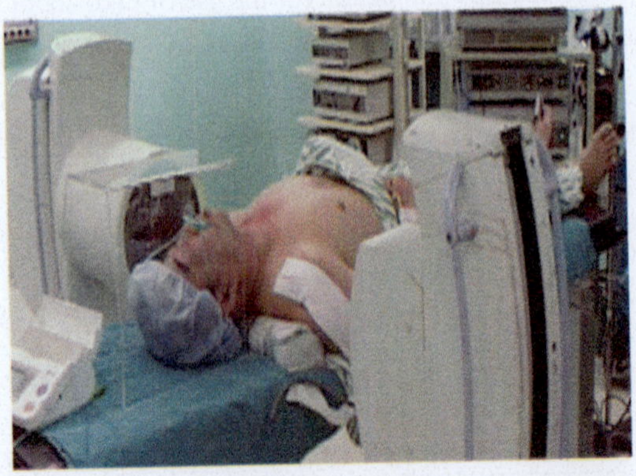

Fig. 15.1 The patient is in a supine position with the neck slightly extended on a radiolucent operating table. Note that the plastic tape is pulling down the patient's shoulder to proper fluoroscopic exposure of the index level, especially the lower cervical spine

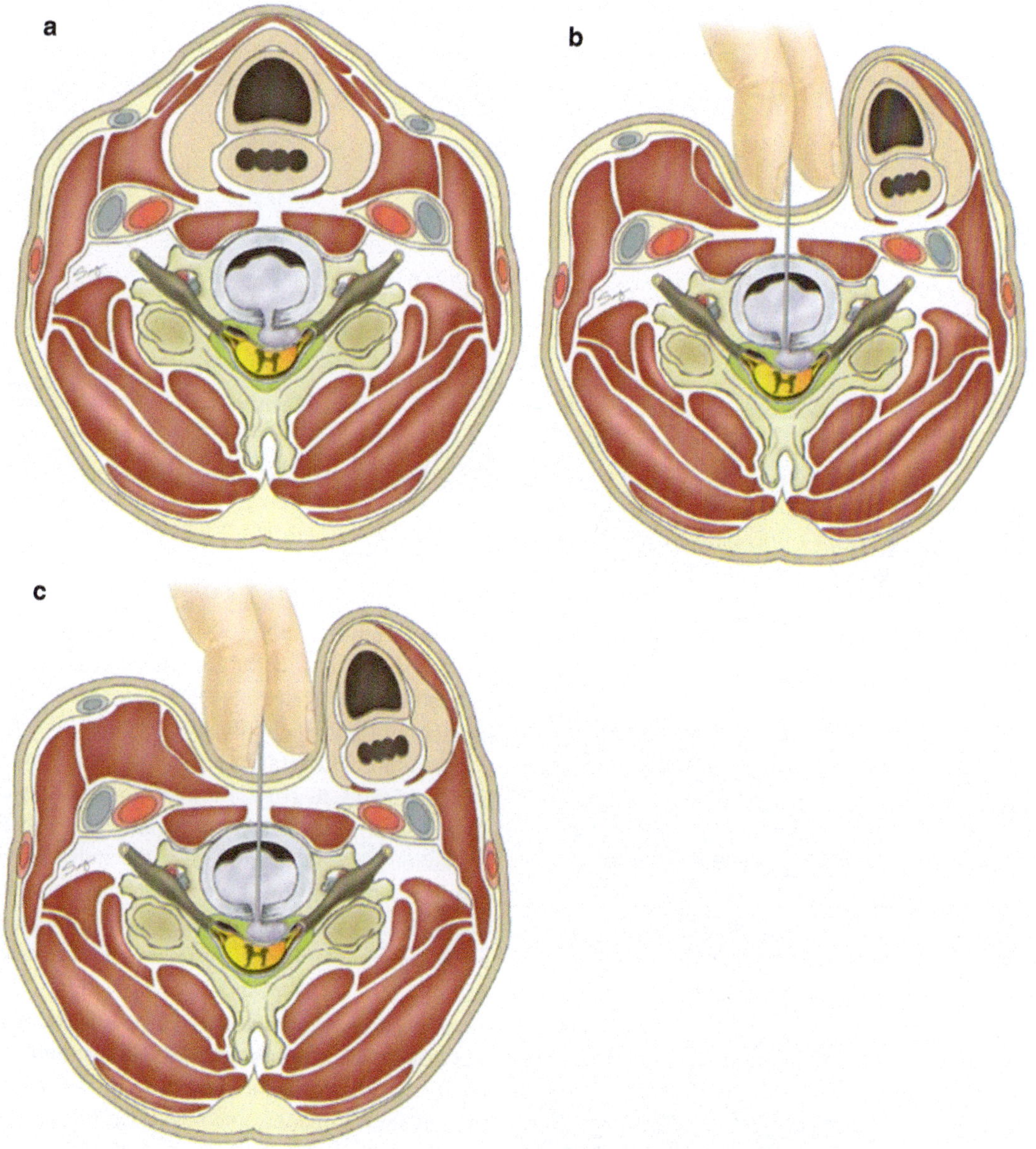

Fig. 15.2 After facilitating the pulsation of the carotid artery, gently move the visceral compartment, including the trachea and esophagus, with the index and third fingers to the opposite side. (**a**, **b**) The access needle is inserted into the disc space between the tips of your fingers. (**c**) Note that the needle is inserted at the midline of the annulus between longus colli muscles to prevent muscle injury

the PLL to approach into the epidural space (Fig. 15.12), (4) resecting of the posterior part of the uncinated process for foraminal decompression, and (5) resecting of foraminal ligament to explore foraminal herniation. It is important to define the fissure of PLL and preserve the normal annulus layer. While opening the fissure of PLL for fragmentectomy, the laser tip should gently sag over the normal PLL and dura using the hernia as a safety barrier. To prevent recurrent herniation, it is important not to expose the dural sac widely (Fig. 15.13).

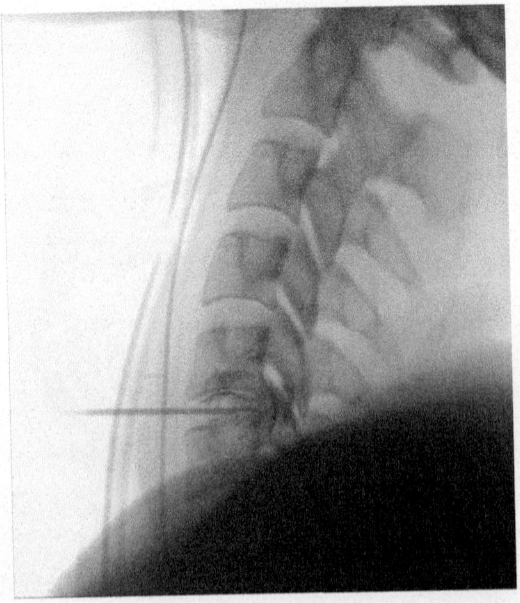

Fig. 15.3 Discography is performed to show the contrast agent leaks into the epidural space

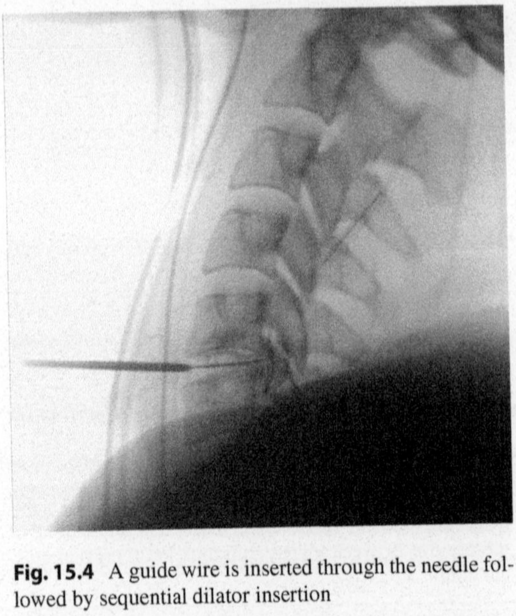

Fig. 15.4 A guide wire is inserted through the needle followed by sequential dilator insertion

15.4 Postoperative Consideration

The working tube and endoscope are removed, and the wound is closed with a subcutaneous stitch and covered with a strip. The patient is observed for 3 h after surgery and must be discharged within 24 h. The patient wears a soft neck collar for 2 weeks after surgery.

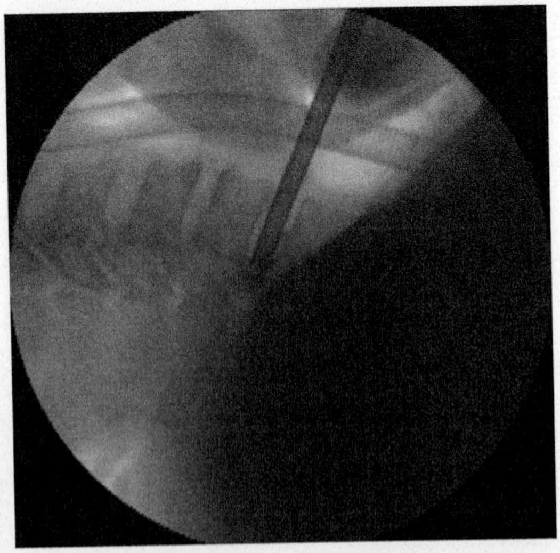

Fig. 15.5 The working tube is introduced to reach the posterior vertebral body

The reported overall success rate varies from 51 to 94.5% [3, 8, 10, 11]. Revision surgery was related with older age, male gender, foraminal herniation, disc degeneration at the index level and the adjacent level, spondylosis, cervical kyphosis, and segmental angle deterioration after index surgery [3]. In case of recurrent herniation and aggravated stenosis, revision surgery by anterior cervical discectomy and fusion or artificial disc replacement is required. There is another report that the foraminal and posterolateral herniation showed better outcomes than the central herniation group [2, 7, 9].

15.5 Case Illustration

15.5.1 Case 1

A 36-year-old male patient presented with neck pain and left radiculopathy. MRI showed soft disc herniation at the C5–6 level. Central disc herniation extended into the left side foraminal area

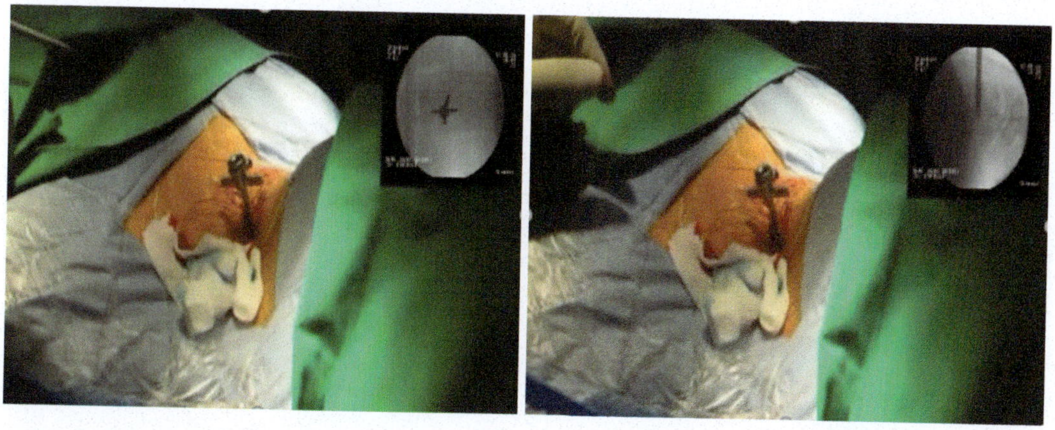

Fig. 15.6 Intraoperative photo showing the working channel is placed at midline on the anteroposterior view and the posterior vertebral body line on the lateral view

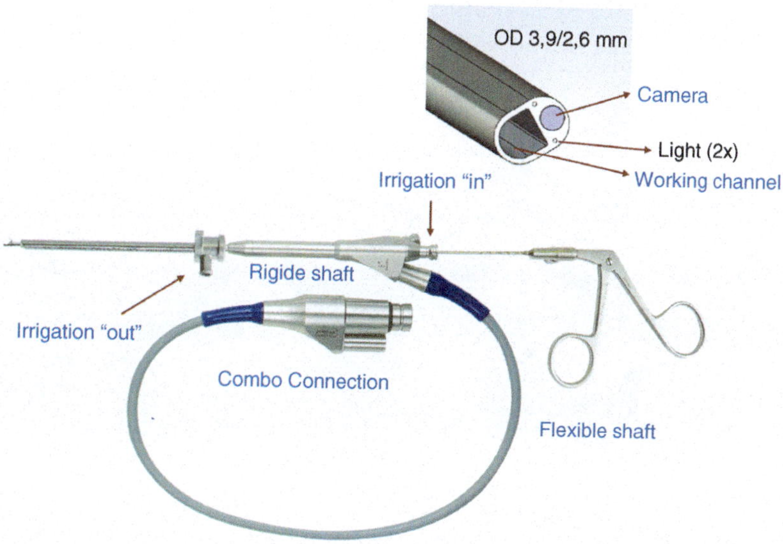

Fig. 15.7 Working channel endoscopy for anterior cervical endoscopic surgery. The oval-shaped endoscopy has a single working channel, camera, and light source

compressing the C6 nerve root (Fig. 15.14a, b). Anterior cervical endoscopic discectomy was performed under awakened anesthesia. After introducing working channel endoscopy at the posterior central disc space, PLL tear portion was visualized, where the herniated fragment extruded into the epidural space (Fig. 15.14c). After removal of hernia, epidural pulsation was identified (Fig. 15.14d). Postoperative MRI shows full decompression of the nerve root (Fig. 15.14e, f).

15.5.2 Case 2

A 44-year-old female patient presented with neck pain and left arm radiating pain caused by disc herniation at the C5–6 level (Fig. 15.15a). After anterior endoscopic cervical discectomy, her pain was relieved (Fig. 15.15b). Twenty-one years after surgery, her follow-up MRI and x-ray showed preservation of disc height and cervical alignment (Fig. 15.15c, d).

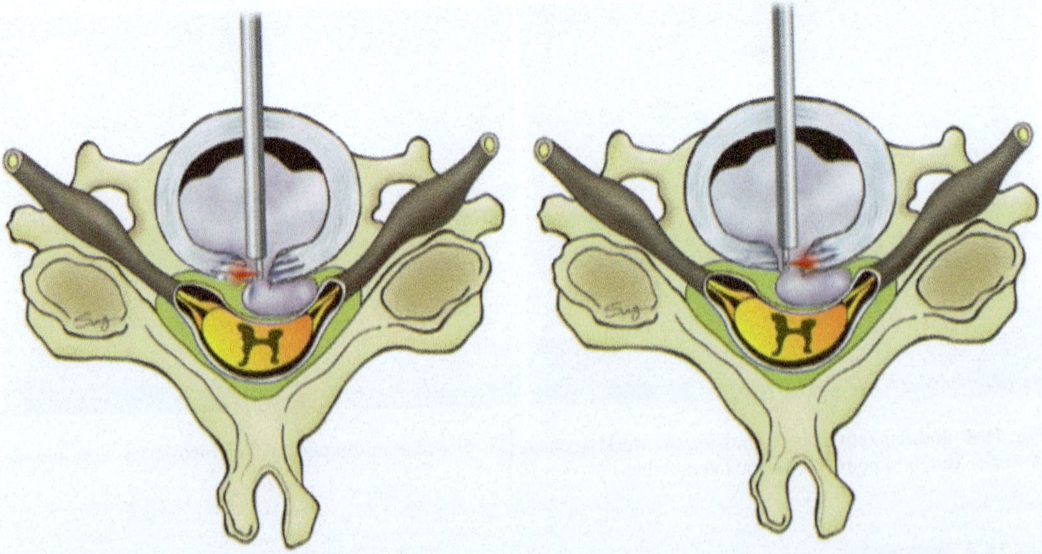

Fig. 15.8 Side-firing Ho:YAG laser is used to release fibrotic anchoring posterior annulus and herniated fragment

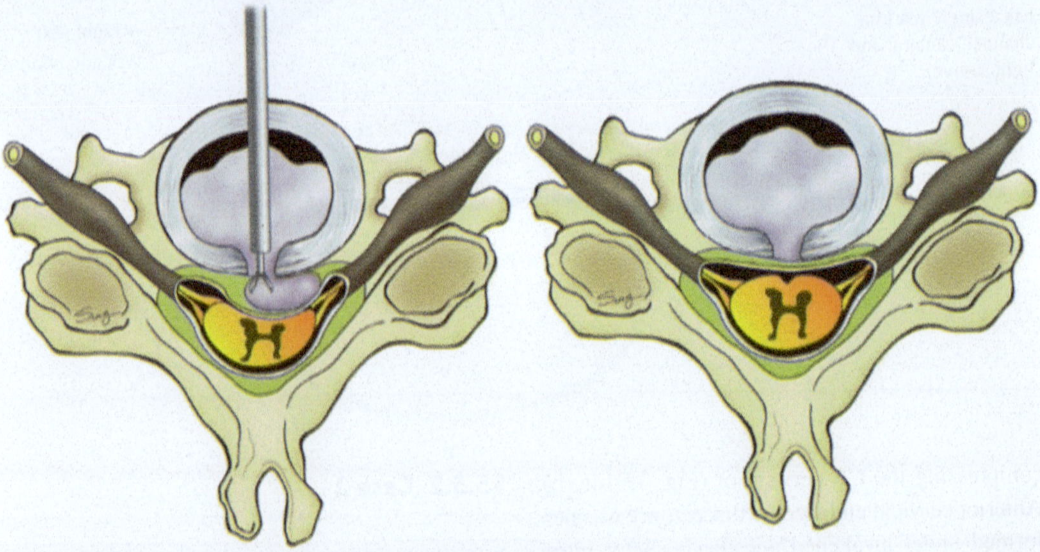

Fig. 15.9 After releasing annular anchoring and opening of the PLL with side-firing laser to expose and mobilize the hernia, herniated fragment can be removed with grabbing forceps

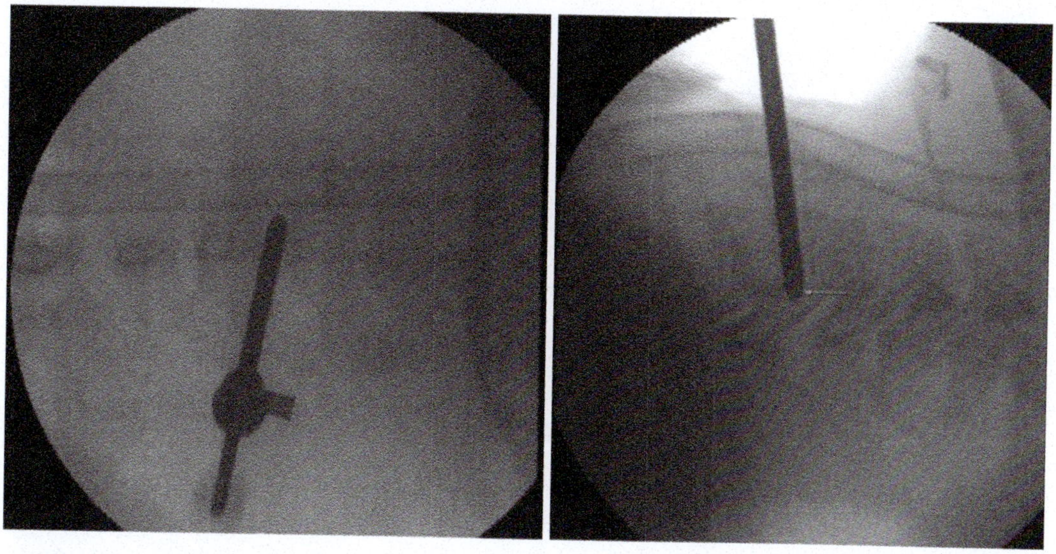

Fig. 15.10 An endoscopic reamer (arrow) is used to remove the posterior part of the uncinated process for foraminal herniation

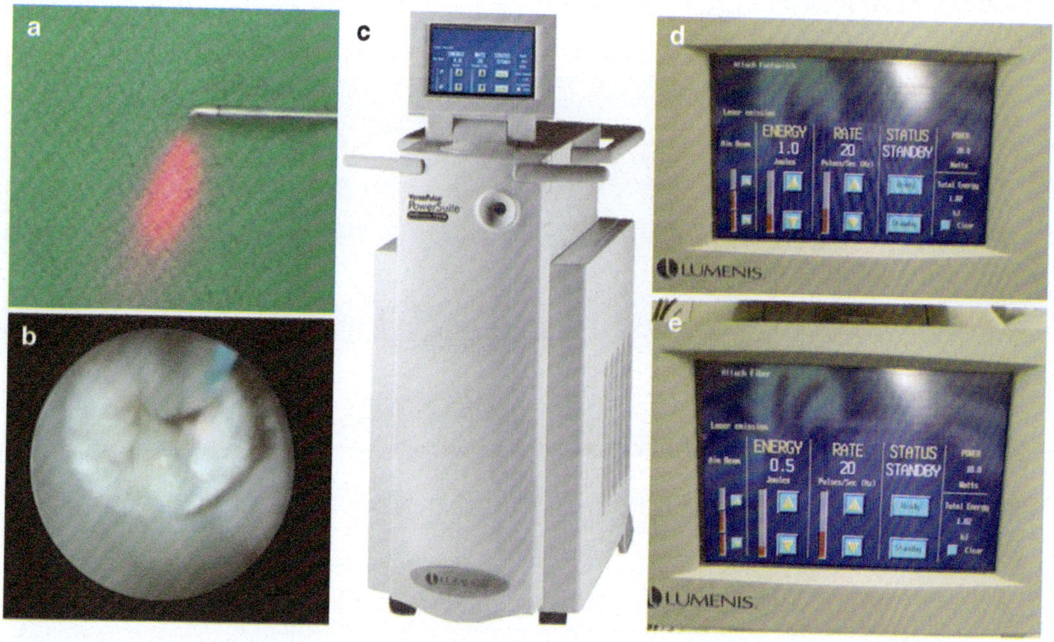

Fig. 15.11 Side-firing Ho:YAG laser tip (**a**) and its usage for evaporating posterior annulus (**b**). Laser machine (**c**) and its setting for initial stage (**d**) and later stage close to neural tissue (**e**)

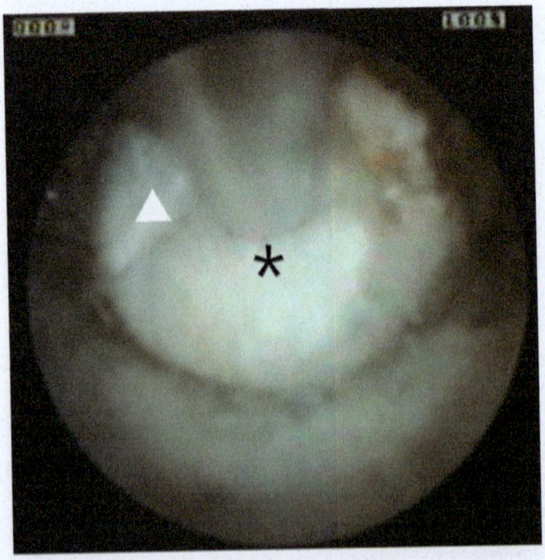

Fig. 15.12 Side-firing laser is opening of the defects in the PLL (arrowhead) to approach into the epidural space. Note that the laser tip is gently sagging over the dura using the hernia (*) as a safety barrier

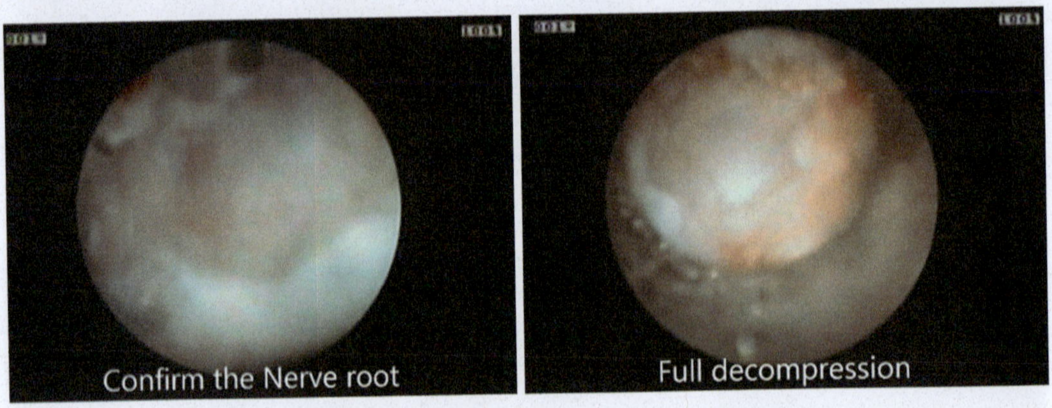

Fig. 15.13 Intraoperative endoscopic view showing root and dural decompression. It is important to preserve the PLL layer as much as possible to prevent recurrent herniation

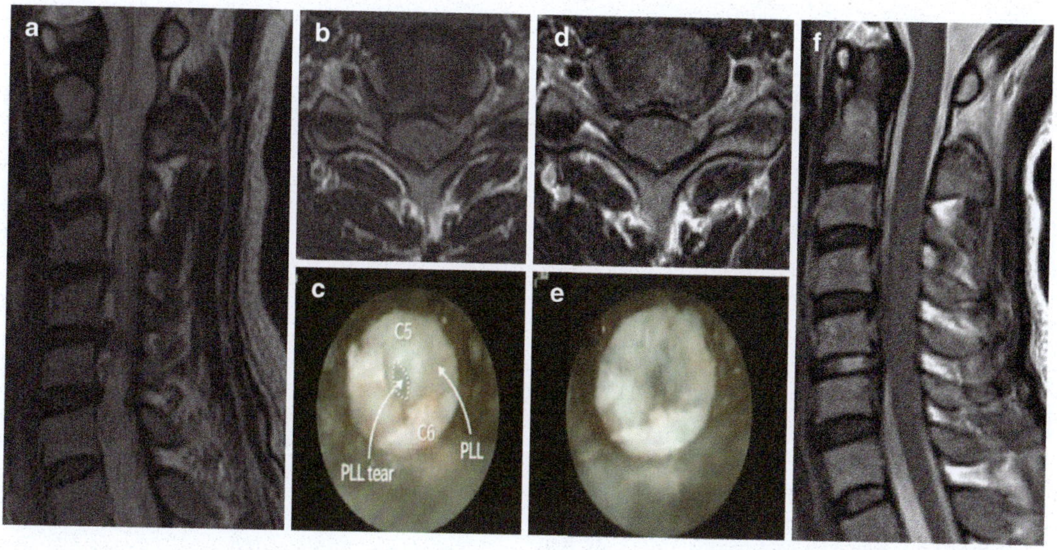

Fig. 15.14 A 36-year-old male patient presented with neck pain and left radiculopathy. MRI showed soft disc herniation at the C5–6 level. Central disc herniation extended into the left side foraminal area compressing C6 nerve root. (**a**, **b**) Anterior cervical endoscopic discectomy was performed under awakened anesthesia. After introducing working channel endoscopy at the posterior central disc space, PLL tear portion was visualized, where the herniated fragment extruded into the epidural space. (**c**) After removal of hernia, epidural pulsation was identified. (**d**) Postoperative MRI shows full decompression of nerve root (**e**, **f**)

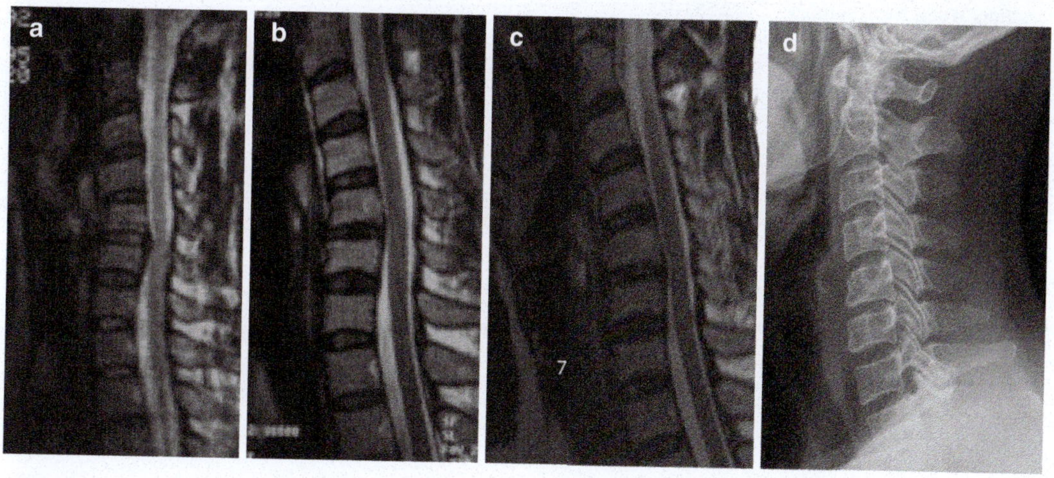

Fig. 15.15 A 44-year-old female patient presented with neck pain and left arm radiating pain caused by disc herniation at the C5–6 level (**a**). After anterior endoscopic cervical discectomy, her pain was relieved (**b**). Twenty-one years after surgery, her follow-up MRI and x-ray showed preservation of disc height and cervical alignment (**c**, **d**)

15.6 Summary

Anterior endoscopic cervical discectomy is an effective and feasible surgical option for soft disc herniation in the cervical spine. Side-firing Ho:YAG laser is an essential instrument for safe and accurate surgery. Although it requires a steep learning curve, the skillful hands with proper surgical instrument will produce reproducible and relevant surgical outcomes.

References

1. Bae DH, Seuk JW, Lee SH, Bae J. Long-term clinical and radiological follow-up after anterior endoscopic cervical discectomy: a case report. AME Case Rep. 2020;4:31.
2. Ahn Y, Keum HJ, Shin SH. Percutaneous endoscopic cervical discectomy versus anterior cervical discectomy and fusion: a comparative cohort study with a five-year follow-up. J Clin Med. 2020;9(2):371.
3. Oh HS, Hwang BW, Park SJ, Hsieh CS, Lee SH. Percutaneous endoscopic cervical discectomy (PECD): an analysis of outcome, causes of reoperation. World Neurosurg. 2017;102:583–92.
4. Choi G, Pophale CS, Patel B, Uniyal P. Endoscopic spine surgery. J Korean Neurosurg Soc. 2017;60(5):485–97.
5. Ahn Y, Lee SH, Chung SE, Park HS, Shin SW. Percutaneous endoscopic cervical discectomy for discogenic cervical headache due to soft disc herniation. Neuroradiology. 2005;47(12):924–30.
6. Ahn Y, Lee SH, Lee SC, Shin SW, Chung SE. Factors predicting excellent outcome of percutaneous cervical discectomy: analysis of 111 consecutive cases. Neuroradiology. 2004;46(5):378–84.
7. Ahn Y. Endoscopic spine discectomy: indications and outcomes. Int Orthop. 2019;43(4):909–16.
8. Lee SH, Ahn Y, Choi WC, Bhanot A, Shin SW. Immediate pain improvement is a useful predictor of long-term favorable outcome after percutaneous laser disc decompression for cervical disc herniation. Photomed Laser Surg. 2006;24(4):508–13.
9. Quillo-Olvera J, Lin GX, Kim JS. Percutaneous endoscopic cervical discectomy: a technical review. Ann Transl Med. 2018;6(6):100.
10. Lee JH, Lee SH. Clinical and radiographic changes after percutaneous endoscopic cervical discectomy: a long-term follow-up. Photomed Laser Surg. 2014;32(12):663–8.
11. Ahn Y, Lee SH, Shin SW. Percutaneous endoscopic cervical discectomy: clinical outcome and radiographic changes. Photomed Laser Surg. 2005;23(4):362–8.

Microscopic OPLL Resection with CO_2 Laser

16

Ji Young Cho and Ho-Yeon Lee

Abstract

Cervical ossification of the posterior longitudinal ligament (OPLL) presents a significant surgical challenge, especially when it involves multiple cervical levels. However, the choice of surgical approach for multilevel cervical OPLL is still a controversial issue. Anterior corpectomy is not easy, but achieved by removing the ossified mass.

OPLL has a tendency to adhere to the underlying dura matter. Besides, it may often be unexpectedly softer than the vertebra body itself. Excessive traction of adhered OPLL with a Kerrison punch may injure the spinal cord because of a dural tear. In the presence of an adhered OPLL, the use of CO_2 laser is helpful. A CO_2 laser was used to lyse any adhesions because of their micropulsation.

This chapter was written for the purpose of describing a technique of direct anterior cervical corpectomy using CO_2 laser for cervical OPLL. As a CO_2 laser at a power setting of 5 Watts is known to penetrate the outer table of the bone, vaporization of an already thinned OPLL or small osteophytes can be sufficiently performed with irradiations of 5 Watts. We demonstrate that a focused laser beam could vaporize the OPLL with protected dural membrane using an angled microdissector.

Keywords

Cervical ossification of the posterior longitudinal ligament · Microscopic · Laser surgery OPLL · Spine surgery

J. Y. Cho (✉) · H.-Y. Lee
Department of Neurosurgery, Gangbuk Wooridul Spine Hospital, Seoul, Republic of Korea
e-mail: george70@wooridul.co.kr

16.1 Introduction

Ossification of the posterior longitudinal ligament (OPLL) is one of the major disorders of cervical spondylotic myelopathy (CSM) [1, 2]. The optimal surgical choice for the treatment of ossification of the posterior longitudinal ligament (OPLL) has been a matter of debate, and controversy about it still exists over using anterior or posterior surgery [3–12]. Anterior cervical corpectomy and OPLL resection provides better therapeutic benefit than posterior decompression surgery. Anterior decompression achieves better neurological outcomes for patients with more significant canal compromise (canal occupying ratio $\geq 60\%$) or if global cervical kyphosis is >10 degrees, or if K-line is negative [13–16]. However, anterior corpectomy is technically demanding and may cause iatrogenic deterioration of the neurological state and unexpected surgery-related complications, including cerebrospinal fluid (CSF) leakage and graft problems [17–19]. Naturally, it will be more technically

J. Bae, S.-H. Lee (eds.), *Laser Spine Surgery*, https://doi.org/10.1007/978-981-16-2206-9_16

demanding if the OPLL is involved at multiple cervical levels, and treatment success will depend heavily on a less traumatic manipulation.

Recent advances in surgical techniques and tools such as the surgical microscope that allows improved vision, the high-speed drill that can cut horizontally rather than vertically, and the carbon dioxide (CO_2) laser that can be attached to the operating microscope have made it feasible and safe to drill the bone to paper-thin thickness and then to completely ablate the OPLL [20, 21].

Here, we described surgical technique and case presentation of laser-assisted corpectomy result in adequate decompression of the spinal canal with less risk of dural injury and with better recovery of neurological deficit. We demonstrated that a focused laser beam could vaporize the OPLL with protected dural membrane using an angled microdissector.

16.2 Indications

Cervical OPLL required anterior decompression (with/without fusion):

- Significant canal compromise (canal occupying ratio ≥ 60%).
- Global cervical kyphosis is >10 degrees.
- K-line is negative.

16.3 Surgical Technique

16.3.1 Choice of Surgical Procedure

Over the last 30 years, surgical techniques for cervical OPLL have significantly changed from a more invasive to a less invasive technique [3–5, 18, 22]. Corpectomy with autobone graft to vertebral graft, allobone, and decompression without fusion were done. Multilevel corpectomy with autobone (iliac bone or fibular bone) was used for multilevel OPLL, but graft problem and donor site discomfort occurred. Cages were used under microsurgical control as a less invasive procedure. A multilevel oblique corpectomy without fusion consisted of a less invasive and more effective ventral approach and yielded favorable results [23, 24]. There were no clear criteria to choose either with or without fusion, so the approach was dependent on surgeon preference. However, multilevel oblique corpectomy without fusion procedure was avoided in those who showed definite instability on plain radiographs.

16.3.2 Surgical Techniques

1. Anterior corpectomy and fusion (ACF)

The patient is placed supine. Prior to induction of general anesthesia, a safe range of cervical motion should be checked to avoid any cord injury during intubation. A lateral plain radiograph is obtained to verify the level of interest. A standard corpectomy procedure using a high-speed drill was performed. It is important to drill out the central portion of the OPLL first and then to drill in a medial to lateral direction to avoid a floating OPLL. When only a tiny shell of cortical bone remains, we generally replace the diamond burr with a match-head burr. Because the match-head burr is blunt at the tip and cuts along its sides, it is relatively safe and does not require excessive pressure while in use. This avoids too much pressure being directed toward the underlying spinal cord. In order to prevent dural tearing and subsequent spinal fluid leakage, a thin layer of the OPLL was left in place, and careful dissection was performed with a microdissector, beginning with the unadhered portion, to separate the OPLL from the dura.

A CO_2 laser system (Sharplan Laser Industries, Tel Aviv, Israel) attached to the operating microscope and a red He-Ne aiming beam enable us to perform this work with safe precision. A CO_2 laser was then used to lyse any adhesions, while a specially designed angled microdissector was inserted through the opening between the OPLL mass and the dura to ablate the remaining OPLL. The superficial layer of the dura was protected by a microdissector (Figs. 16.1 and 16.2). Ossification of the posterior longitudinal ligament can be vaporized by a focused laser beam with a spot size of 0.46–0.85 mm. A 5-Watt pulser-single pulse mode laser is sufficient to

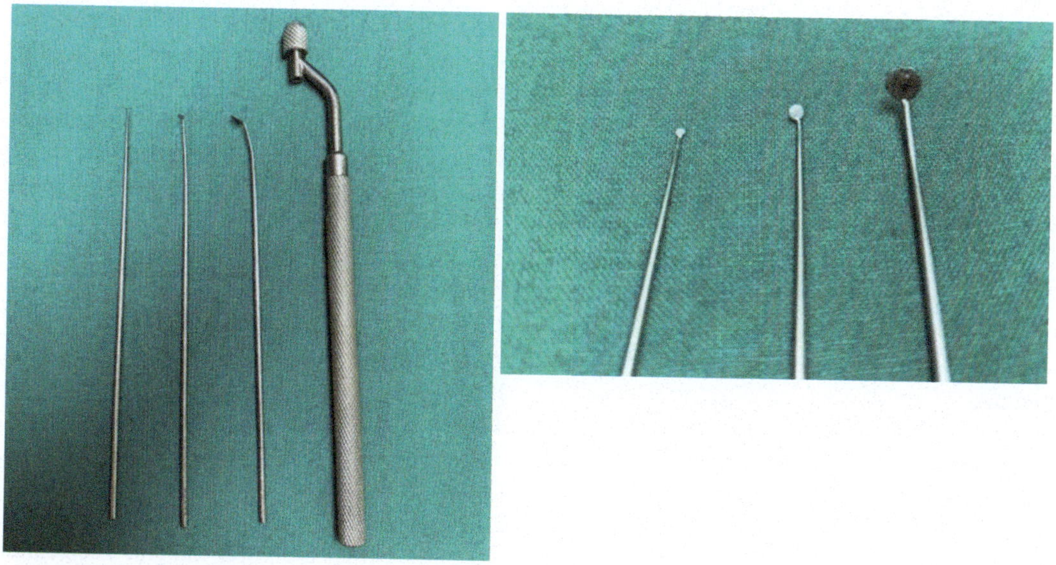

Fig. 16.1 Specially designed angle microdissector. Because it has round flat head, it is placed under the OPLL to protect the spinal cord during the use of CO_2 laser

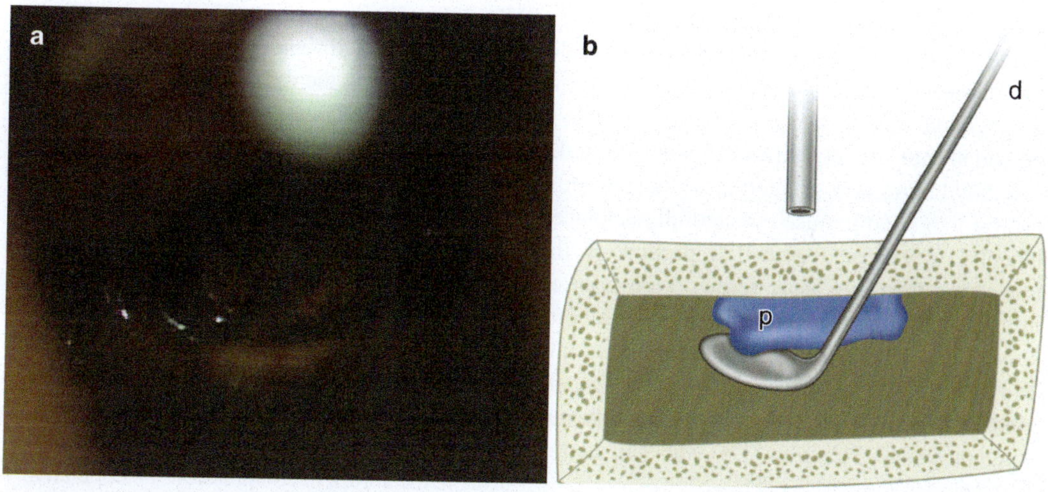

Fig. 16.2 Intraoperative photo taken by a microscope (**a**). The left side of photograph indicated a cephalad direction, and the bottom side indicated a lateral direction. An illustration showing the surgical technique for removal of densely adhered OPLL using CO_2 laser and angled microdissector located between OPLL and the dura mater (**b**)

vaporize a thinned OPLL or an osteophyte. Keeping the surgical field moistened during the use of CO_2 laser is important to minimize the risk of inadvertent injuries, as water can be absorbed by the energy of CO_2 laser immediately. An adapter was used to attach the laser to the operating microscope, making possible micromanipulations of the laser with a joystick. Using the method, the OPLL could be lysed and removed completely, leaving the underlying dura intact.

A few areas of the OPLL that were associated with incompetent dura could be removed along with the dura. In such cases, we usually performed temporary cerebrospinal fluid drainage later in the procedure. After complete removal of the OPLL, we performed foraminotomies and undercut the vertebral bodies laterally using burrs and a 1-mm Kerrison punch until the lateral margins of the spinal cord could be discerned. Once decompression revealed adequate pulsation of the re-expanded dura, the anterior lip of the upper vertebra and spurs were removed to make flat surfaces for the graft bed. Instead of using a peg-in-hole technique, we retained a small posterior lip to prevent dorsal graft displacement. A fibular bone allograft or cylindrically shaped mesh cages filled with cadaveric bone chips were used for osseous fusion. After a gentle placement of graft, a lateral radiograph is obtained to confirm the position of the graft and the alignment of the spine. Properly contoured plates are fixed with screws.

2. Multilevel oblique corpectomy (MOC) without fusion

After satisfactory general anesthesia, the patient was placed in a supine position with the neck in extension. A transverse skin incision was made, and the prevertebral space was exposed in the usual Smith-Robinson approach from the more compressive and more symptomatic side. Soft tissue dissection was performed by pulling the trachea and esophagus medially and toe carotid sheath laterally. After the exposure of the vertebral bodies and ipsilateral longus colli muscle, the longus colli muscle is carefully displaced laterally to expose the medial portion of the transverse process. Caspar screws were inserted into the midpoint of operative segment vertebral bodies. The navigation system (StealthStation® TREON™ system, Medtronic Sofamor Danek, Memphis, TN) based on O-arm® (Medtronic Sofamor Danek, Memphis, TN) was activated to confirm operative levels [25].

A transcorporeal bony window was made on the approached side of the upper vertebral body using a drill. We started drilling with a diamond burr at the upper edge of the anterior surface of the upper vertebral body. We usually use a diamond burr, because it considerably causes less bleeding from the cancellous portion of vertebral bodies. Drilling proceeded posteriorly toward the OPLL mass and was stopped at the posterior part of the disc space. Then the bony window was expended obliquely via lateral undercutting of the upper vertebral body and into the upper portion of the lower vertebral body. The vertebral body is drilled obliquely from the lateral side toward the opposite posterolateral corner. This decompression is achieved through limited bone resection (<50% of the VB). Bony and discal trough was expanded to trapezoid working space in axial and sagittal planes, with careful application of sharp dissection technique on disc to avoid thermal or vibration injury from high-speed drill. During bone resection, drilling and then irrigation was better than continuous irrigation to control bone bleeding. Then the central portion of exposed OPLL was peeled off with swinging high-speed burr till bilateral skirts were exposed. Usually, the less adherent portion was present at the lower level, so dissection of OPLL from dura was started from the lower margin. The central portion of OPLL was removed with a burr to complete floating of main OPLL mass and OPLL mass was removed. A CO_2 laser was also used to lyse any adhesions, while an angled microdissector was inserted through the opening between the OPLL mass and the dura to ablate the remaining OPLL to prevent dural injury.

In case of severely invaded dura by OPLL without dissection margin, dura was cut to preserve arachnoid to prevent cord herniation. And an artificial dural patch larger than dural defect was put between the subdural spaces to cover the hole [26]. After full decompression, the restoration of the cord pulsation should be confirmed on both ipsilateral and contralateral sides, and a single layer of the surgical sponge was onlayed over the dura to prevent excessive anterior thecal sac swelling following the abrupt decompression. Postoperatively, the patients were advised to wear neck brace 2 to 4 weeks and to do bed rest for 3 days. Cerebrospinal fluid leakage was controlled with epidural drainage and 7 days of bed rest.

16.4 Postoperative Consideration

1. CSF leakage; a volume-controlled wound drain for CSF leakage or lumbar drain.
2. Graft problem; in some cases, additional posterior fixation may be needed (Fig. 16.3).

3. Instability; vertebral body resected more than 50% during MOC, impractical extension of decompression revealed instability and compression fracture. As a result, instability may occur, which may be needed to be addressed by placement of body graft with posterior instrumentation.

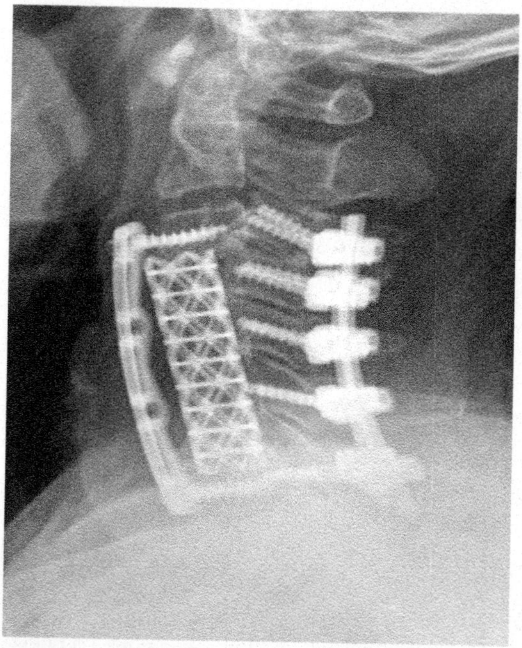

Fig. 16.3 In case of multisegmental OPLL, anterior corpectomy and fusion followed by posterior fusion. Graft problem and non-fusion were reduced

16.5 Case Illustration

16.5.1 Case 1

A 45-year-old male patient presented with neck pain and both arm numbness and weakness. He had had walking difficulty aggravated after falling down. Preoperative images show cervical OPLL at C3–C4–C5–C6–C7 with cord compression. We performed corpectomy and OPLL removal with fibular graft (Fig. 16.4).

16.5.2 Case 2

A 39-year-old man presented with both arm pain and weakness. Preoperative MR and CT revealed a cervical OPLL at C3–C4–C5–C6 with maximal cord compression at the C3–C4 level and associated cord compression. We performed corpectomy and OPLL removal with internal fixation. OPLL mass was totally removed, and kyphotic cervical curvature was corrected and more lordotic (Fig. 16.5).

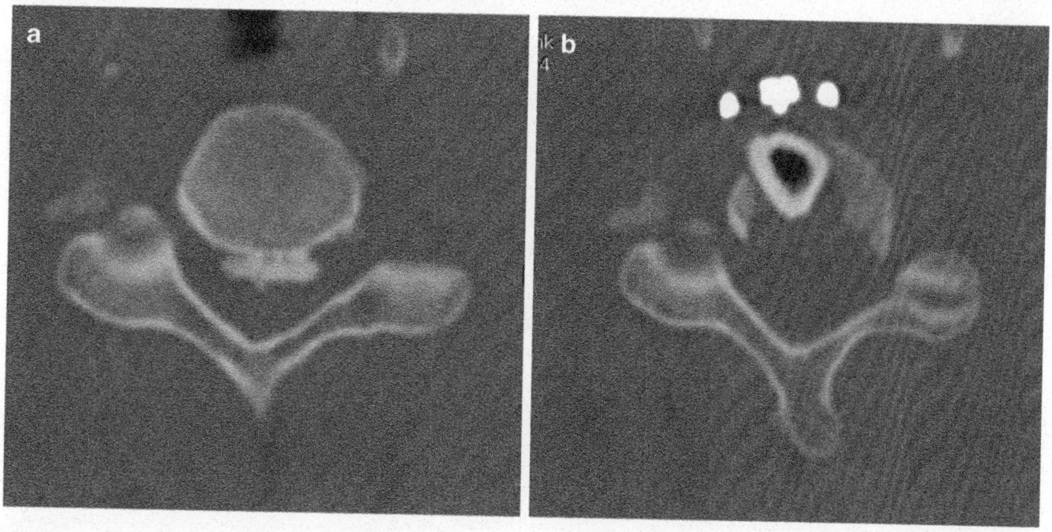

Fig. 16.4 A 45-year-old male patient who had neck pain, walking difficulty, and arm weakness underwent corpectomy and fusion using laser-assisted microsurgical techniques. A preoperative axial CT image showed OPLL (**a**). A postoperative axial CT image demonstrated full decompression of the spinal canal (**b**)

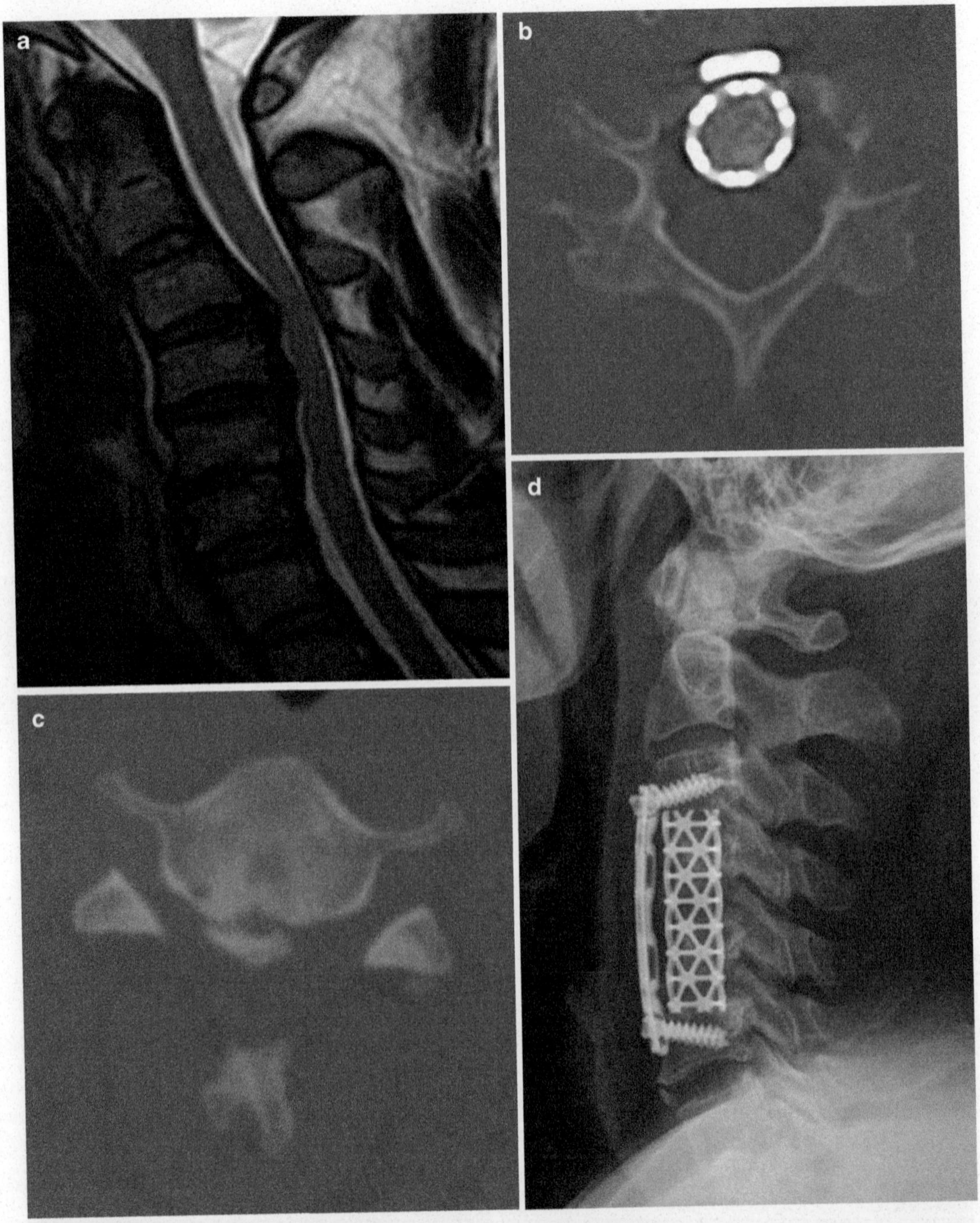

Fig. 16.5 Preoperative MR and CT revealed a cervical OPLL at C3–C4–C5–C6 with maximal cord compression at the C3–C4 level and associated cord compression (**a**, **b**). We performed corpectomy and OPLL removal with internal fixation. OPLL mass was totally removed (**c**), cervical curvature is more lordotic (**d**)

16.5.3 Case 3

A 54-year-old woman presented with neck pain and cervicogenic headache. She also had both arm numbness and pain. Preoperative MR and CT revealed a cervical OPLL at C3–C4. Relatively small size OPLL mass was removed using oblique corpectomy without fusion technique. The level and direction of the oblique corpectomy were confirmed and guided by navigation. OPLL mass was removed completely without any complication (Fig. 16.6).

16.5.4 Case 4

A 46-year-old man presented with myelopathy. He complained both arms and legs weakness and numbness with rigidity. Preoperative MR and CT revealed a cervical OPLL at C2–C3. We performed OPLL removal via multilevel oblique corpectomy without fusion using navigation system. Postoperative T2-weighted sagittal MRI and axial image showed complete extirpation of the C2–3 OPLL mass. A small long hole was seen at C2–3 anterior portion at 3D reconstructed CT image (Fig. 16.7).

16.5.5 Case 5

A 53-year-old woman presented with a 2-year history of neck and chest pain with dyspnea. Preoperative MRI and CT revealed a hard, calcified cervicothoracic OPLL at C3 to T2 with cord compression. We performed modified MOC technique without fusion with navigation system. The patient reported immediate postoperative relief from neck and chest pain. Postoperative CT scans showed complete removal of the OPLL (Fig. 16.8).

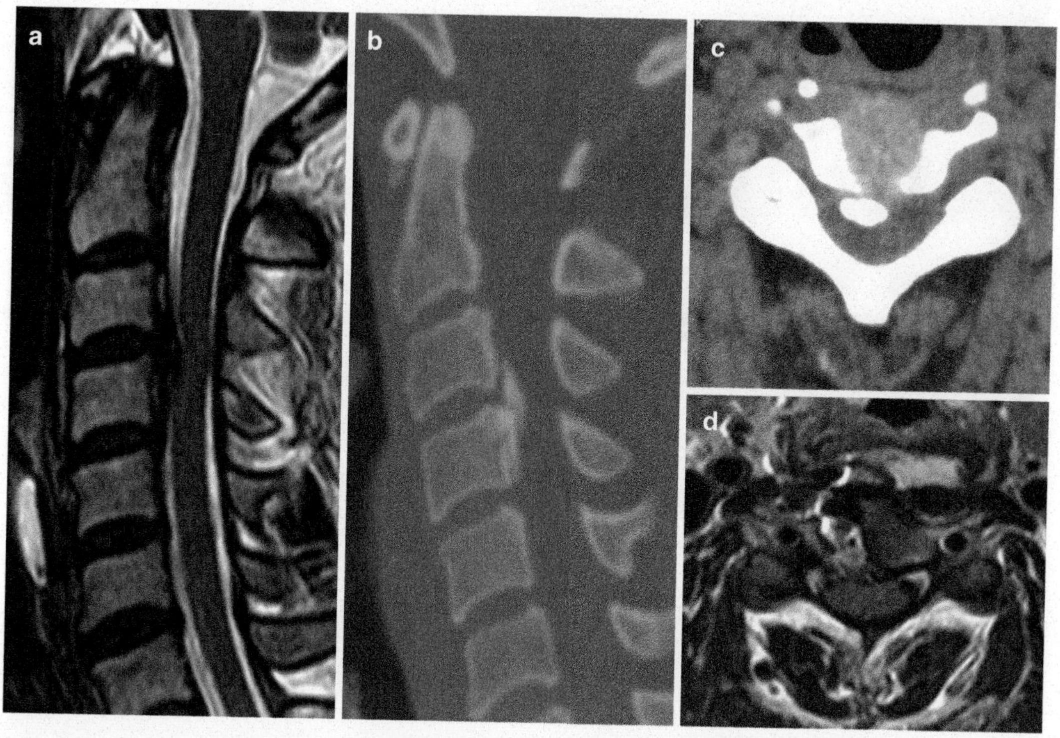

Fig. 16.6 Preoperative MR and CT revealed a cervical OPLL at C3–C4 (**a**–**c**). Relatively small size segmental type OPLL mass was removed using oblique corpectomy without fusion technique. OPLL mass was removed completely (**d**). The level and direction of the oblique corpectomy were confirmed and guided by navigation (**e**)

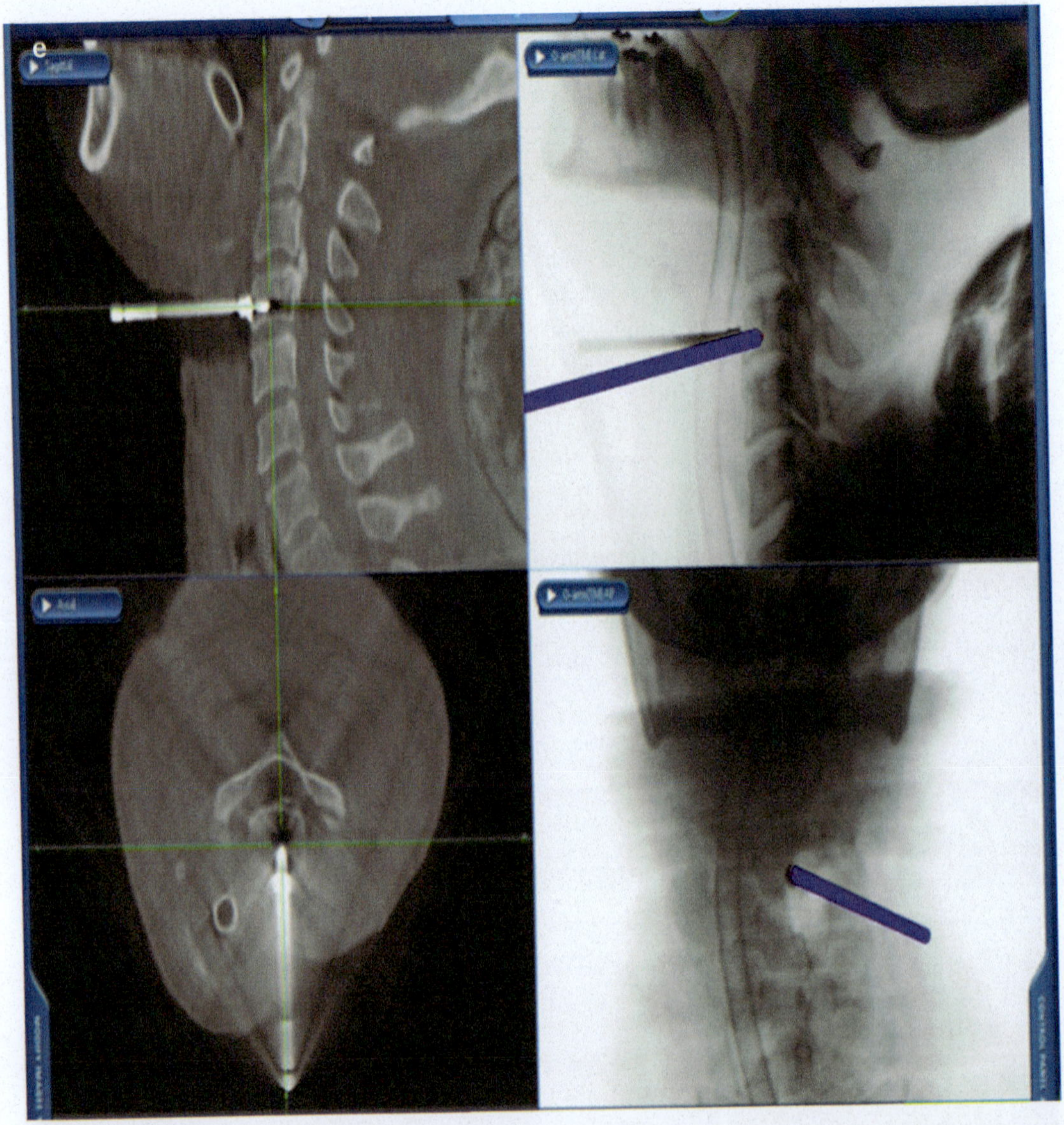

Fig. 16.6 (continued)

16.5.6 Case 6

A 72-year-old man presented with myelopathy. Preoperative images revealed OPLL at C3–C4–C5 with cord compression. We performed multi-level oblique corpectomy from C3 to C5 without fusion. This patient has ossification of the anterior longitudinal ligament (OALL). Postoperative images show complete removal of OPLL mass without instability after 3 years (Fig. 16.9).

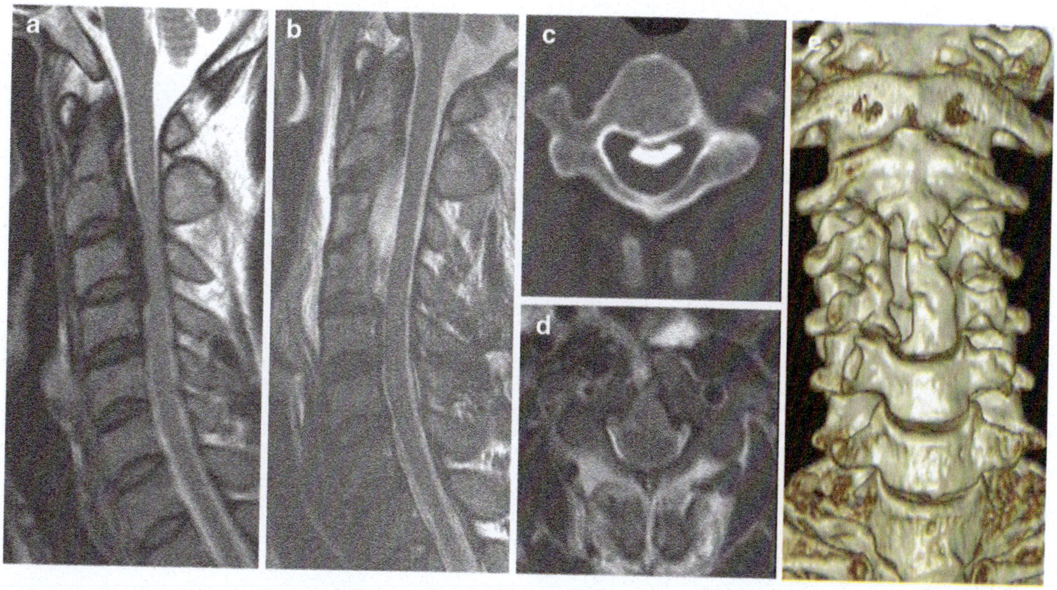

Fig. 16.7 Preoperative MR and CT revealed a continuous type cervical OPLL at C2–C3 (**a**, **c**). Postoperative T2-weighted sagittal MRI (**b**) and axial image (**d**) showing the complete extirpation of the C2–3 OPLL mass. A small long hole was seen at C2–3 anterior portion at 3D reconstructed CT image (**e**)

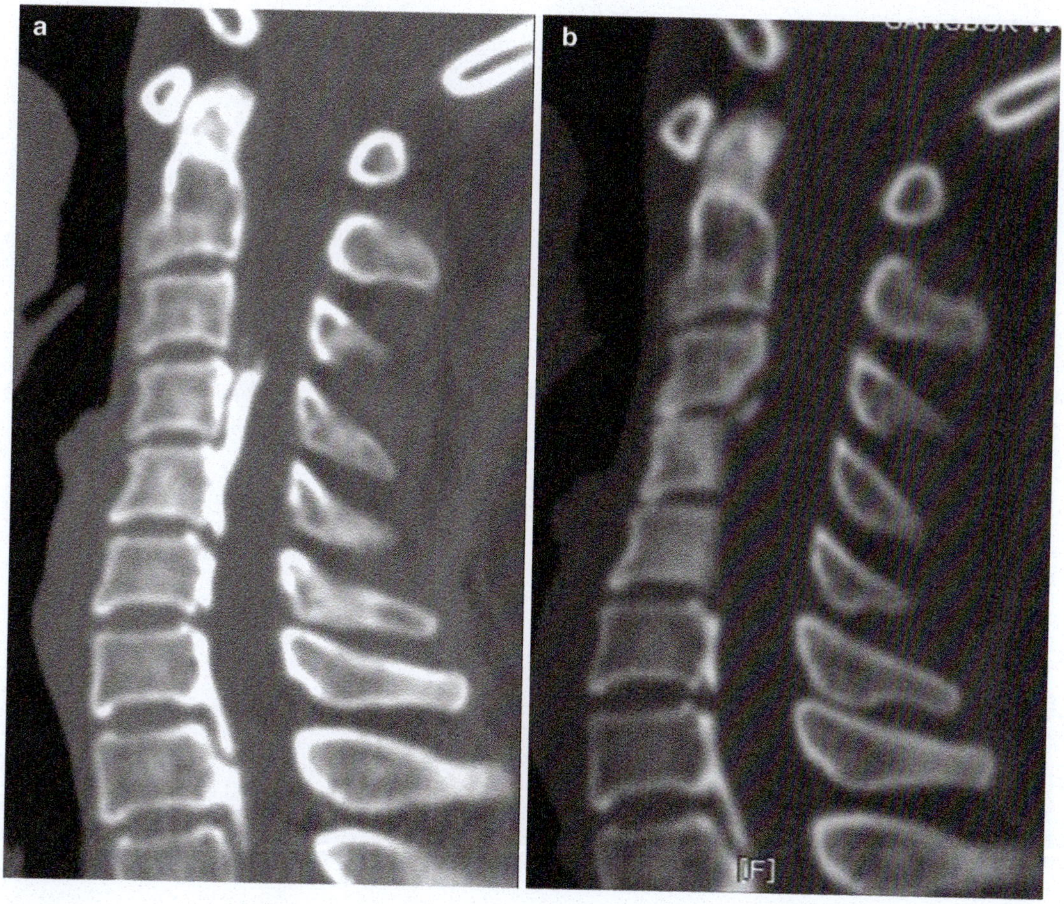

Fig. 16.8 Pre- (**a**) and postoperative (**b**) sagittal CT images. Mixed type OPLL mass at C4–C5 was removed via oblique corpectomy without fusion

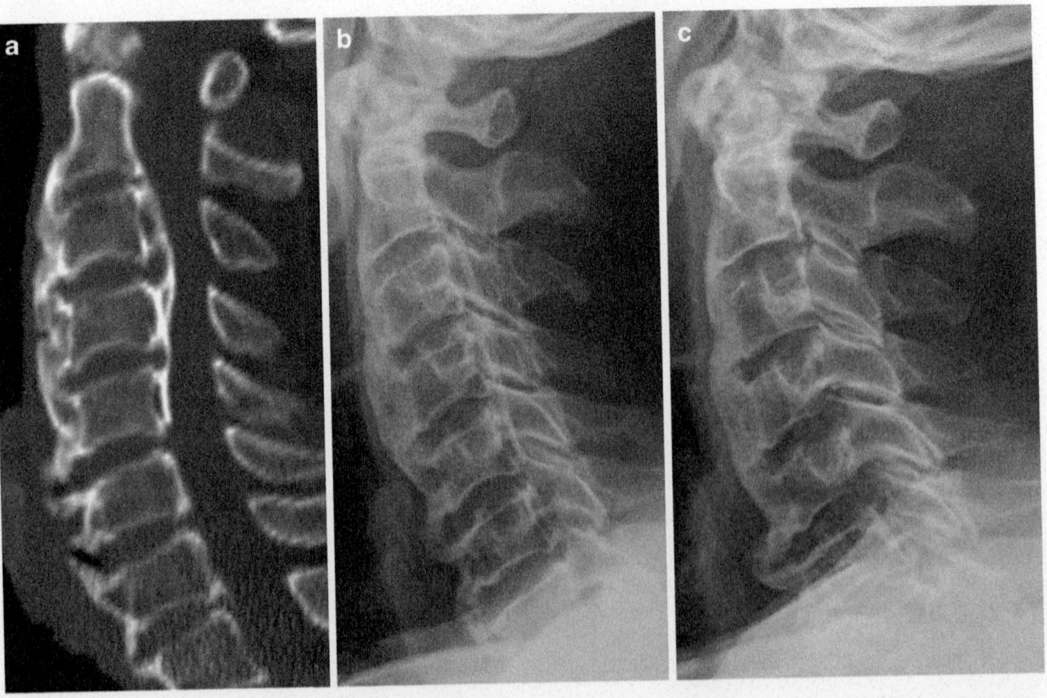

Fig. 16.9 Preoperative CT revealed a cervical OPLL at C3–C4–C5–C6 with OALL (**a**). OPLL mass seen in preoperative radiograph (**b**) was removed postoperatively and stable during 3 years (**c**)

16.6 Summary

This chapter describes a technique of direct anterior cervical corpectomy using CO_2 laser for cervical OPLL. The laser-assisted corpectomy results in inadequate decompression of the spinal canal with less risk of dural injury and with better recovery of neurological deficit.

References

1. Epstein N. Diagnosis and surgical management of cervical ossification of the posterior longitudinal ligament. Spine J. 2002;2:436–49.
2. Matsunaga S, Sakou T. Ossification of the posterior longitudinal ligament of the cervical spine: etiology and natural history. Spine (Phila Pa 1976). 2012;37:E309–14.
3. Banerji D, Acharya R, Behari S, Chhabra DK, Jain VK. Corpectomy for multi-level cervical spondylosis and ossification of the posterior longitudinal ligament. Neurosurg Rev. 1997;20:25–31.
4. Belanger TA, Roh JS, Hanks SE, Kang JD, Emery SE, Bohlman HH. Ossification of the posterior longitudinal ligament. Results of anterior cervical decompression and arthrodesis in sixty-one North American patients. J Bone Joint Surg Am. 2005;87:610–5.
5. Epstein N. Anterior approaches to cervical spondylosis and ossification of the posterior longitudinal ligament: review of operative technique and assessment of 65 multilevel circumferential procedures. Surg Neurol. 2001;55:313–24.
6. Herkowitz HN. A comparison of anterior cervical fusion, cervical laminectomy, and cervical laminoplasty for the surgical management of multiple level spondylotic radiculopathy. Spine. 1988;13:774–80.
7. Hirabayashi K, Miyakawa J, Satomi K, Maruyama T, Wakano K. Operative results and postoperative progression of ossification among patients with ossification of posterior longitudinal ligament. Spine. 1981;6:354–64.
8. Kimura I, Shingu H, Nasu Y. Long-term follow-up of cervical spondylotic myelopathy treated by canal-expansive laminoplasty. J Bone Joint Surg Br. 1995;77:956–61.
9. Onari K, Akiyama N, Kondo S, Toguchi A, Mihara H, Tsuchiya T. Long-term follow-up results of anterior interbody fusion applied for cervical myelopathy due to ossification of the posterior longitudinal ligament. Spine. 2001;26:488–93.
10. Satomi K, Nishu Y, Kohno T, Hirabayashi K. Long-term follow-up studies of open-door expansive lami-

noplasty for cervical stenosis myelopathy. Spine. 1994;19:507–10.
11. Tani T, Ushida T, Ishida K, Iai H, Noguchi T, Yamamoto H. Relative safety of anterior microsurgical decompression versus laminoplasty for cervical myelopathy with a massive ossified posterior longitudinal ligament. Spine. 2002;27:2491–8.
12. Wada E, Suzuki S, Kanazawa A, Matsuoka T, Miyamoto S, Yonenobu K. Subtotal corpectomy versus laminoplasty for multilevel cervical spondylotic myelopathy. Spine. 2001;26:1443–8.
13. Chen Z, Liu B, Dong J, et al. Comparison of anterior corpectomy and fusion versus laminoplasty for the treatment of cervical ossification of posterior longitudinal ligament: a meta-analysis. Neurosurg Focus. 2016;40:E8.
14. Edwards CC 2nd, Heller JG, Murakami H. Corpectomy versus laminoplasty for multilevel cervical myelopathy: an independent matched-cohort analysis. Spine (Phila Pa 1976). 2002;27:1168–75.
15. Liu X, Min S, Zhang H, et al. Anterior corpectomy versus posterior laminoplasty for multilevel cervical myelopathy: a systematic review and meta-analysis. Eur Spine J. 2014;23:362–72.
16. Shin JH, Steinmetz MP, Benzel EC, et al. Dorsal versus ventral surgery for cervical ossification of the posterior longitudinal ligament: considerations for approach selection and review of surgical outcomes. Neurosurg Focus. 2011;30:E8.
17. Epstein N. The surgical management of ossification of the posterior longitudinal ligament in 43 North Americans. Spine. 1994;19:664–72.
18. Kojima T, Waga S, Kubo Y, Kanamaru K, Shimosaka S, Shimizu T. Anterior cervical vertebrectomy and interbody fusion for multi-level spondylosis and ossification of the posterior longitudinal ligament. Neurosurgery. 1989;24:864–72.
19. Smith MD, Bolesta MJ, Leventhal M, Bohlman HH. Postoperative cerebrospinal-fluid fistula associated with erosion of the dura. Findings after anterior resection of ossification of the posterior longitudinal ligament in the cervical spine. J Bone Joint Surg Am. 1992;74, 270:–277.
20. Lee SH, Choi S. Laser-assisted microsurgical techniques for the treatment of cervical ossification of the posterior longitudinal ligament. Joint Dis Rel Surg. 2005;16:77–81.
21. Lee SH, Ahn Y, Lee JH. Laser-assisted anterior cervical corpectomy versus posterior laminoplasty for cervical myelopathic patients with multilevel ossification of the posterior longitudinal ligament. Photomed Laser Surg. 2008;26(2):119–27.
22. Abe H, Tsuru M, Ito T, Iwasaki Y, Koiwa M. Anterior decompression for ossification of the posterior longitudinal ligament of the cervical spine. J Neurosurg. 1981;55:108–16.
23. Bruneau M, Cornelius JF, George B. Multilevel oblique corpectomies: surgical indications and technique. Neurosurgery. 2007 Sep;613(3 Suppl):106–12.
24. Chibbaro S, Mirone G, Makiese O, George B. Multilevel oblique corpectomy without fusion in managing cervical myelopathy: long-term outcome and stability evaluation in 268 patients. J Neurosurg Spine. 2009 May;10(5):468–5.
25. Jang SH, Cho JY, Choi WC, Lee HY, Lee SH, Hong JT. Novel method for setting up 3D navigation system with skin-fixed dynamic reference frame in anterior cervical surgery. Comput Aided Surg. 2015;20(1):24–8.
26. Cho JY, Chan CK, Lee SH, Choi WC, Maeng DH, Lee HY. Management of cerebrospinal fluid leakage after anterior decompression for ossification of posterior longitudinal ligament in the thoracic spine: the utilization of a volume-controlled pseudomeningocele. J Spinal Disord Tech. 2012;25(4):E93–102.

17 Percutaneous Endoscopic Laser Annuloplasty with Ho:YAG Laser for Discogenic Back Pain

Shih Min Lee and Junseok Bae

Abstract

Patients with chronic low back pain, not responsding to the conservative treatment experience severe impact on their the economic, psychological, and social activities. There are several treatment options for chronic low back pain for over 6 months, ranging from conservative treatment, local procedures, and microscopic surgery to fusion surgery. Percutaneous endoscopic laser annuloplasty (PELA), an extremely minimally invasive technique, uses laser-assisted spinal endoscopy (LASE) kit to directly coagulate the inflamed disc granulation tissue associated with annular tears. In this chapter, the authors sought to describe and demonstrate the safety and efficacy of PELA for controlling chronic discogenic low back pain due to abnormal disc tissues, new vessels, and nerves in the central torn posterior annulus such as intra-annular granulation tissue syndrome.

Keywords

Chronic lower back pain · Discogenic lower back pain · Intra-annular granulation tissue syndrome · Percutaneous endoscopic laser annuloplasty (PELA) · Laser-assisted spinal endoscopy (LASE)

Supplementary Information The online version of this chapter (https://doi.org/10.1007/978-981-16-2206-9_17) contains supplementary material, which is available to authorized users.

S. M. Lee · J. Bae (✉)
Department of Neurosurgery, Chungdam Wooridul Spine Hospital, Seoul, Republic of Korea

17.1 Introduction

Multiple biomechanical etiologies for low back pain have been suggested in the literature such as degenerative disc disease, annular fissures, compressive herniated nucleus pulposus, and internal disc disruption [1–5]. Among patients with low back pain, 39% had an internal disc disruption, with concordant pain provocation at discography indicating the discogenic origin of their pain [6]. As can be seen, the pathophysiology of discogenic back pain is granulation tissue ingrowth into the disc space via an annular defect (fissure, tear, or cleft) resulting from either degenerative disease or trauma. Granulation tissue causes angiogenesis, free nerve growth, and chronic inflammatory processes in the disc that irritate free nerve endings in the area [7, 8]. It is notable that patients with this "interannular granulation" status (Fig. 17.1) have back pain rather than leg pain.

The era of intradiscal treatment began in 1975, when Hijikata et al. reported on percutaneous posterolateral intradiscal nuclear resection for indirect nerve root decompression [9] and

J. Bae, S.-H. Lee (eds.), *Laser Spine Surgery*, https://doi.org/10.1007/978-981-16-2206-9_17

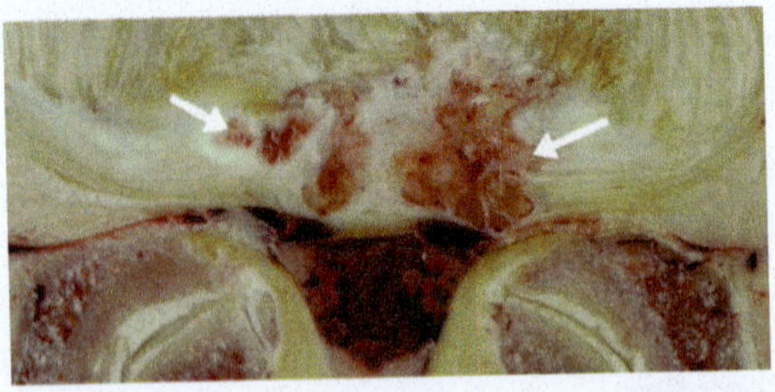

Fig. 17.1 Granulation tissue observed (white arrows) in disc with annular tear (courtesy of Dr. Wolfgang Rauschning, Academic University Hospital, Uppsala, Sweden)

advanced again in 1983 with a report on the outcome of percutaneous lateral discectomy by Kambin et al. [10]. The non-visualization method continued to be developed by many surgeons [7, 11–13]. After the introduction of endoscopy, many spinal surgeons applied and developed endoscopic spinal treatment, including Kambin et al., who used arthroscopy for microdiscectomy in 1997 [14]; Yeung et al., who introduced transforaminal endoscopic decompression in 2002 [15, 16]; and Choi et al., who introduced percutaneous endoscopic discectomy via the interlaminar approach in 2005 [17]. This led to the concept of using endoscopic procedures to treat discogenic back pain by direct visualization of the annular defect and posterior part of the nucleus pulposus, removal of the nucleus and nucleoplasty to manage inflammation, and annuloplasty to narrow the annular defect. In 2002, Yeung et al. introduced thermal discoplasty and annuloplasty using the YESS endoscope via a transforaminal approach [16]. They were followed in the same year by Tsou et al.'s description of the surgical technique for posterolateral transforaminal discectomy and annuloplasty for chronic lumbar discogenic back pain [15] and in 2010 by Lee's introduction of the use of laser for nucleoplasty and annuloplasty [18]. In addition, Lee et al. defined "intra-annular granulation tissue syndrome" as a disease with chronic low back pain of over 6 months and HIZ (high-intensity zone) on MRI findings. The Ho:YAG laser was then used to perform the thermal treatment of the damaged annulus [19]. Park CH et al. reported that transforaminal laser annuloplasty is more effective in treating discogenic low back pain than intradiscal radiofrequency annuloplasty in 2019 [20]. The general course of discogenic pain is controversial, but the pain is known to be due to internal disc destruction, degenerative disc changes, and damage to the annulus. Percutaneous endoscopic laser annuloplasty procedure cauterizes the granulation tissue related to the damaged annulus. The greatest advantage of this procedure is to preserve a healthy nucleus pulposus by minimizing damage to the center of disc.

17.2 Diagnosis

Discogenic back pain is difficult to diagnose accurately. In particular, it is important to identify the exact cause and select patients who will definitely benefit from percutaneous endoscopic laser annuloplasty (PELA). The causes of back pain vary from mechanical instability, intervertebral disc pathology, posterior joint pain, neurogenic pain, and others, but in general, 40% of back pain is known as discogenic pain [6]. If the patient has chronic discogenic back pain and mechanical instability, stabilization surgery should be considered. Interbody fusion is inevitable for patients with disc collapse, and Bae et al. recommended interlaminar dynamic spacer (IntraSPINE®) for chronic low back pain with mild segmental instability [21].

As shown in Table 17.1, the clinical manifestations of discogenic back pain include sitting intolerance, difficulty in lifting heavy objects, extension catch, increased pain after a hard work, and loss of ability to maintain a posture for 30 min, and all of these symptoms are mostly nonspecific. Because of this, provocative discography and MRI are very useful diagnostic tests for discogenic back pain. In the case of discogenic back pain, sharp and shooting-like pain is experienced during discography. And MRI findings can be seen as follows: annular defect on both T1 and T2, thickening of the posterior portion of the annulus, and the disk trapped inside the defect. The HIZ (high-intensity zone) is also a helpful finding in T2 MRI (Fig. 17.2).

Invasive provocative discography is performed if the patient's clinical features and MRI results are consistent with discogenic back pain. If there is a defect or tear in the posterior annulus, contrast leakage can be seen in real time during discography. In addition, as the intradiscal pressure increases, the nerve ending is stimulated, causing pain at the pathologic level. Certainly, if the provocation test is positive, percutaneous endoscopic laser annuloplasty (PELA) is performed on the lesion in the same position.

Table 17.1 Diagnostic criteria of discogenic back pain

Diagnostic tool	Positive finding
Clinical symptoms	Sitting intolerance Difficulty lifting heavy objects Extension catch Increased pain after a hard day's work Cannot maintain posture for over 30 min
MRI	Annular defect with both T1 and T2 images Thickening of posterior annulus HIZ on T2
Provocative discography	Positive with sharp, shooting pain

17.3 Indications

Since there are many causes of discogenic back pain, there is still controversy about which procedure is better for treating discogenic back pain, but the general relative indications for surgery include:

1. Chronic low back pain and no improvement from conservative treatment for 6 months
2. High-intensity zone (HIZ) on magnetic resonance imaging (MRI)
3. Discogenic back pain and annular tear were confirmed by provocative discography

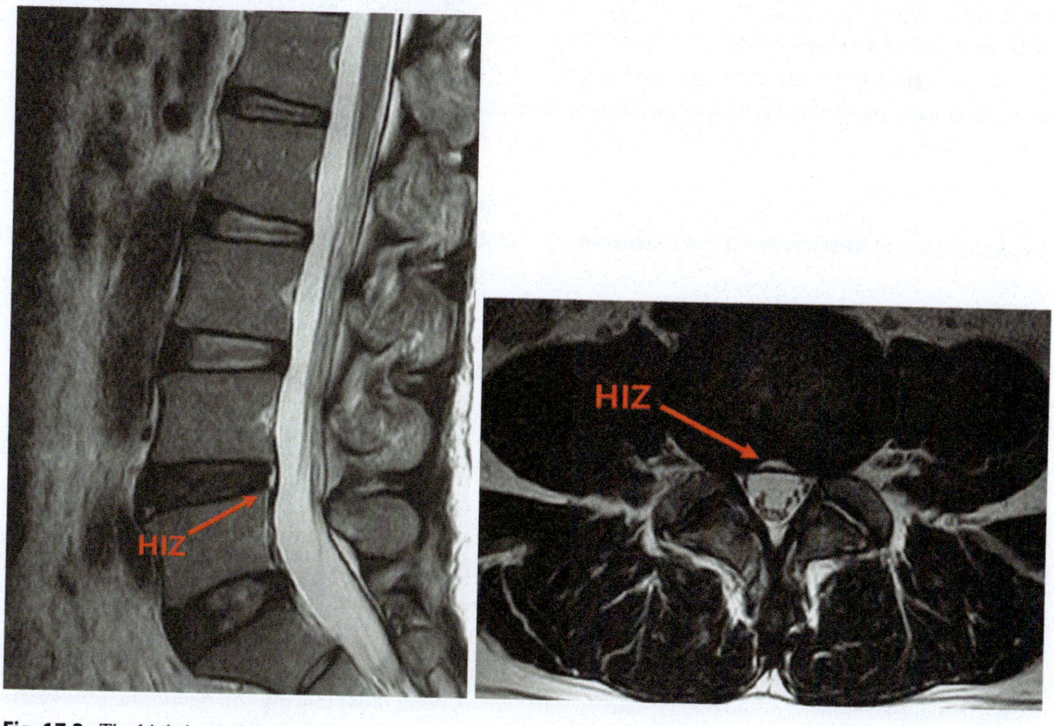

Fig. 17.2 The high-intensity zone (HIZ) is shown at the L4–5 level

17.4 Exclusion Criteria

Disc herniation, fragments, instability of a segment, and multi-segment disc degeneration, tumor, and infectious lesion

17.5 Surgical Technique

17.5.1 Instrument

The holmium:yttrium-aluminum-garnet (Ho:YAG) laser has become widely used in minimally invasive surgical procedures, and laser-assisted spinal endoscopy (Clarus Medical, LASE®) kit and working cannula (Elliquence, Disc-FX® System) have been used for discogenic pain (Fig. 17.3(1 to 3)). The Ho:YAG laser, owing to its close approximation to the intense 2.0 μm absorption band of water, appears to be safer for clinical trials of laser discectomy. Being also a pulsed laser, in contrast to the continuous-wave, near-infrared lasers, it has the advantage of producing minimal amounts of heat in adjacent tissues. The flexible endoscopic Ho:YAG laser has a very small diameter, and the length of the laser tip can also be actively adjusted (Fig. 17.4). It can be flexibly adjusted even in a very small space, and it enables treatment by targeting to the desired location.

17.5.2 Step 1: Setting and Anesthesia

It is important to know before the PELA procedure how will we approach and how we prepare the operating room. First, the direction of approach is for the patient to proceed from prone position to the posterolateral side. The operating surgeon should always stand on the symptomatic side, and the intraoperative image intensifier should be located on the opposite side. Level marking with intraoperative fluoroscopy (C-arm) guide and draping are done. Make sure the patient is comfortable and prepare for anesthesia (Fig. 17.5). We recommend conscious sedation using benzodiazepine (midazolam) and local anesthesia with skin infiltration by 2 to 3 mL of 1% lidocaine and paraspinal muscle infiltration by 6 to 8 mL; wait 1 min for full effect. The most painful points in the procedure are skin entry and annulus penetration; therefore, we also recommend infiltration with another 2 to 3 mL of 1% lidocaine just before penetrating the annulus; this will be enough to minimize the pain. Stronger concentrations (e.g., 2% lidocaine) can paralyze motor function; if it occurs, confusion can arise whether this is a lidocaine side effect or a direct needle injury.

17.5.3 Step 2: Discography and Tube Insertion

Patients received provocative discography preoperatively or just before the operative procedure. Provocative discography was performed with manual injection of indigo carmine, contrast, and normal saline solution in a 2:1:2 ratio. It can be checked for leakage of contrast through annular tear and positive provocation test. The procedure was canceled if there was no concordant pain or annular tear in fluoroscopy.

Needle insertion is considered the most important step for establishing the working channel and for optimal visualization. Our recommendation is use of the 18-G spinal needle introduced under fluoroscopic guidance according to the location of pathology. The entry point is calculated preoperative axial MR and CT image. That was made at the meeting point of two lines crossing the facet joint (lateral view) and horizontal to the disc space (anteroposterior [AP] view) under intraoperative fluoroscopy.

Because the target is not a nucleus pulposus, but an ingrowth annulus, the approach pathway should be made shallower, and it is recommended to start from the lateral side more than the traditional PELD procedure. Therefore, the usual skin entry point was 12 to 15 cm lateral from the midline. The surgeon advanced the needle on a trajectory that approached the facet joint, and the usual axial angle of the needle was below 22° so as not to touch the anterior and central nucleus. During the needle insertion, the surgeon can communicate with a conscious patient's and know in real time whether the nerve is damaged through the patient's reaction. Discography is done after needle insertion, followed by guide wire insertion through the needle. Skin incision is needed before putting in the working cannula. The working cannula is inserted to establish the endoscope under intraoperative image guidance. After the cannula passes the medial pedicular border, gentle hammering is possible to reach the point just past midline. During cannula insertion, make sure that it is facing dorsally (Fig. 17.6(1 to 3)).

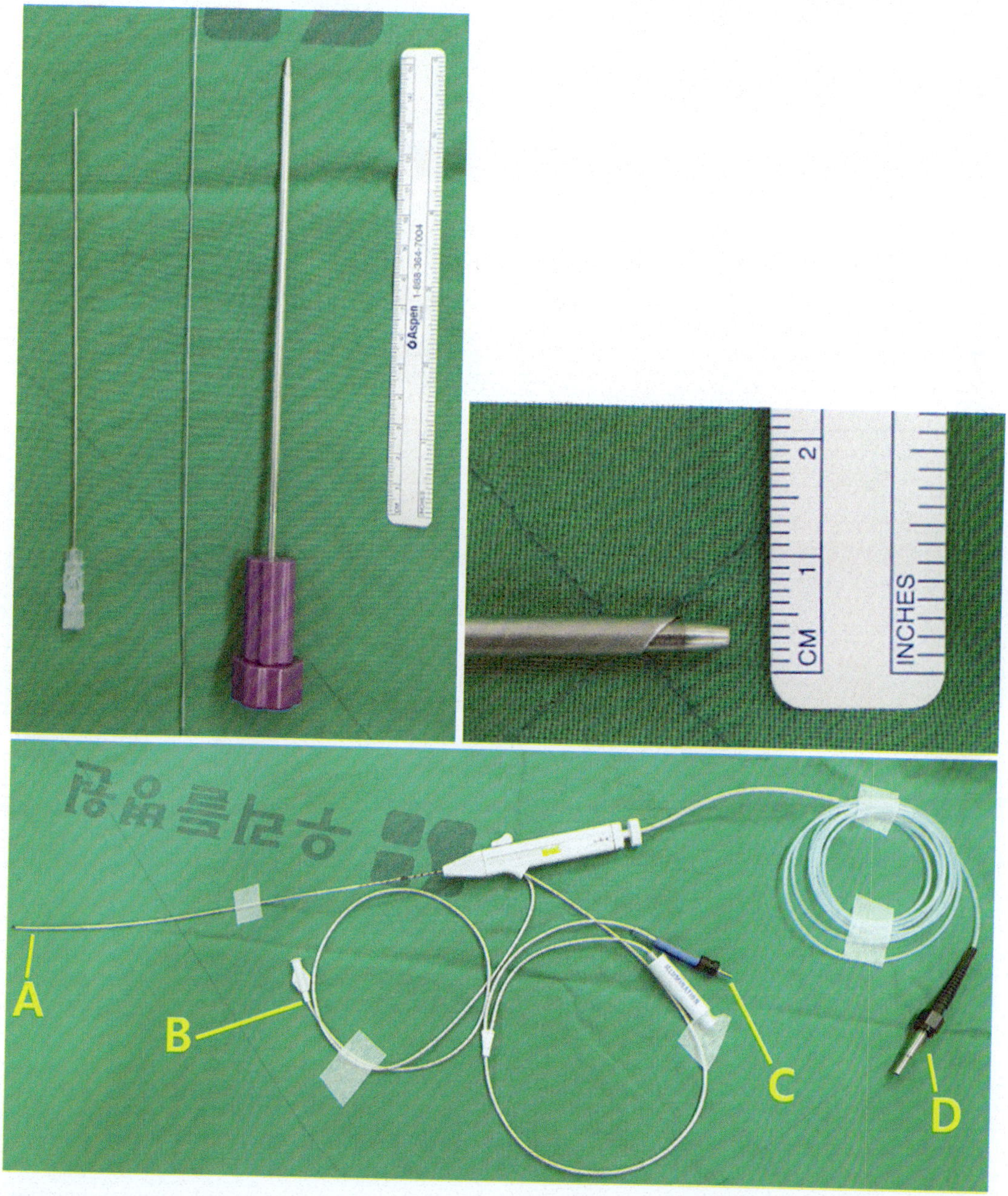

Fig. 17.3 (1) Working cannula. There is no need for another dilator because the obturator is in the inlet. (2) Laser-assisted spinal endoscope set (A: laser tip. B: Irrigation line. C: Endoscopic line. D: Laser line.). (3) Tip of the flexible Ho:YAG laser scope (A: Image fiber. B: Illumination fiber. C: Irrigation. D: Laser fiber)

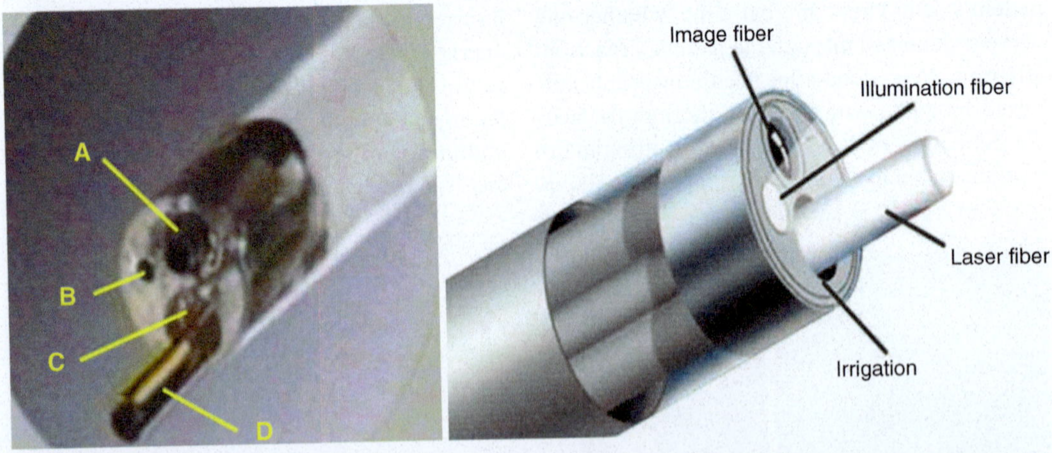

Fig. 17.3 (continued)

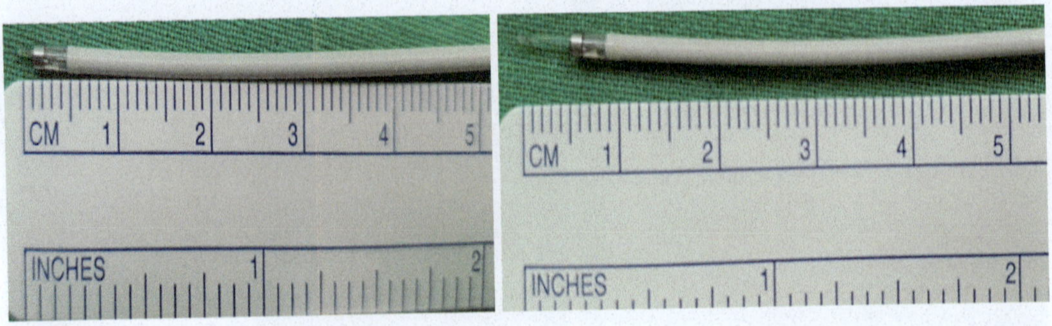

Fig. 17.4 The laser tip can be lengthened and reduced by 1–5 mm

Fig. 17.5 C-arm on the opposite side of the surgeon and the scrub nurse stands on the right side

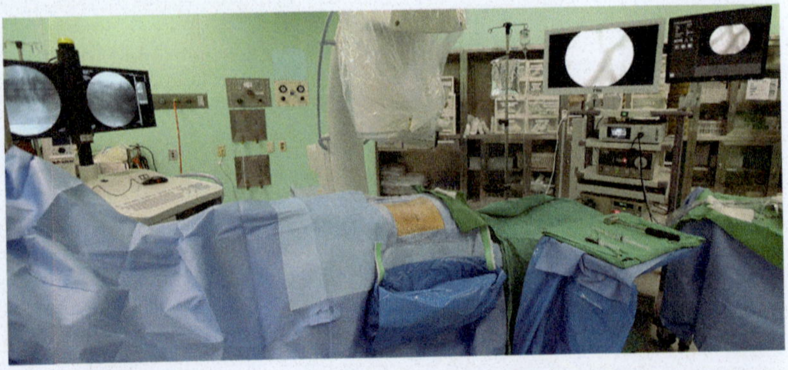

17.5.4 Step 3: Annuloplasty

After the proper working channel is established, the posterior rim of the annulus has been reached. The endoscope and the beveled cannula make visualization of the inner part of the posterior annulus possible. The annular defect can be located, and some trapped nucleus pulposus stained by indigo carmine can be visualized inside the defect. At this point, because disco-

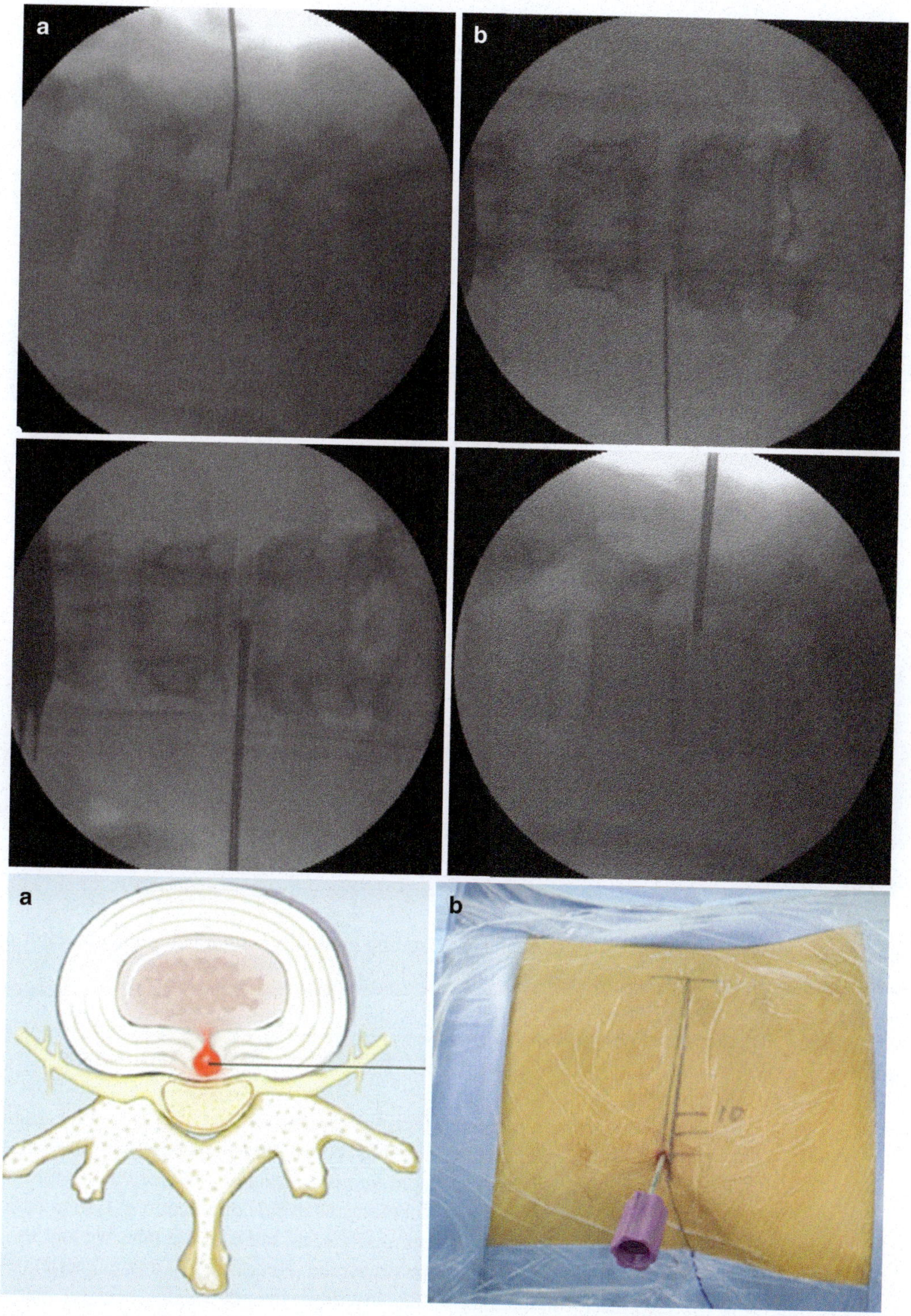

Fig. 17.6 (1) Fluoroscopic view of facet joint on lateral view (A) and disc space on AP view (B). (2) Schematic representation of location of working cannula within annulus pulposus. (3) A. Needle was placed in the posterior annulus. B. Cannula establishment is completed. (4) Disc was removed using endoscopic forceps. (5) (A) Endoscopic view of inflamed nuclear material dyed blue with indigo carmine. (B) High-pressured annulus was found during the procedure

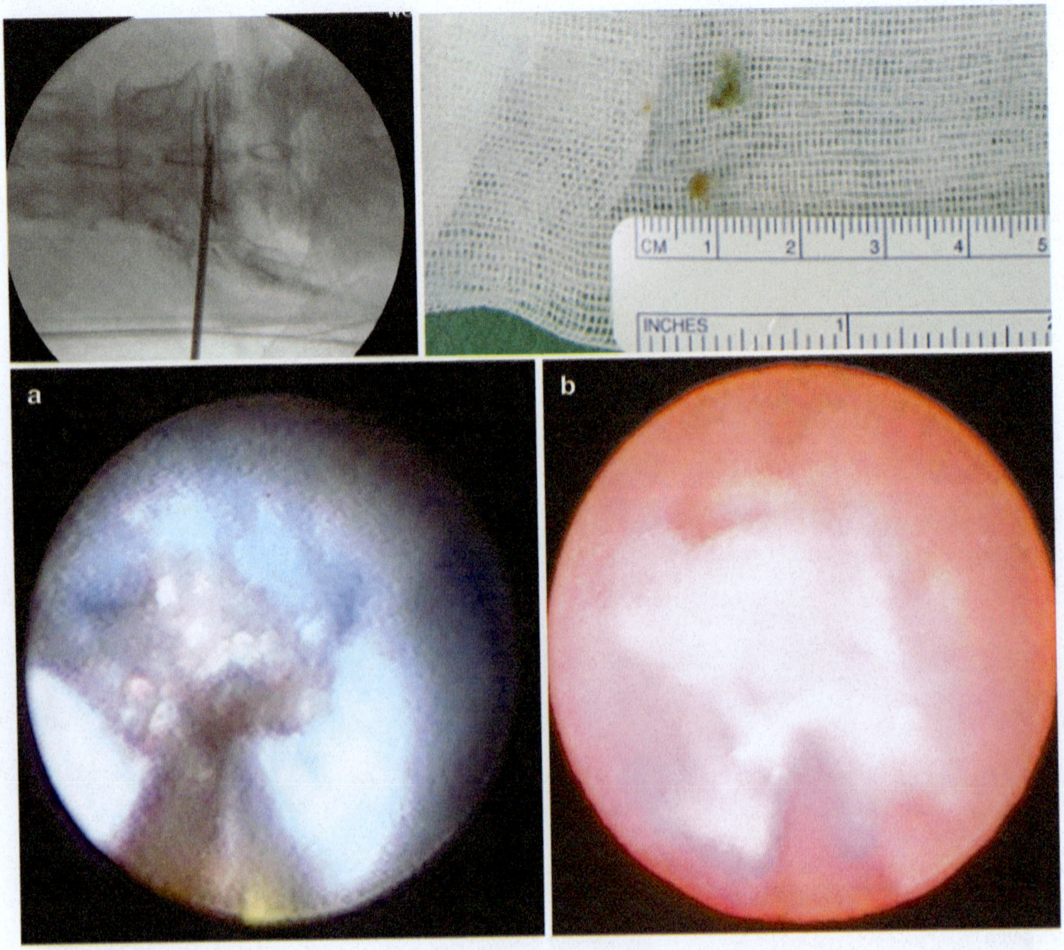

Fig. 17.6 (continued)

genic back pain is the result of inflammation and granulation tissue ingrowth, intradiscal bleeding can be seen. This sign confirms the diagnosis and indicates that the outcome of the procedure will be beneficial to the patient. After identification of the annular defect and trapped disc material, the disc is removed using endoscopic forceps (Fig. 17.6(4)). If the trapped disc is too large, the opening of the defect can be widened using a side-firing holmium:yttrium-aluminum-garnet (Ho:YAG) laser to accommodate the removal. After the disc is removed, annuloplasty is done using the side-firing Ho:YAG laser. Inflamed tissue and bleeding are managed using the side-firing Ho:YAG laser. Finally, if needed, the traversing root and epidural space can be visualized by gradually withdrawing the obturator and endoscope.

17.6 Complication Avoidance

During the procedure, because the patient remains conscious, the operating surgeon can continuously evaluate the patient's neurologic function and avoid complications. Complications are rarely seen, but they are possible and should be prevented. Neural injury due to careless needle insertion occurs rarely, because patients themselves are the best neuromonitoring system. Since irrigation fluid is continuously used during the procedure, headache and neck pain may occur due to an increase in intracranial pressure. However, unlike other endoscopic procedures, the diameter of the cannula is very small and the flow rate is low, so there are few complications due to pressure. Dural tear is possible but is rarely seen in this procedure, because the tip of the cannula is anchored in the annulus and epidural content does not need to be visualized. And since continuous intraoperative irrigation with antibiotic-infused saline was used during the procedure, there has been no surgical infection so far.

Persistent symptoms after surgery are avoided by strictly selecting only patients who have discogenic back pain. We strongly recommend the use of provocative discography for diagnosis of discogenic back pain. If inflammation and intradiscal bleeding are observed intraoperatively, we can confirm that the patient will improve after the procedure.

17.7 Case Illustration

A 30-year-old female Korean patient who is a professional golf player (Ladies Professional Golf Association) was unable to drive for more than 30 minutes due to a pain in her back when sitting for a long time. She had been suffering from severe back pain two or three times a year. Particularly after competing in the game, she had a back pain attack that made it difficult for her to swing.

She traveled to several hospitals in the United States and tried oriental medical treatment or pain injection treatment, but the effect was only for a while. Discectomy was recommended at the university hospital. She visited our hospital and confirmed the L4–5 high-intensity zone (HIZ) on MRI (Fig. 17.7). PELA was performed under conscious anesthesia. Presumptive skin entry and needle track were infiltrated with 1% lidocaine. A

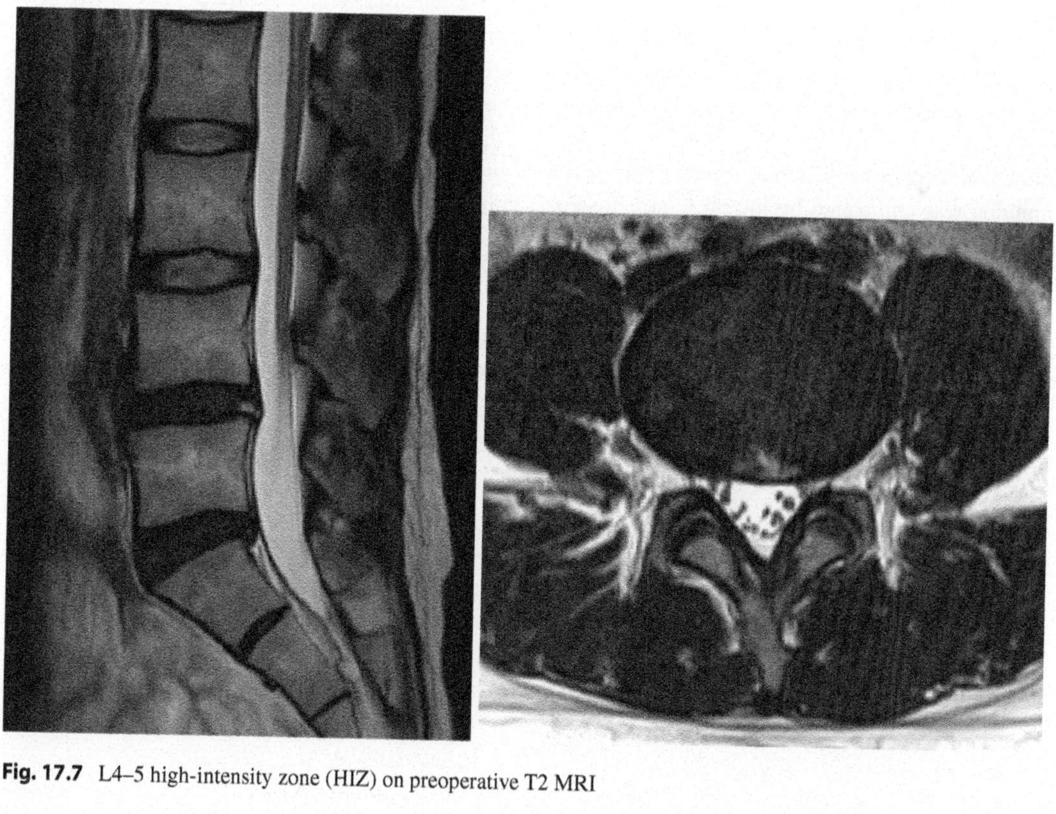

Fig. 17.7 L4–5 high-intensity zone (HIZ) on preoperative T2 MRI

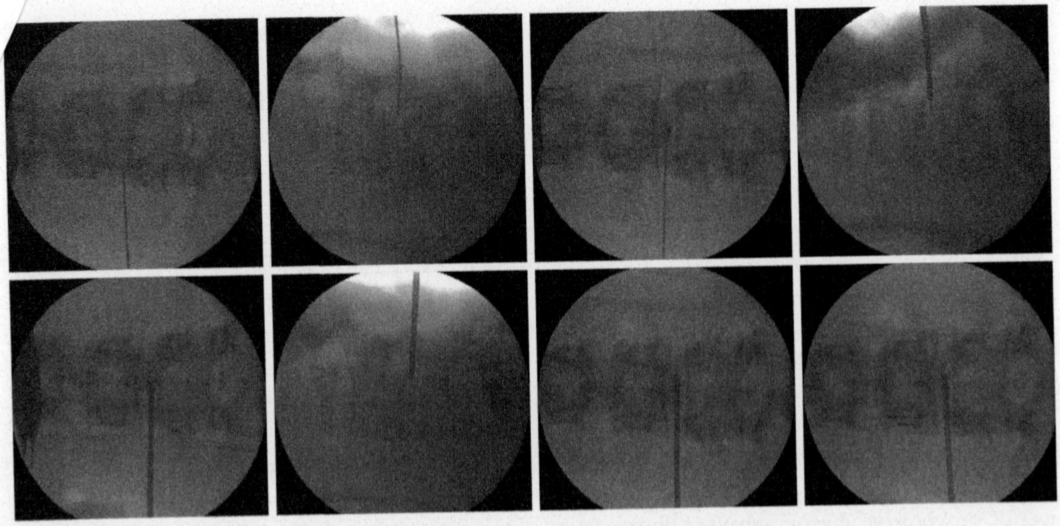

Fig. 17.8 Schematic representation of PELA procedure

15-gauge spinal needle was inserted just lateral to the superior articular pillar (SAP) toward the target level. A guide wire was inserted and a small incision (0.3 cm) was made in the overlying skin. A cannula and a soft tissue dilator were then advanced over the guide wire into the ventral epidural space under fluoroscopic monitoring. After cannula placement, the endoscope was introduced, and placement in the posterior rim of the annulus was confirmed by lateral C-arm fluoroscopic view. Forceps removal and laser ablation of the interposed granulation and nucleus pulposus were performed through the annular puncture (Ho:YAG laser with side-firing fiber side, set at 2.5 to 10 W) (Fig. 17.8). The nucleus flowed through the annular tears, which lasted for a long time and became a scar. It was transformed like calluses. Her treatment ended safely, and after rehabilitation, she successfully returned to LPGA (Fig. 17.9).

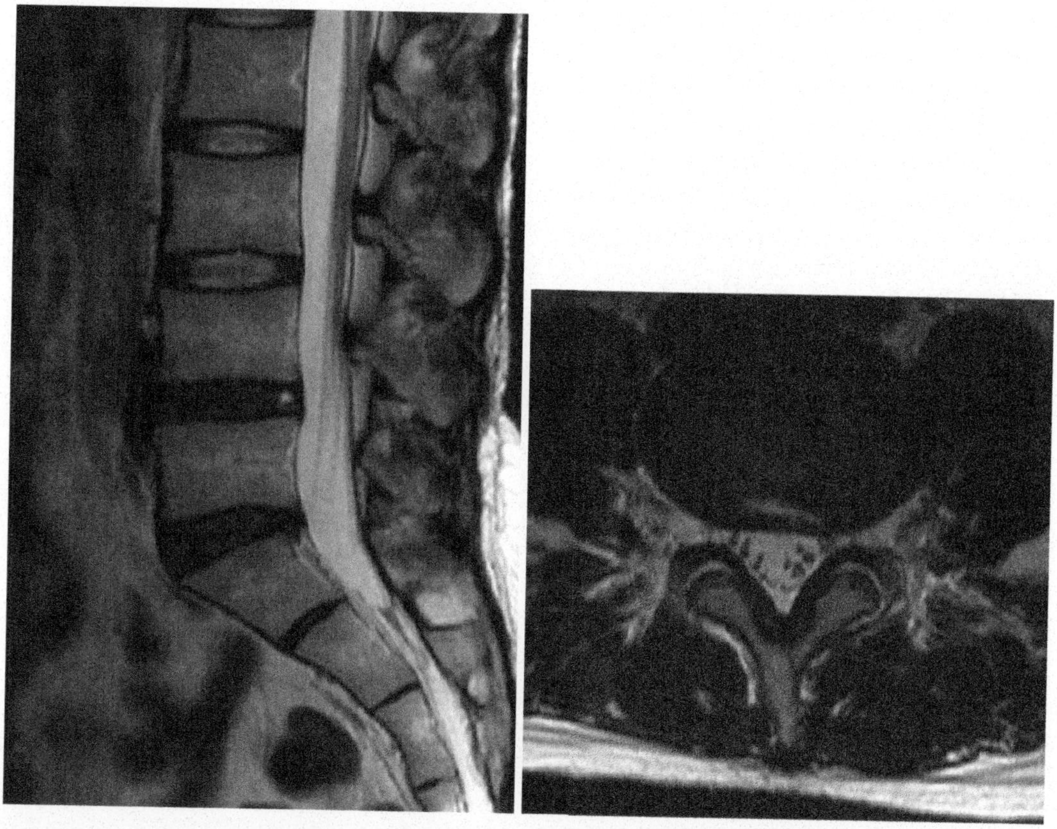

Fig. 17.9 High-intensity zone (HIZ) and bulging disc were removed on postoperative MRI

17.8 Summary

Percutaneous endoscopic laser annuloplasty/ nucleoplasty (PELA) has the benefit of visualization of intradiscal pathology and removal of the entrapped fragment that is the main cause of chronic inflammation leading to discogenic back pain. The clear visualization and the use of the Ho:YAG laser with a side-firing probe allow the surgeon to accomplish both annuloplasty and nucleoplasty in the same procedure.

References

1. Bogduk N, Windsor M, Inglis A. The innervation of the cervical intervertebral discs. Spine (Phila Pa 1976). 1988;13:2–8.
2. Bogduk N, Tynan W, Wilson AS. The nerve supply to the human lumbar intervertebral discs. J Anat. 1981;132:39–56.
3. Malinsky J. The ontogenetic development of nerve terminations in the intervertebral discs of man. (Histology of intervertebral discs, 11th communication). Acta Anat (Basel). 1959;38:96–113.
4. Groen GJ, Baljet B, Drukker J. Nerves and nerve plexuses of the human vertebral column. Am J Anat. 1990;188:282–96.
5. Yoshizawa H, O'Brien JP, Smith WT, Trumper M. The neuropathology of intervertebral discs removed for low-back pain. J Pathol. 1980;132:95–104.
6. Schwarzer AC, Aprill CN, Derby R, et al. The prevalence and clinical features of internal disc disruption in patients with chronic low back pain. Spine. 1995;20(17):1878–83.
7. Saal JA, Saal JS. Intradiscal electrothermal treatment for chronic discogenic low back pain: prospective outcome study with a minimum 2-year follow-up. Spine. 2002;27(9):966–73.

8. Hermantin FU, Peters T, Quartararo L, Kambin P. A prospective, randomized study comparing the results of open discectomy with those of video-assisted arthroscopic microdiscectomy. J Bone Joint Surg Am. 1999 Jul;81(7):958–65.
9. Hijikata S, Yamagishi M. Percutaneous nucleotomy: a new treatment method for lumbar disc herniation. J Toden Hosp. 1975;5:5–13.
10. Kambin P, Gellman H. Percutaneous lateral discectomy of the lumbar spine: a preliminary report. Clin Orthop Relat Res. April 1983;174:127–32.
11. Onik G, Helms CA. Percutaneous lumbar diskectomy using a new aspiration probe: porcine and cadaver model. Radiology. 1985;155(1):251–2.
12. Hayashi K, Thabit G III, et al. The effect of nonablative laser energy on the ultrastructure of joint capsular collagen. Arthroscopy. 1996;12(4):474–81.
13. Hermantin FU, Kambin P. A prospective, randomized study comparing the results of open discectomy with those of video-assisted arthroscopic microdiscectomy. J Bone Joint Surg Am. 1999;81(7):958–65.
14. Kambin P. Arthroscopic microdiscectomy. In: Frymoyer JW, editor. The adult spine principle and practice. 2nd ed. Philadelphia: Lippincott-Raven Publishers; 1997. p. 2023–36.
15. Tsou PM, Yeung AT. Transforaminal endoscopic decompression for radiculopathy secondary to non-contained intracanal lumbar disc herniation. Spine. 2002;2:41–8.
16. Yeung AT, Tsou PM. Posterolateral endoscopic excision for lumbar disc herniation: surgical technique, outcome, and complications in 307 consecutive cases. Spine. 2002;27(7):722–31.
17. Choi G, Lee SH. Percutaneous endoscopic interlaminar discectomy for intracanalicular disc herniations at L5-S1 using a rigid working channel endoscope. Neurosurgery. 2006;58
18. Lee SH, Kang HS. Percutaneous endoscopic laser annuloplasty for discogenic low back pain. World Neurosurg. 2010;73(3):198–206.
19. Lee SH, Kumar R, Bae JS. Intra-annular granulation tissue syndrome: clinico-histological study of high intensity zones and the role of percutaneous endoscopic lumbar annuloplasty as therapy with two years follow-up. Med Lasers. 2014;3(2):75–83.
20. Park CH, Lee KK, Lee SH. Efficacy of transforaminal laser annuloplasty versus intradiscal radiofrequency annuloplasty for discogenic low back pain. Korean J Pain. 2019 April;32(2):113–9.
21. Bae JS, Lee SM. The likelihood of reaching substantial clinical benefit after an interlaminar dynamic spacer for chronic low back pain: a clinical and radiologic analysis of a prospective cohort. World Neurosurg. May 2017;101:589–98.

Trans-sacral Epiduroscopic Laser Adhesiolysis with Ho:Yag Laser

18

Dongho Seo, Ki-Hyoung Moon, and Oon-ki Baek

Abstract

Lumbar intervertebral disc herniation (LDH) is a clinically symptomatic condition caused by compression of the spinal nerve root by protruded disc material. LDH can be treated with various endoscopic procedures. Recently, trans-sacral epiduroscopic laser decompression (SELD) using epiduroscopy and laser is one of the preferred options for minimally invasive treatment in lumbar disc diseases. Epiduroscopy has been employed because of the smaller diameter of the access portal and the flexible fiber when compared with transforaminal endoscopic lumbar discectomy. It allows treatment of a symptomatic herniated disc that has failed to respond to conservative treatment. SELD showed rapid improvement of back pain and radiculopathy with significant differences in the visual analog scale (VAS) and Oswestry Disability Index (ODI) scores between preoperative and postoperative data in the present study. The advantages of the SELD are direct decompression by laser and targeted mechanical adhesiolysis through direct visualization and very low complication rates. SELD is a safe and effective treatment for lower back and leg pain which arise from a herniated lumbar disc.

Keywords

SELD · Lumbar disc herniation · Annular tear syndrome

18.1 Introduction

Lumbar disc herniation is a very common disease that causes sciatica or backache. With the development of the endoscope and the laser system, PELD through the transforaminal or interlaminar approach has become an important alternative minimally invasive spine procedure for the treatment of a herniated disc. However, because PELD employs a rigid endoscope with a large diameter (6.5–8.0 mm), it may impede the ability to work in the epidural space. Recently, epiduroscopy has been employed because of the smaller diameter of the access portal and the flexible fiber when compared with PELD. This new technique is also known as epidural spinal endoscopy and requires the insertion of a fiberoptic endoscope into the epidural space through the sacral hiatus. It allows treatment of a symptomatic herniated disc that has failed to respond to conservative treatment [1]. In 1931, Burmann [2] introduced

Supplementary Information The online version of this chapter (https://doi.org/10.1007/978-981-16-2206-9_18) contains supplementary material, which is available to authorized users.

D. Seo · K.-H. Moon (✉) · O.-k. Baek
Seoul Gimpo Airport Wooridul Spine Hospital, Seoul, Republic of Korea

J. Bae, S.-H. Lee (eds.), *Laser Spine Surgery*, https://doi.org/10.1007/978-981-16-2206-9_18

the concept of epiduroscopy, and in 1993, Leu reported on peridural intraductal endoscopies via the sacral approach technique [3]. In 1996, the US Food and Drug Administration (FDA) approved epiduroscopy using the Myelotec fiber-optic endoscope (Myelotec, Inc., Roswell, GA) to visualize the epidural space [1]. Ruetten reported on the clinical application of epiduroscopically assisted laser therapy for postnucleotomy syndrome in 2002 [4]. After 1 year, Ruetten used epiduroscopy to guide intervention in 93 patients with chronic back-leg pain syndrome [5], and in 2007, Graziotti reported on 300 cases of epiduroscopic interventions [6]. Lee et al. reported the effect of trans-sacral epiduroscopic laser decompression (SELD) for 250 cases of back pain related to lumbar disc herniation [1]. Kim et al. reported complications of lumbar disc herniations following trans-sacral epiduroscopic lumbar decompression [7] and compared the clinical results of microscopic open interlaminar approach and SELD [8]. As a result of these studies, SELD began to be considered as an alternative minimally invasive spine procedure for the treatment of a lumbar herniated disc. In particular, approaches to the ventral side of the dural sac by the epiduroscope can ease the access and aid in the diagnosis and treatment of annulus pathology anterior to the dural sac. This chapter focuses on the neural decompression of a lumbar disc herniation by the use of a laser epiduroscope through the sacral hiatus.

The advantages of the SELD are:

- Direct decompression by laser compared with chemical adhesiolysis by epidural neuroplasty
- Targeted mechanical adhesiolysis by manipulation of the catheter and laser
- Direct visualization of lumbar epidural pathology by the epiduroscope

18.2 Indication

With this approach, various types of disc disease can be treated [1, 5, 9–18]:

- Small lumbar disc herniation, particularly those with a small protrusion or extrusion known as an "iceberg lesion"—the smaller the better.
- Migrated lumbar disc herniation; it is possible to remove either upward- or downward-migrated disc herniation, with removal of the downward-migrated herniated disc being easier than the upward type as the SELD procedure accesses the spinal canal from distal to rostral in the direction of the downward-migrated fragment.
- Annular tear syndrome.
- Recurrent disc herniation.
- Remnant disc herniation after open surgery or endoscopic procedures.
- Discal cyst.
- Failed back surgery syndrome.

18.3 Surgical Technique

The epiduroscopic equipment consisted of an epidural endoscope, a video camera system, and a video monitor (Figs. 18.1, 18.2, 18.3, 18.4, and 18.5).

The procedure was performed with the patient under local anesthesia, utilizing lidocaine with epinephrine over the sacral hiatus, and patients were monitored by an anesthesiologist. All patients were awake, allowing them to converse freely throughout the procedure. Each patient was placed in the prone position on a radiolucent operating table with a Wilson's frame to decrease lumbosacral lordosis. A 5-mm skin incision was made over the sacral hiatus using a No. 11 blade. The sacrococcygeal ligament was punctured with a Tuohy needle under fluoroscopic guidance followed by a guidewire and dilator, and a video-guided catheter (VGC) was inserted into the sacrococcygeal ventral epidural space. Subsequently, a 3-mm steerable VGC was introduced. A C-arm fluoroscope with image intensification was used to provide images in both the anterior/posterior and lateral views to verify the position of the catheter in the ventral epidural

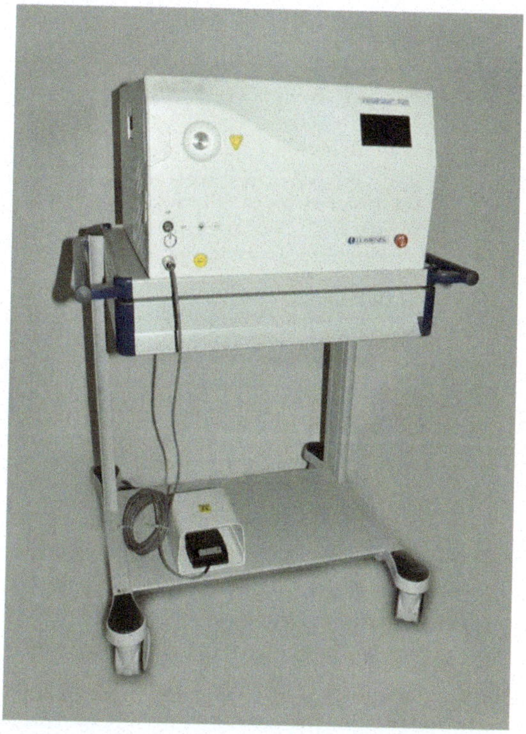

Fig. 18.1 The procedures were performed using a holmium:yttrium-aluminum-garnet (Ho:YAG) laser (Versa-Pulse P20; Lumenis, Yokneam, Israel)

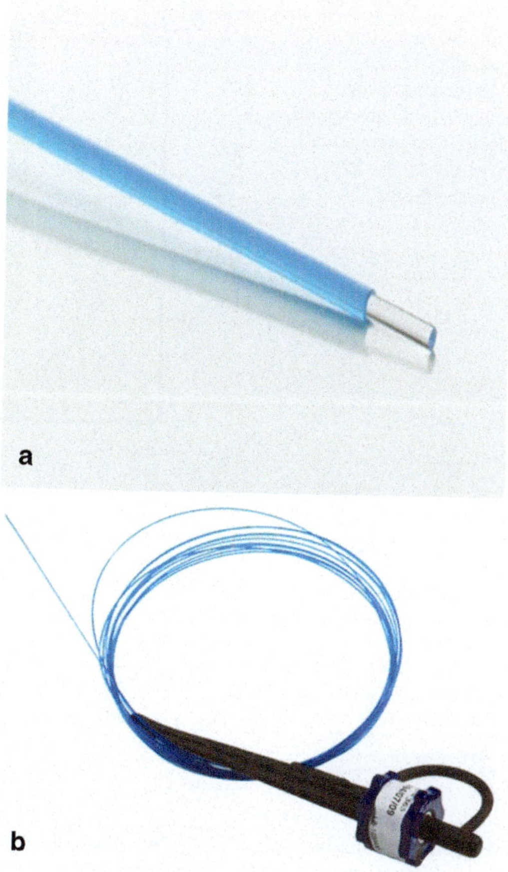

Fig. 18.2 (**a**) Ho:YAG laser has an end-firing fiber, which contains a 2.3-F outer diameter optic fiber. (**b**) Ho:YAG laser fiber and connecter

space (Fig. 18.6). Through the VGC, the epiduroscope and Ho:YAG laser were advanced into the end of the catheter to visualize the epidural space and perform herniated nucleus pulposus (HNP) ablation (Fig. 18.7). A Ho:YAG laser was used because of the high quality of its ablation of the disc: it does not cause significant thermal injury to the neural structures, with HNP ablation limited to between the posterior longitudinal ligament (PLL) and the posterior annulus. On the epiduroscopic view, the upper half of the view must be the ventral dura and the lower half of the annulus as shown in Fig. 18.7. If fibrous adhesion between the ventral dura and annulus is severe (Fig. 18.8), mechanical adhesiolysis can be performed by steering the catheter or laser firing. After introducing the VGC, fluoroscopy and epiduroscopy were used to confirm that the tip of the catheter was located at the most inferior part of the targeted disc, covering the PLL. Radio-opaque dye was then injected to obtain an epidurogram, showing the outline of the herniation and the flow obstruction caused by the HNP and adhesion at the pathologic level. After identification of the herniated disc, perform a cauterization and decompression using the Ho:YAG laser (Fig. 18.9). The peripheral portion of the herniated disc is initially targeted because mechanical adhesiolysis between the herniated disc and attached dura is easy after shrinkage around the herniated disc. Central decompression is then performed by laser, using energies from 2.5 Watts (0.5 J, 5 Hz) to 8 Watts (0.8 J, 10 Hz). If the impinged root is decompressed, the catheter can

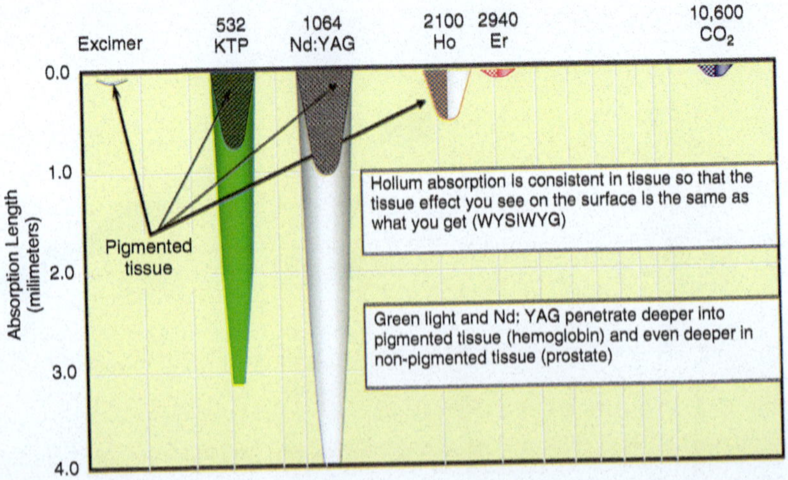

Fig. 18.3 Laser absorption depth. The Ho:YAG laser (black oval shape) has a 2100-nm wavelength and a 0.4-mm absorption depth (with permission from VersaPulse P20; Lumenis Korea

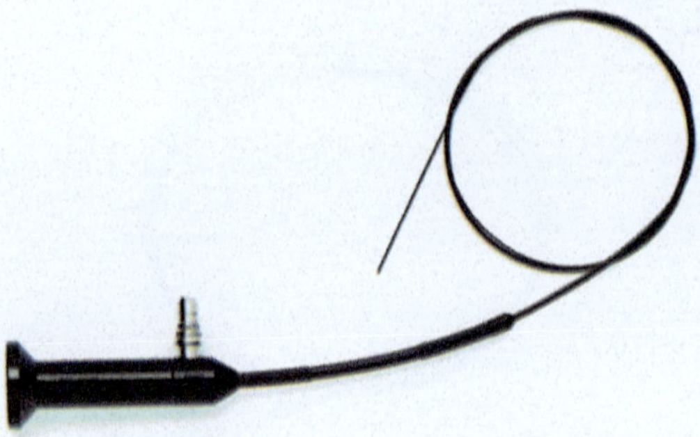

Fig. 18.4 Epiduroscope is a 15-kilopixel flexible fiber-optic endoscope with a 1.2-mm diameter

be advanced easily between the impinged root and the annulus. Before the SELD, there was narrow epidural space between the dura and bulging PLL with an underlying HNP (Fig. 18.10a). The epidurogram after SELD showed a flattened outline of the herniation and a wide epidural space at the previous pathologic level (Fig. 18.10b).

During the procedure, the total volume of injected saline should generally not exceed 200 mL, to avoid increasing intracranial pressure. The surgery is performed under monitored anesthesia care.

18.4 Case Illustration

A 35-year-old man was presented with chief complaints of left buttock and leg pain. He also had paresthesia on the left thigh and posterior calf area. Symptom has developed 2 weeks ago. The imaging studies showed L5/S1 left paracentral disc rupture. We have performed L5/S1 SELD. After surgery, his symptoms have improved without any complications. The pre- and postoperative images are shown in Fig. 18.11.

18.5 Postoperative Consideration

18.5.1 Complication

There were some but rare complications along the SELD. Increased intracranial pressure due to the saline injection into the spinal canal for improved visualization during the procedure may occur, and patients may develop headache, neck stiffness, seizure, and retinal hemorrhage as a result.

Other complications include dural puncture, which can occur when there are excessive ventral dural adhesions from prior surgery, annular tears, or extruded disc herniations [19]. Bed rest typically suffices and no additional treatment is required in most cases. Large cerebrospinal fluid (CSF) leaks are uncommon since the leak is usually minimal due to the small confines of the spinal canal that become quickly filled. The resulting focal increase in hydrostatic pressure may also minimize further leakage. There was a report of decreased CSF pressure with a chronic subdural hematoma after dural puncture [20].

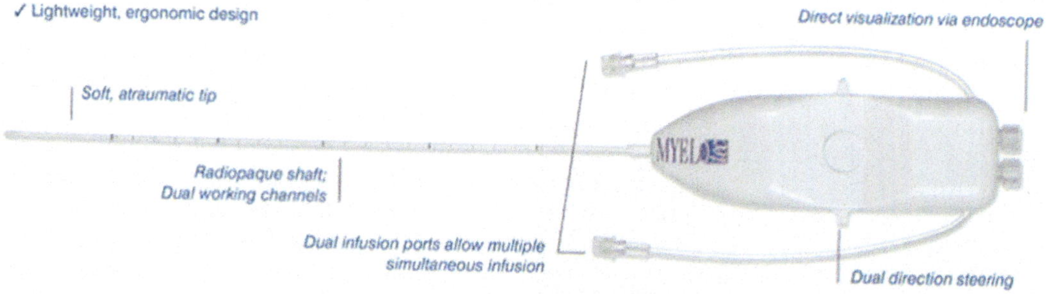

Fig. 18.5 3-mm video-guided catheter (VGC) with a 3.0-mm outer diameter for trans-sacral epiduroscopic laser decompression (with permission form Myelotec Inc., Roswell, GA). The VGC has a radiopaque shaft with 1.3-mm dual working channels. It also has dual infusion ports for infusing saline for irrigation

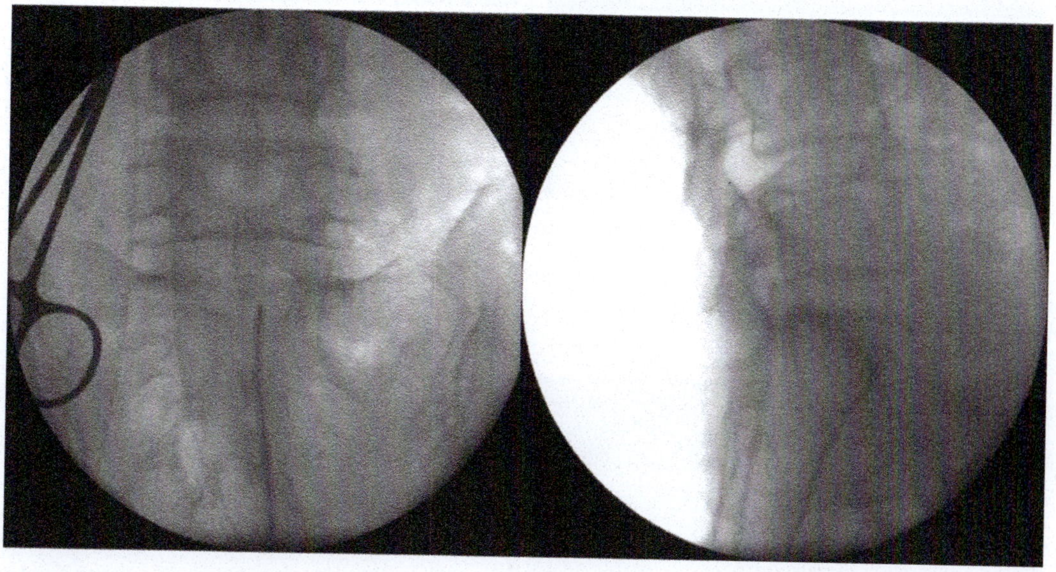

Fig. 18.6 C-arm fluoroscopic image intensification shows (**a**) access to the ventral epidural space of the video-guided catheter in the anteroposterior and (**b**) lateral views

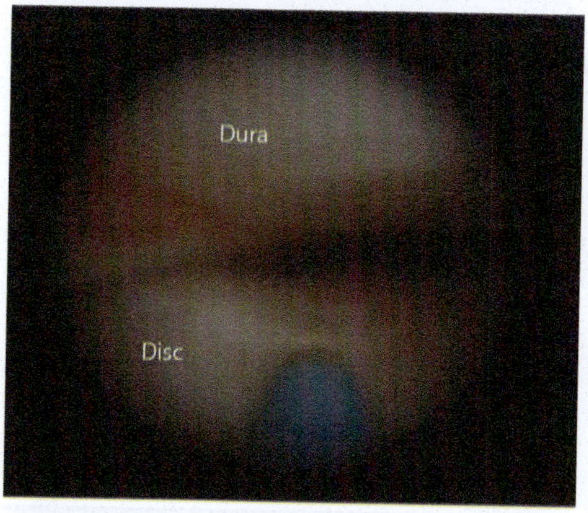

Fig. 18.7 The upper half is the ventral dura of the thecal sac, and the bottom half is the bulging posterior longitudinal ligament (PLL) underlying the herniated lumbar disc (HLD)

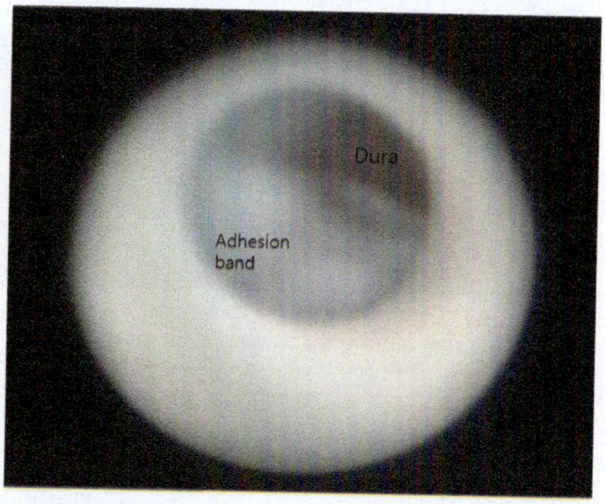

Fig. 18.8 Adhesion bands are shown in epiduroscope

Transient neurologic deficits have been reported. Generally, these deficits are resolved spontaneously (motor weakness or perineal numbness) [19, 21, 22]. Permanent neurologic deficits after SELD are extremely rare. A case of sacral root damage has been reported after using a Nd:YAG laser [23].

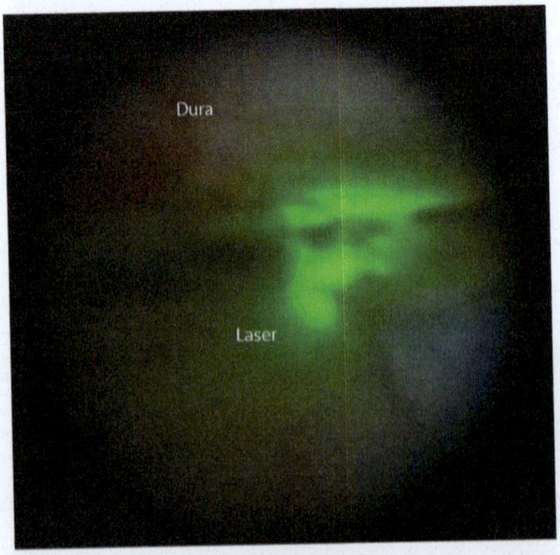

Fig. 18.9 Herniated nucleus pulposus are decompressed by Ho:YAG laser

Infection or epidural hematoma is very rare. Jung et al. reported a rare case of bacterial meningitis with cauda equina syndrome [24]. Also, Yeonkyu et al. reported a case of epidural hematoma [25].

Recurrence postoperatively is caused by multiple factors. Known risk factors for recurrent LDH include sex, smoking, body mass index, and diabetes [26]. The primary cause of recurrent LDH is continued degeneration of the surgically treated disc. Kim et al. propose that multiple vaporization holes and exogenic action may be precipitating causes of recurrent LDH [7]. It is very likely that annular tear was exacerbated by multiple vaporization holes, and it can lead to RLDH.

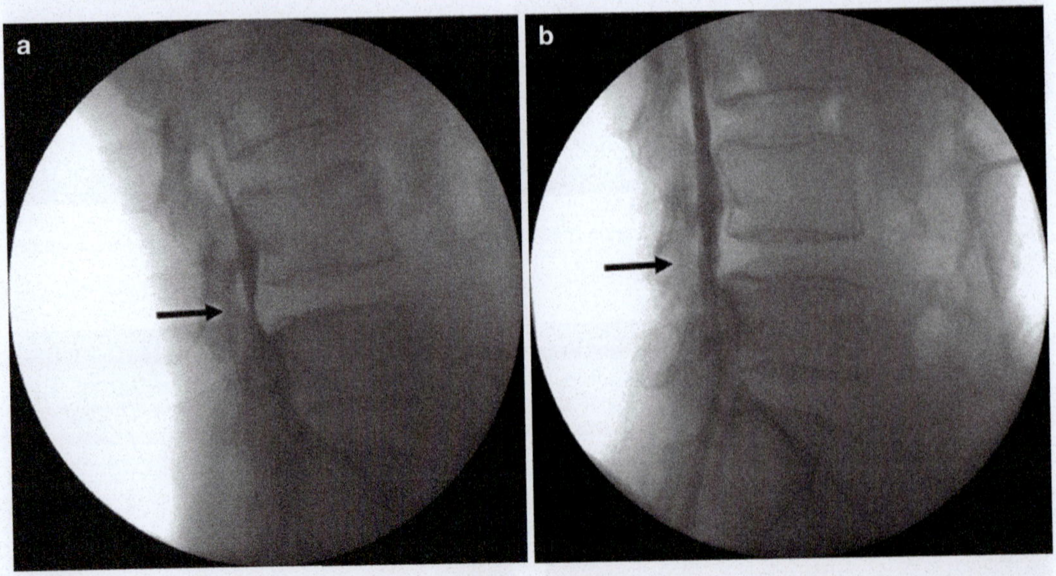

Fig. 18.10 (**a**) Before the sacral epiduroscopic laser decompression (SELD), there was a narrow epidural space between the dura and bulging posterior longitudinal ligament with an underlying herniated nucleus pulposus. (**b**) Epidurogram after SELD showed a flattened outline of the herniation and a wide epidural space at the previous pathologic level

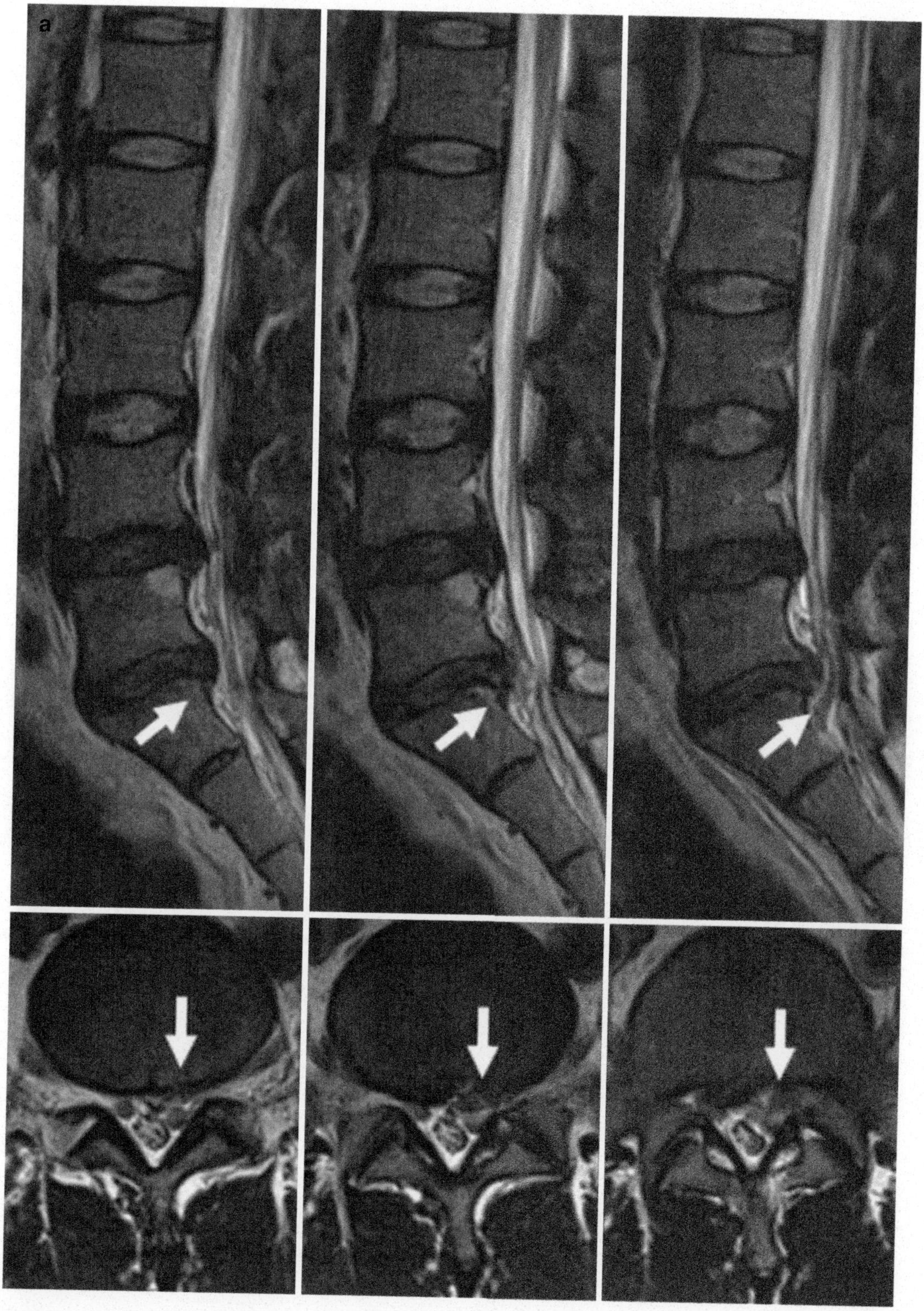

Fig. 18.11 (**a**) Preoperative MRI. (**b**) Postoperative MRI

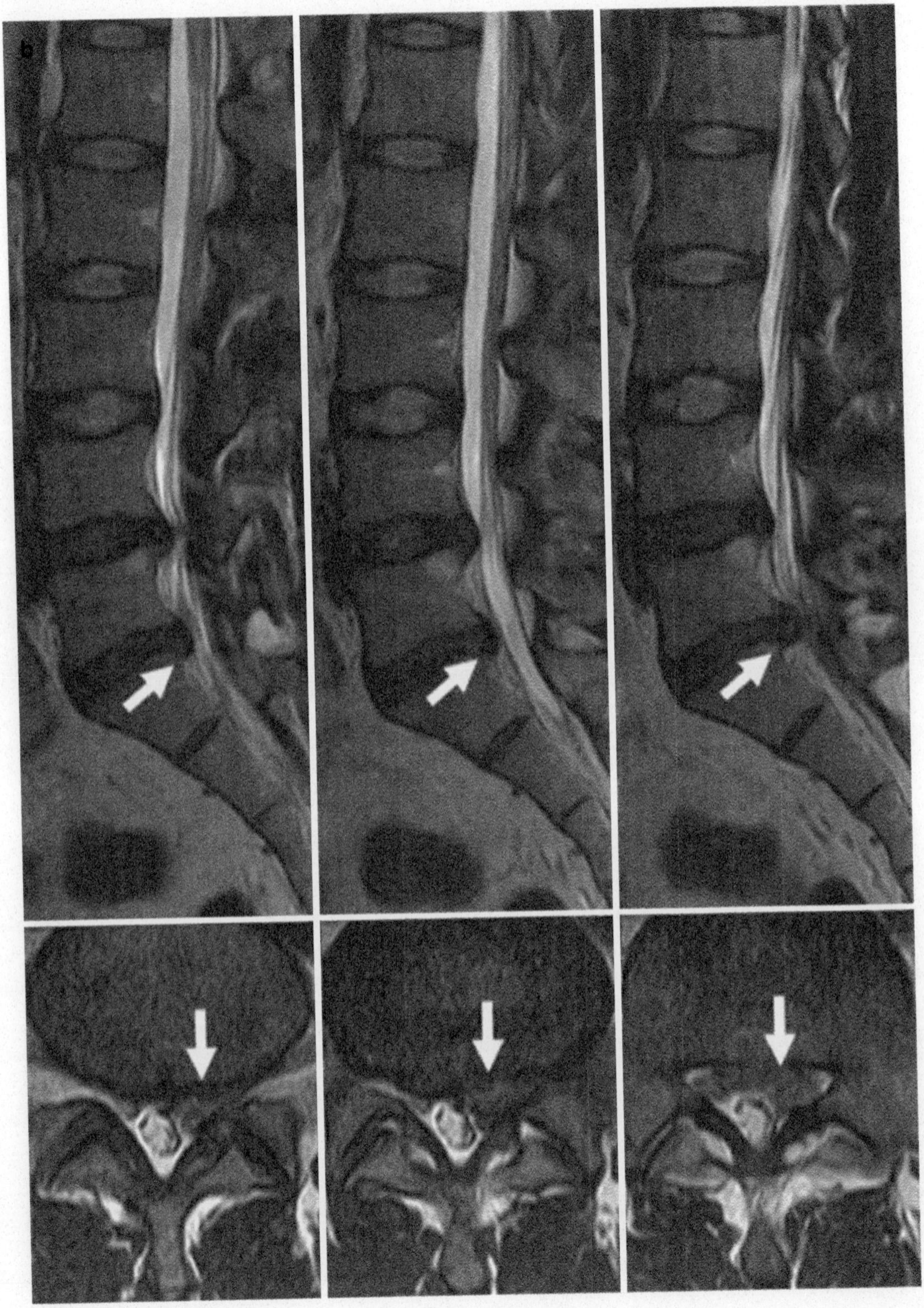

Fig. 18.11 (continued)

18.6 Summary

SELD has gained popularity for the treatment of LDH, with both spine surgeons and patients, due to its noninvasive nature, short postoperative hospital stay, use of local anesthesia, and high level of effectiveness [8]. Additionally, SELD can treat multiple levels of annular tears simultaneously.

SELD enables vaporization of the protruded part of the disc, cauterization of the sinuvertebral nerve, lysis of adhesions near the nerve root, and irrigation of inflamed areas [1]. Initial improvement of low back and radicular symptoms after SELD has been suggested to be due to a reduction in inflammatory mediators (e.g., TNF-α, PLA2) caused by the normal saline lavage of the surgical site. In addition, mechanical lysis of perineural adhesions can play a role in symptom relief because diminished epidural fibrosis could interfere with the motion of the dura and spinal roots and cause radicular pain. Laser ablation also enables a contained herniated disc to be physically changed to an uncontained herniated disc. This allows mononuclear cells entering along the margins of the extruded disc to express inflammatory mediators and induce angiogenesis, causing persistent inflammation [27]. An uncontained herniated disc has a possibility of absorption due to dehydration and the inflammation-mediated resorption response because the water content of the disc is higher [28].

During SELD with the epiduroscopy and the laser device, decompression of the ruptured lumbar disc and adhesiolysis in the epidural space are performed [1].

Several previous reports stated that the clinical outcomes of SELD were favorable even compared with those of open discectomy, as there was a significant decrease of low back pain or radiating leg pain, patient satisfaction higher than 70%, low rates of incomplete decompression, and a low recurrence rate [1, 7, 8, 29–31]. But Son et al. reported the clinical results of the patients were not all favorable. Although the mean VAS of low back pain and leg pain decreased significantly, the satisfaction and surgical failure rates were not all favorable [32].

A low absorption of laser energy results in the vaporization of an insufficient amount of soft tissue, but a high energy can increase the risk of tissue burning [33]. The Ho:YAG laser strongly absorbs water molecules because the optimal wavelength is close to the absorption of water (2000 nm), it has a 350-μs pulse duration, it absorbs <0.4 mm of fluid, and there is little to no danger of injuring normal anatomical structures [33].

The Ho:YAG laser is based on the vaporizing effect to destroy the disc, which is influenced by energy absorption by water. Because the laser light is transmitted through flexible fibers, this technique is especially suited for minimally invasive endoscopic procedures. Moreover, because of the fast absorbing wavelength, which does not extend beyond 0.4 mm [34] of depth, precise hemostatic cutting and ablation of tissue with minimal thermal damage can be achieved [35]. The herniated disc is therefore removed effectively and safely.

However, SELD is difficult to remove large LDH, foraminal LDH, and iceberg lesion. Since the Ho:YAG laser does not extend to more than 0.4 mm, it is very difficult to treat large LDH. Foraminal LDH is difficult to treat because the catheter cannot pass through the foramen. And iceberg lesion is also difficult to treat since it requires manipulation in the epidural space. When treating annular tears with SELD, care must be taken because application of Ho:YAG laser can cause recurrent LDH by widening the annular tear.

Incomplete decompression always results in persistent postoperative radiating pain, without a pain-free interval after surgery [36, 37]. Zhao et al. [38] suggested that herniations with stenosis (degeneration) and high-grade migration of the nucleus are associated with the highest rate of incomplete decompression. The presence of a high-grade migration of the disc, especially in the upward direction, significantly decreases the mobility of the epiduroscope, increasing the difficulty of the decompression. Therefore, preoperative identification of degeneration findings and migration should be taken into consideration to achieve sufficient decompression.

Decompression of the root by de-bulking of the HNP is the most important objective of the procedure, and this is where some limitations of the SELD procedure become apparent. The two major disadvantages of the technique are the narrow epiduroscopic view and unclear image quality in the narrow epidural space, which occasionally impairs visibility and limits the ablation of soft tissue with the end-firing laser. To resolve this matter in the future, epiduroscopy will require the development of high-definition optics with a wider angle of view. There is also a limit as to how much the laser can burn away with end-firing, as the herniated disc cannot be completely cauterized. In contrast, a side-firing laser can be a more effective delivery source of energy to the disc.

References

1. Lee SH, Lee SH, Lim KT. Trans-sacral epiduroscopic laser decompression for symptomatic lumbar disc herniation: a preliminary case series. Photomed Laser Surg. 2016;34(3):121–9.
2. Burman MS. Myeloscopy or the direct visualization of the spinal canal and its contents. J Bone Joint Surg. 1931;13:695–6.
3. Leu H. Percutaneous techniques: decompression and intradiscal laser in discoscopy, external pedicular fixation, percutaneous interbody fusion, peridural endoscopy with discoscopy. 12th Course for Percutaneous Endoscopic Spinal Surgery. Balgrist, 1993.
4. Ruetten S, Meyer O, Godolias G. Application of holmium:YAG laser in epiduroscopy: extended practicabilities in the treatment of chronic back pain syndrome. J Clin Laser Med Surg. 2002;20:203–6.
5. Ruetten S, Meyer O, Godolias G. Endoscopic surgery of the lumbar epidural space (epiduroscopy): results of therapeutic intervention in 93 patients. Minim Invasive Neurosurg. 2003;46(1):1–4.
6. Schutze G. Epiduroscopy: spinal endoscopy. Berlin: Springer; 2009.
7. Kim SK, et al. Complications of lumbar disc herniations following trans-sacral epiduroscopic lumbar decompression: a single-center, retrospective study. J Orthop Surg Res. 2017;12:187.
8. Kim SK, Lee SC, Park SW. Trans-sacral epiduroscopic laser decompression versus the microscopic open interlaminar approach for L5-S1 disc herniation. J Spinal Cord Med. 2018;43(1):46–52.
9. Igarashi T, Hirabayashi Y, Seo N, Saitoh K, Fukuda H, Suzuki H. Lysis of adhesions and epidural injection of steroid/local anaesthetic during epiduroscopy potentially alleviate low back and leg pain in elderly patients with lumbar spinal stenosis. Br J Anaesth. 2004;93(2):181–7.
10. Dashfield AK, Taylor MB, Cleaver JS, Farrow D. Comparison of caudal steroid epidural with targeted steroid placement during spinal endoscopy for chronic sciatica: a prospective, randomized, double-blind trial. Br J Anaesth. 2005;94(4):514–9.
11. Donato AD, Fontana C, Pinto R, Beltrutti D, Pinto G. The effectiveness of endoscopic epidurolysis in treatment of degenerative chronic low back pain: a prospective analysis and follow-up at 48 months. Acta Neurochir Suppl. 2011;108:67–73.
12. Jo DH, Yang HJ. The survey of the patient received the epiduroscopic laser neural decompression. Korean J Pain. 2013;26(1):27–31.
13. Jo DH, Yang HJ, Kim JJ. Approach for epiduroscopic laser neural decompression in case of the sacral canal stenosis. Korean J Pain. 2013;26(4):392–5.
14. Jo DH, Kim ED, Oh HJ. The comparison of the result of epiduroscopic laser neural decompression between FBSS or not. Korean J Pain. 2014;27(1):63–7.
15. Lee GW, Jang SJ, Kim JD. The efficacy of epiduroscopic neural decompression with Ho:YAG laser ablation in lumbar spinal stenosis. Eur J Orthop Surg Traumatol. 2014;24(1):231–7.
16. Jeon S, Lee GW, Jeon YD, Park I-H, Hong J, Kim J-D. A preliminary study on surgical navigation for epiduroscopic laser neural decompression. Proc Inst Mech Eng H J Eng Med. 2015;229(10):693–702.
17. Kim SK, Lee BH, Song MB, Lee SC. A novel technique for managing symptomatic spinal cysts using epiduroscopic neural laser decompression: technical note and preliminary results. J Orthop Surg Res. 2018;13(1):136.
18. Ceylan A, Aşık İ, Özgencil GE, Erken B. Evaluation of the efficacy of epiduroscopic adhesiolysis in failed back surgery syndrome. Turk J Med Sci. 2019;49(49):249–57.
19. Veihelmann A, Devens C, Trouillier H, Birkenmaier C, Gerdesmeyer L, Refior HJ. Epidural neuroplasty versus physiotherapy to relieve pain in patients with sciatica: a prospective randomized blinded clinical trial. J Orthop Sci. 2006;11:365–9.
20. Kim SB, Kim MK, Kim KD, Lim YJ. Unintended complication of intracranial subdural hematoma after percutaneous epidural neuroplasty. J Korean Neurosurg Soc. 2014;55:170–2.
21. Ho KY, Manghnani P. Acute monoplegia after lysis of epidural adhesions: a case report. Pain Pract. 2008;8:404–7.
22. Lim YS, Jung KT, Park CH, Wee SW, Sin SS, Kim J. Acute motor weakness of opposite lower extremity after percutaneous epidural neuroplasty. Korean J Pain. 2015;28:144–7.
23. Chang MC. Sacral root injury during trans-sacral epiduroscopic laser decompression: A case report. Medicine. 2017;96:42.

24. Jung YJ, Chang MC. Bacterial meningitis and cauda equina syndrome after trans-sacral epiduroscopic laser decompression: a case report. Medicine. 2019;98:11.
25. Yeonkyu YU, et al. Epidural hematoma after trans-sacral epiduroscopic laser decompression: a case report. Photobiomodul Photomed Laser Surg. 2020 Feb;38(2):112–4. https://doi.org/10.1089/photob.2019.4664.
26. Huang W, Han Z, Liu J, Yu L, Yu X. Risk factors for recurrent lumbar disc herniation: a systematic review and meta-analysis. Medicine. 2016;95:e2378.
27. Doita M, Kanatani T, Harada T, Mizuno K. Immunohistologic study of the ruptured intervertebral disc of the lumbar spine. Spine. 1996;21(2):235–41.
28. Orief T, Orz Y, Attia W, Almusrea K. Spontaneous resorption of sequestrated intervertebral disc herniation. World Neurosurg. 2012;77(1):146–52.
29. Jo D, Lee DJ. The extent of tissue damage in the epidural space by Ho/YAG laser during epiduroscopic laser neural decompression. Pain Phys. 2016;19(1):E209–14.
30. Hazer DB, Acarbas A, Rosberg HE. The outcome of epiduroscopy treatment in patients with chronic low back pain and radicular pain, operated or non-operated for lumbar disc herniation: a retrospective study in 88 patients. Korean J Pain. 2018;31(2):109–15.
31. Oh J, Jo D. Epiduroscopic laser neural decompression as a treatment for migrated lumbar disc herniation: case series. Medicine. 2018;97(14):e0291.
32. Son S, et al. Clinical outcomes of trans-sacral epiduroscopic laser decompression (SELD) in patients with lumbar disc herniation. Pain Res Manag, Article ID. 2020:1537875, 8 pages.
33. Buchelt M, Schlangmann B, Schmolke S, Siebert W. High power Ho:YAG laser ablation of intervertebral discs: effects on ablation rates and temperature profile. Lasers Surg Med. 1995;16:179–83.
34. Casper GD, Hartman VL, Mullins LL. Results of a clinical trial of the holmium:YAG laser in disc decompression utilizing a side-firing fiber: a two-year follow-up. Lasers Surg Med. 1996;19:90–6.
35. Bader MJ, Tilki D, Gratzke C, Sroka R, Stief CG, Reich O. Ho:YAG-laser: treatment of vesicourethral strictures after radical prostatectomy. World J Urol. 2010;28:169–72.
36. Singh V, Manchikanti L, Benyamin RM, Helm S, Hirsch JA. Percutaneous lumbar laser disc decompression: a systematic review of current evidence. Pain Phys. 2009;12:573–88.
37. Ahn Y. Transforaminal percutaneous endoscopic lumbar discectomy: technical tips to prevent complications. Expert Rev Med Devices. 2012;9:361–6.
38. Zhao XL, Fu ZJ, Xu YG, Zhao XJ, Song WG, Zheng H. Treatment of lumbar intervertebral disc herniation using C-arm fluoroscopy guided target percutaneous laser disc decompression. Photomed Laser Surg. 2012;30:92–5.

19 Transforaminal Epiduroscopic Annuloplasty with Nd:YAG Laser for Discogenic Low Back Pain

Chan Hong Park

Abstract

Transforaminal epiduroscopic annuloplasty with Nd:YAG laser (TEA) is a reasonable treatment option for carefully selected patients with discogenic back pain (Schwarzer et al., Spine (Phila Pa 1976) 20(17):1878–1883, 1995).

Keywords

Discogenic pain · Laser · Annuloplasty · Transforaminal · Epiduroscope

19.1 Introduction

Chronic low back pain (LBP) is a common clinical problem among patients. Chronic LBP can be caused by structure-specific etiology, including facet joint abnormality, disc pathology, and sacroiliac joint dysfunction, and discogenic pain has been postulated as an important and common cause [1].

Abnormal nerve ingrowth and the expression of pain nociceptors are reported to be the primary etiological factors in discogenic pain [2, 3]. Thus, despite the treatment challenges, the modulation of in-growing nociceptors originating from the outer annulus fibrosus for patients with discogenic back pain shows promising results.

Numerous studies have investigated the efficacy of the minimally invasive intradiscal procedures, intradiscal electrothermal therapy [4, 5], laser-assisted annuloplasty [6], and intradiscal radiofrequency annuloplasty (IDRA). IDRA combines percutaneous manual discectomy with nuclear ablation and annular modification using radiofrequency equipment. Transforaminal epiduroscopic annuloplasty with Nd:YAG laser (TEA) is another recent development enabling thermal annuloplasty in patients with discogenic low back pain. Park et al. [7] reported that TEA is superior to IDRA in patients with discogenic low back pain.

19.2 Indication

1. Discogenic low back
2. Herniated intervertebral disc

19.3 Surgical Technique

TELA was likewise performed with patients prone, under local anesthesia. Prior to procedure, point of entry (usually 12–14 cm in spinal midline) was determined by measuring from midline on MR imaging. A conventional posterolateral approach on the side of pathology was used.

C. H. Park (✉)
Department of Anesthesiology and Pain Medicine, Wooridul Spine Hospital of Daegu, Daegu, Republic of Korea

J. Bae, S.-H. Lee (eds.), *Laser Spine Surgery*, https://doi.org/10.1007/978-981-16-2206-9_19

Presumptive skin entry and needle track was infiltrated with 1% lidocaine and then inserting 15-G spinal needle just lateral to the superior articular pillar (SAP) toward the target level (Figs. 19.1 and 19.2). After touching SAP with needle, the needle slipped down from SAP toward the ventral epidural space. Confirmed needle placement in anterior epidural space, as shown in anteroposterior and lateral radiographic views (Figs. 19.3 and 19.4), was followed by guide wire insertion and incision (0.7 cm) of the overlying skin. Both the cannula and soft tissue dilator were then inserted along the guide wire into ventral epidural space, under continuous fluoroscopic monitoring (anteroposterior and lateral views). Once the cannula was placed, an epiduroscope (Needle viewCH, outer diameter, 3.4 mm) was introduced, carrying Nd:YAG laser with side-firing fiber. C-arm fluoroscopy yielded

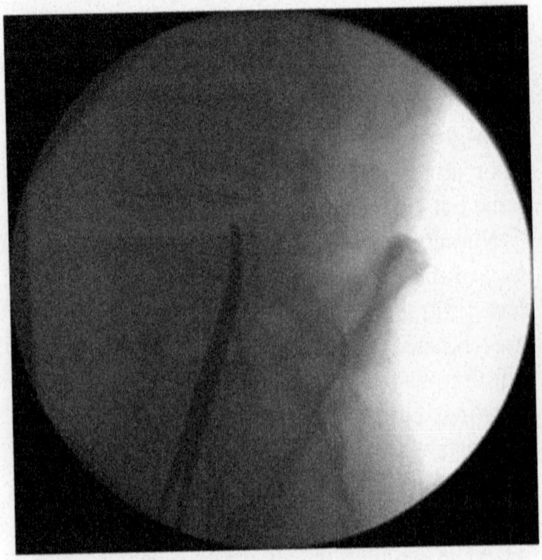

Fig. 19.1 Oblique views of target vertebral level

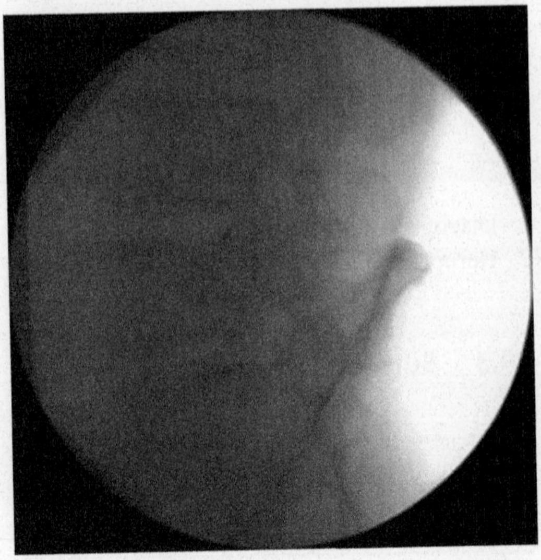

Fig. 19.2 The needle was inserted at the previously identified entry point and directed lateral to the superior articular pillar toward the target lesion

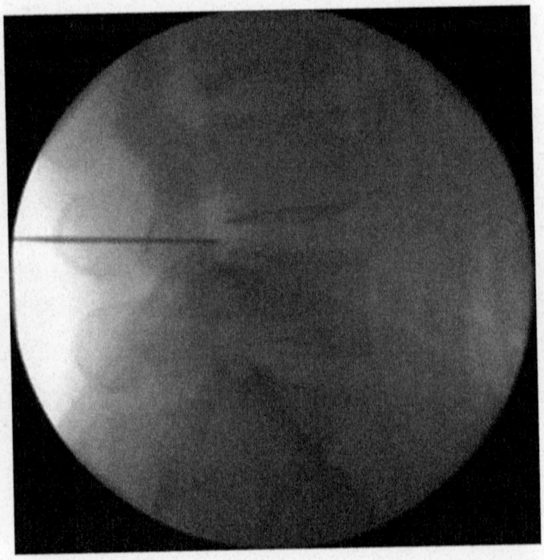

Fig. 19.3 Confirmed needle placement in lateral radiographic views

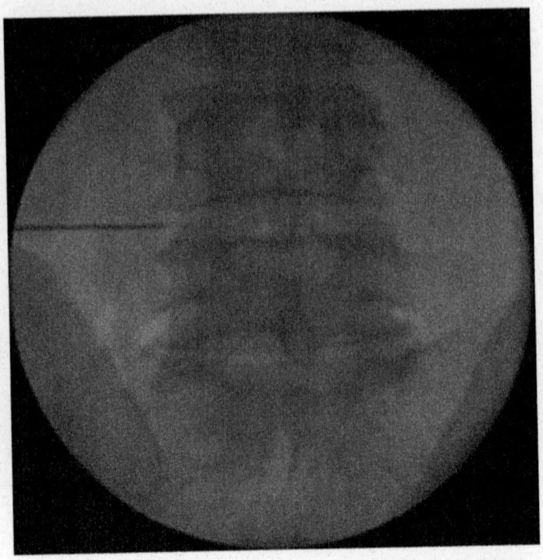

Fig. 19.4 AP view during needle insertion into the disc

images in lateral view, verifying epiduroscopic position in the ventral epidural space and confirming appropriate locations near targeted disc (Figs. 19.5 and 19.6). And then check any neural injury such as dual puncture or traversing or exiting nerve injury through the epiduroscopic views. Epidural fat and transforaminal ligament were first removed (via forceps) to ensure anatomic visualization (Fig. 19.7). Once the laser tip had entered below PLL, Nd:YAG laser treated the annulus, with unit set at 8 W (0.5–0.8 J, 5–10 Hz) (Fig. 19.8).

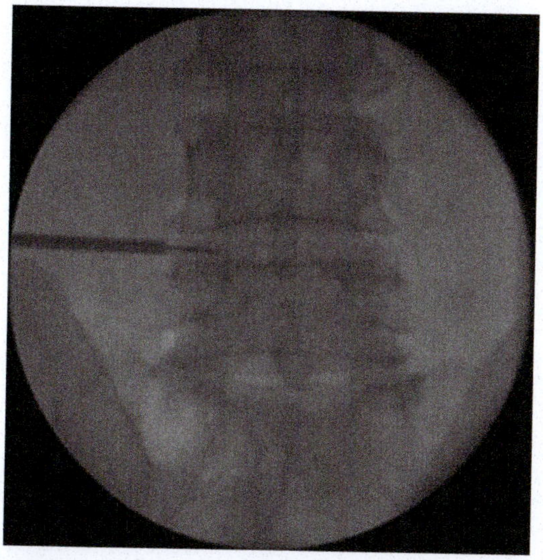

Fig. 19.5 Verifying in ventral epidural space and confirming appropriate locations near targeted disc in AP view

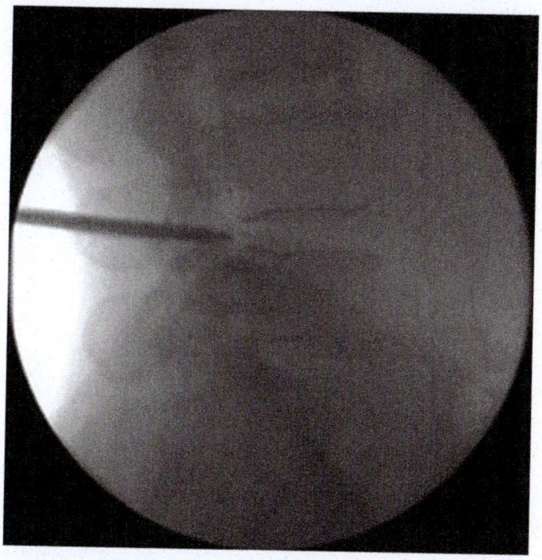

Fig. 19.6 Verifying in ventral epidural space and confirming appropriate locations near targeted disc in lateral view

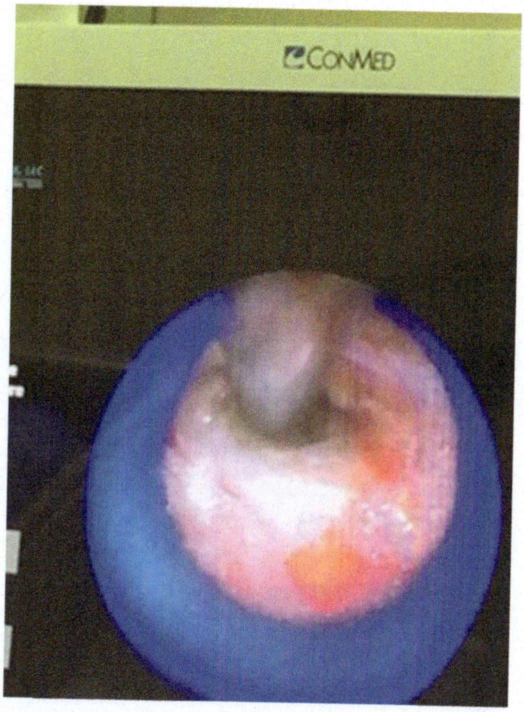

Fig. 19.7 Epidural fat and transforaminal ligament were first removed (via forceps) to ensure anatomic visualization

1. Intradiscal procedure
   The annulus was then punctured at the annular foraminal zone with a sharpened wire. Forceps removal and laser ablation of interposed granulation or nucleus pulposus was performed through the annular puncture (Nd:YAG laser with side-firing fiber side, set at 2.5 to 10 W (0.5 J, 5 to 20 Hz).
2. Extradiscal procedure
   The epiduroscope was bended and the epidural space was dissected beyond the midline to the contralateral annulus followed by extradiscal laser annuloplasty (Nd:YAG laser with side-firing fiber side, set at 2.5 to 10 W (0.5 J, 5 to 20 Hz).

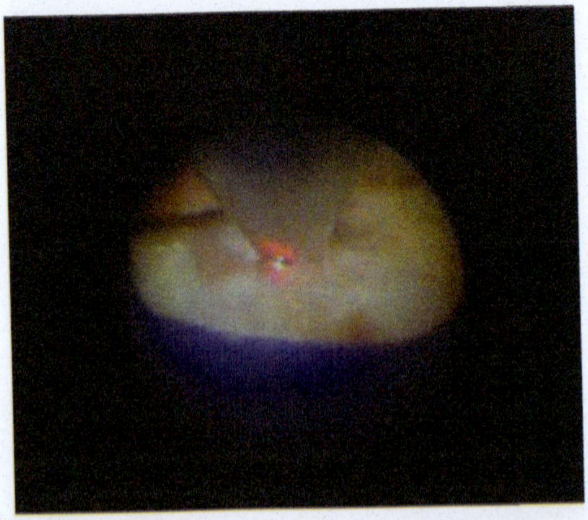

Fig. 19.8 Laser tip had entered below posterior longitudinal ligament and fired to annulus

19.4 Summary

We conclude that the application of TEA with Nd:YAG laser is effective for the treatment of discogenic LBP.

References

1. Schwarzer AC, Aprill CN, Derby R, Fortin J, Kine G, Bogduk N. The prevalence and clinical features of internal disc disruption in patients with chronic low back pain. Spine (Phila Pa 1976). 1995;20(17):1878–83.
2. Freemont AJ, Peacock TE, Goupille P, Hoyland JA, O'Brien J, Jayson MI. Nerve ingrowth into diseased intervertebral disc in chronic back pain. Lancet. 1997;350(9072):178–81.
3. Freeman BJ, Fraser RD, Cain CM, Hall DJ, Chapple DC. A randomized, double-blind, controlled trial: intradiscal electrothermal therapy versus placebo for the treatment of chronic discogenic low back pain. Spine (Phila Pa 1976). 2005;30(21):2369–77. discussion 78
4. Assietti R, Morosi M, Migliaccio G, Meani L, Block JE. Treatment of discogenic low back pain with Intradiscal Electrothermal Therapy (IDET): 24 months follow-up in 50 consecutive patients. Acta Neurochir Suppl. 2011;108:103–5.
5. Kloth DS, Fenton DS, Andersson GB, Block JE. Intradiscal electrothermal therapy (IDET) for the treatment of discogenic low back pain: patient selection and indications for use. Pain Phys. 2008;11(5):659–68.
6. Lee SH, Kang HS. Percutaneous endoscopic laser annuloplasty for discogenic low back pain. World Neurosurg. 2010;73(3):198–206.
7. Park CH, Lee KK, Lee SH. Efficacy of transforaminal laser annuloplasty versus intradiscal radiofrequency annuloplasty for discogenic low back pain. Korean J Pain. 2019;32(2):113–9.

20 Percutaneous Endoscopic Cervical Annuloplasty with Ho:YAG Laser for Discogenic Neck Pain

Junseok Bae

Abstract

Anterior endoscopic cervical annuloplasty is an effective treatment in alleviating cervical discogenic headache or neck pain caused by the degenerated annulus with contained disc herniation. In particular, Ho:YAG laser is the most important surgical tool for efficient and accurate surgery under the endoscopic visualization. In this chapter, we will describe tips and pearls for the use of endoscopic laser in anterior cervical endoscopic annuloplasty.

Keywords

Discogenic neck pain · Cervicogenic headache · Cervical disc degeneration · Cervical endoscopic annuloplasty · Ho:YAG laser

20.1 Introduction

Cervical discogenic axial pain or cervicogenic headache due to soft disc herniation or cervical disc degeneration with or without annular tear are often refractory to conservative treatments such as physical therapy or medications [1–4]. The International Headache Society defined cervicogenic headache as a clinical and/or imaging evidence of a disorder or lesion within the cervical spine or soft tissues of the neck, known to be able to cause headache with at least two of the following symptoms: (1) headache has developed in temporal relation to the onset of the cervical disorder or appearance of the lesion, (2) headache has significantly improved or resolved in parallel with improvement in or resolution of the cervical disorder or lesion, (3) cervical range of motion is reduced and headache is made significantly worse by provocative maneuver, and (4) headache is abolished following diagnostic blockade of a cervical structure or its nerve supply [5, 6]. Although there remains some controversy, provocative discography that shows concordant pain with dye leak into the spinal canal has diagnostic value [4]. Discography can discriminate painful, symptomatic discs from asymptomatic degenerated discs. There's some reports that cervical disc degeneration is attributing intractable dizziness as well as chronic neck pain due to ingrowth of Ruffini corpuscle into the annulus fibrosis [2, 7]. Anterior cervical discectomy and fusion (ACDF) is a gold standard treatment for cervical disc degeneration with excellent outcome and good recovery [8]. Cervical endoscopic annuloplasty with laser is also effective in alleviating cervical discogenic neck pain/headache arising from the damaged annulus of contained cervical disc herniation as

Supplementary Information The online version of this chapter (https://doi.org/10.1007/978-981-16-2206-9_20) contains supplementary material, which is available to authorized users.

J. Bae (✉)
Department of Neurosurgery, Chungdam Wooridul Spine Hospital, Seoul, Republic of Korea

J. Bae, S.-H. Lee (eds.), *Laser Spine Surgery*, https://doi.org/10.1007/978-981-16-2206-9_20

well as preserving normal segmental motion and minimizing surgery-related morbidity [3, 9, 10].

20.2 Indications

Cervical discogenic axial pain or cervicogenic headache due to soft disc herniation or cervical disc degeneration with annular tear that are refractory to appropriate conservative treatments is indicated. Contraindications are calcified disc herniation, sequestrated disc herniation, severe spondylosis with disc space narrowing (disc space <3 mm), cervical myelopathy, spondylolisthesis, instability, fracture, tumor, or infection [3, 9, 10].

20.3 Surgical Technique

Patient position, surgical approach, and anesthesia are the same as anterior cervical endoscopic discectomy (see Chap. 15). Local anesthesia is recommended during the procedure to confirm concordant pain on discography procedure and to monitor patient's response (Fig. 20.1). After introducing endoscopy (CESSYS, joimax GmbH, Germany) into the working channel, blue-stained degenerated nucleus can be observed. Annular tear along with degenerated disc fragment is usually located in the midline of the posterior annulus. Posterior leakage of radiopaque dye is seen during the discography. Side-firing Ho:YAG laser

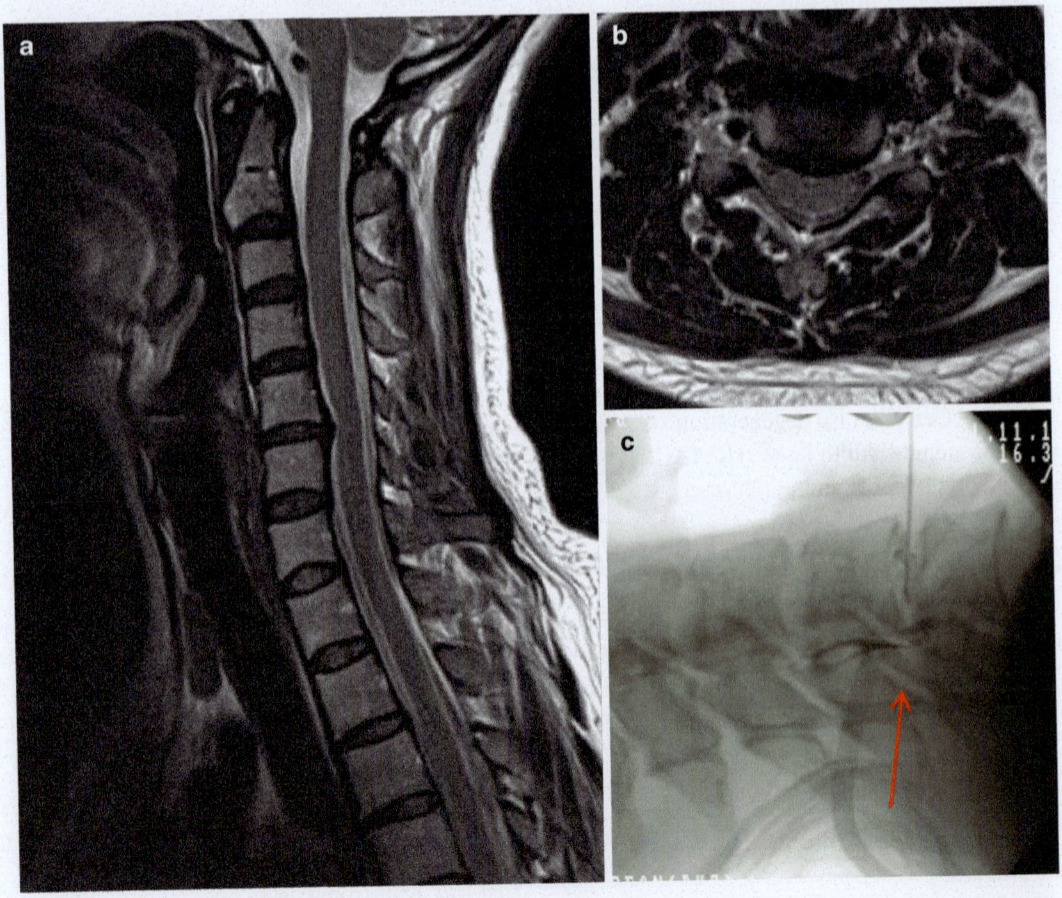

Fig. 20.1 A 41-year-old female patient suffering from chronic neck pain and occipital headache was diagnosed as having cervical disc degeneration with central protrusion at the C5–6 level. (**a**, **b**) Discography showed epidural leakage of radiopaque dye with provocation of concordant pain (**c**)

is used to shrink thickened posterior annulus and subligamentous hernia and to thin the degenerated PLL (Fig. 20.2). By rotation and tilting of the endoscopy, the central protrusion needs to be decompressed with laser (Fig. 20.3a). It is important to be aware of the location of endoscopy in the posterior disc space during the procedure. Because the working channel of the endoscopy for the laser tip is located eccentric of the endoscopy and the laser tip is facing laterally, manipulation of endoscopy is mandatory for complete decompression (Fig. 20.3b). Resection of the PLL is not necessary for annuloplasty procedure. Thorough decompression from cranial to caudal posterior endplate in the central disc space is the goal of the surgery (Fig. 20.3c).

20.4 Postoperative Consideration

The working tube and endoscope are removed, and the wound is closed with a subcutaneous stitch and covered with a strip. The patient is observed for 3 h after surgery and must be discharged within 24 h. The patient wears a soft neck collar for 2 weeks after surgery.

20.5 Case Illustration

20.5.1 Case 1

A 57-year-old female patient presented with chronic axial neck pain with occipital headache. After conservative treatment including epidural block and physical therapy for a few years, her pain was sustained. MRI shows central disc protrusion compressing spinal cord at the C4–5 level. After endoscopic annuloplasty and decompression of protruded hernia, her pain has subsided (Fig. 20.4).

20.5.2 Case 2

A 37-year-old female patient presented with chronic axial neck pain that failed to improve with intensive conservative treatment for 5 years.

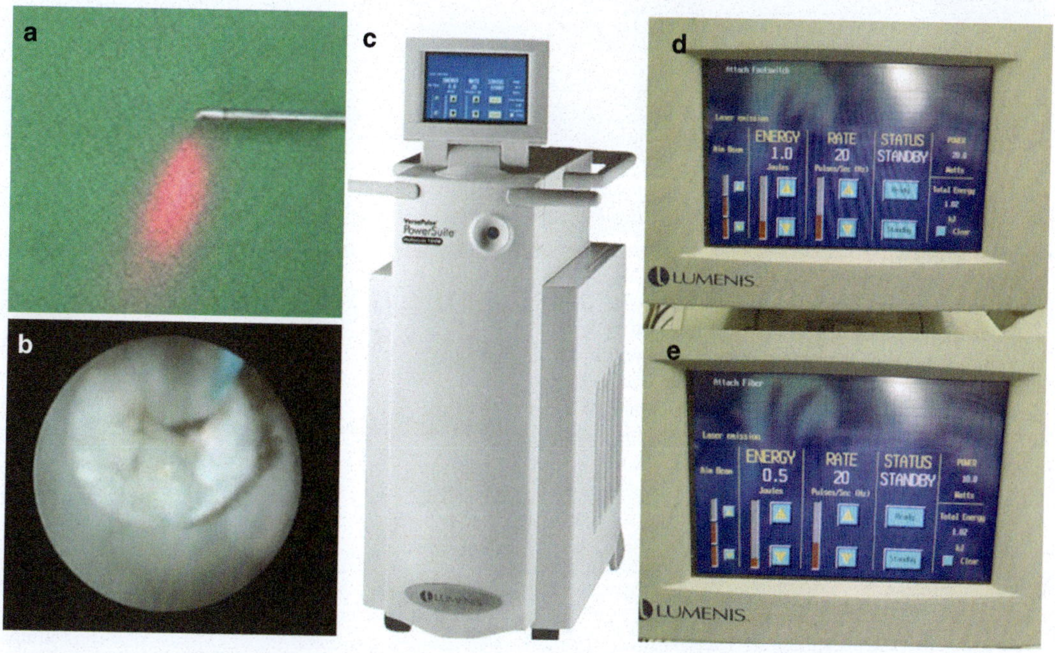

Fig. 20.2 Side-firing Ho:YAG laser tip (**a**) and its usage for evaporating posterior annulus (**b**). Laser machine (**c**) and its setting for initial stage (**d**) and later stage close to neural tissue (**e**)

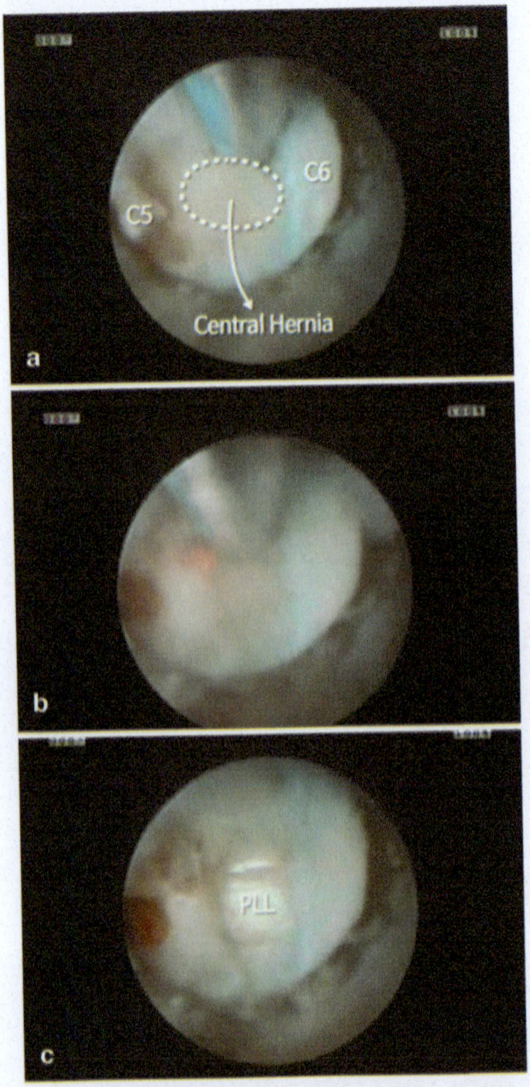

Fig. 20.3 Subligamentous central disc protrusion is identified under the endoscopic visualization. (**a**). By tilting and rotating the endoscope, side-firing laser can evaporate central hernia and thickened posterior annulus. (**b**). Resection of the PLL is not necessary for annuloplasty procedure. Thorough decompression from cranial to caudal posterior endplate in the central disc space is the goal of the surgery (**c**)

MRI showed central disc protrusion compressing spinal cord at the C4–5, C5–6, and C6–7 level with partial signal block on MR-myelography. Endoscopic annuloplasty was performed at the three levels where concordant pain was provoked with discography. After endoscopic annuloplasty and decompression of protruded hernia, her pain was improved (Fig. 20.5).

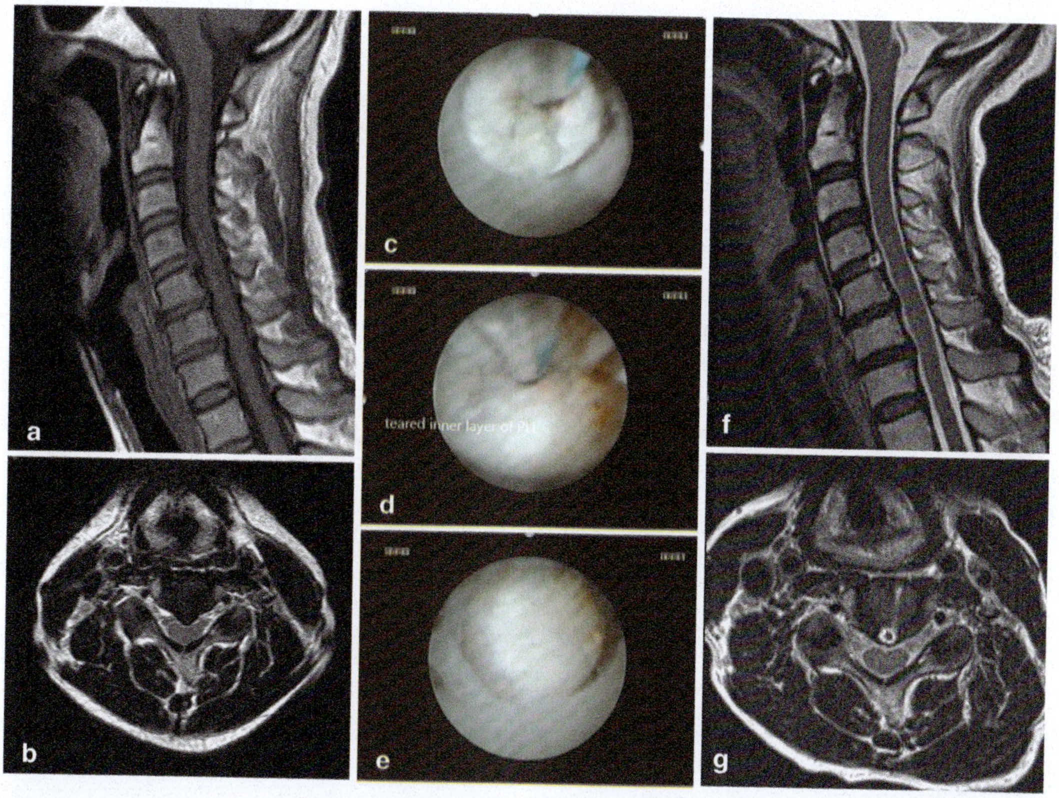

Fig. 20.4 A 57-year-old female patient presented with chronic axial neck pain with occipital headache. Preoperative MRI showing central disc protrusion compressing the spinal cord (**a, b**). After resecting the thickened posterior annulus with Ho:YAG laser (**c**), the teared inner layer of the posterior longitudinal ligament was identified (**d**). Full decompression of epidural space along with intact outer layer of PLL was achieved (**e**). Postoperative MRI showing full decompression of spinal cord (**f, g**)

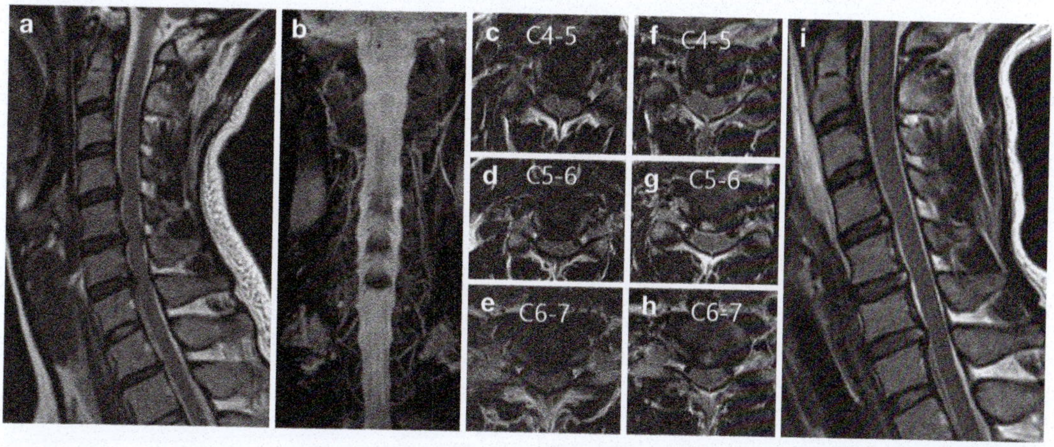

Fig. 20.5 A 37-year-old female patient presented with chronic axial neck pain. MRI showed central disc protrusion compressing the spinal cord at the C4–5, C5–6, and C6–7 level with partial signal block on MR-myelography. (**a–e**) Endoscopic annuloplasty was performed at the three levels where concordant pain was provoked with discography. After endoscopic annuloplasty and decompression of protruded hernia, full decompression of the spinal cord was achieved (**f–i**)

20.6 Summary

Direct decompression using the combined manual decompression with endoscopic forceps and the thermal effect of Ho:YAG laser under direct endoscopic visualization is a safe and effective treatment for cervical discogenic headache and neck pain [11]. Advancement of high-resolution imaging endoscopy and the availability of the side-firing laser have facilitated motion-preserving endoscopic annuloplasty.

References

1. He L, Ni J, Wu B, Yue J, Cao G, Guo Y, et al. Coblation annuloplasty in cervical discogenic pain without radiculopathy. Wideochir Inne Tech Maloinwazyjne. 2020;15(2):305–12.
2. Wu B, Yang L, Peng B. Ingrowth of nociceptive receptors into diseased cervical intervertebral disc is associated with discogenic neck pain. Pain Med. 2019;20(6):1072–7.
3. Ahn Y, Lee SH, Chung SE, Park HS, Shin SW. Percutaneous endoscopic cervical discectomy for discogenic cervical headache due to soft disc herniation. Neuroradiology. 2005;47(12):924–30.
4. Motimaya A, Arici M, George D, Ramsby G. Diagnostic value of cervical discography in the management of cervical discogenic pain. Conn Med. 2000;64(7):395–8.
5. Avijgan M, Thomas LC, Osmotherly PG, Bolton PS. A systematic review of the diagnostic criteria used to select participants in randomised controlled trials of interventions used to treat cervicogenic headache. Headache. 2020;60(1):15–27.
6. Al Khalili Y, Ly N, Murphy PB. Cervicogenic headache. Treasure Island, FL: StatPearls; 2020.
7. Yang L, Chen J, Yang C, Pang X, Li D, Wu B, et al. Cervical intervertebral disc degeneration contributes to dizziness: a clinical and immunohistochemical study. World Neurosurg. 2018;119:e686–e93.
8. Pang X, Liu C, Peng B. Anterior cervical surgery for the treatment of cervicogenic headache caused by cervical spondylosis. J Pain Res. 2020;13:2783–9.
9. Ahn Y. Endoscopic spine discectomy: indications and outcomes. Int Orthop. 2019;43(4):909–16.
10. Choi G, Pophale CS, Patel B, Uniyal P. Endoscopic spine surgery. J Korean Neurosurg Soc. 2017;60(5):485–97.
11. Lee SH, Ahn Y, Choi WC, Bhanot A, Shin SW. Immediate pain improvement is a useful predictor of long-term favorable outcome after percutaneous laser disc decompression for cervical disc herniation. Photomed Laser Surg. 2006;24(4):508–13.

21 Potential Complications of Laser Spine Surgery

Jeong Hoon Choi

Abstract

Complications after laser spine surgery are very rare, but in some cases, they can become more serious. The success of laser spine surgery depends on keeping the basic surgical principle, appropriate patient selection, attention to preoperative radiology, careful surgical approach, and careful use of laser.

Keywords

Complication · Laser spine surgery · Injury Hematoma · Infection

21.1 Introduction

Laser spine surgery is a minimally invasive treatment and a generally very safe and effective procedure, and it may reduce morbidity and recovery time. It is generally used in open microscopic laser surgery (CO_2 laser) and percutaneous endoscopic laser surgery (Ho:YAG laser). Complications after laser spine surgery are very rare, but in some cases, they can become more serious, include nerve root injuries and dural sac injuries, and can cause damage to retroperitoneal structures and abdominal vessel/organ injury [1–5]. Damage to retroperitoneal structures and abdominal vessel/organ injury causes serious bleeding and morbidity. Postoperative hematoma at the epidural and retroperitoneal space, delayed infections, and injury to the vertebral body and paraspinal/epidural soft tissues may occur as well [1–5]. The success of laser spine surgery depends on keeping the basic surgical principle, appropriate patient selection, attention to preoperative radiology, careful surgical approach, and careful use of laser. Assuming the appropriate patient selection, complications in laser spine surgery may be related to operative complication.

21.2 Discitis

Sterile discitis after laser spine surgery is related to an inflammatory response to the thermal injury. Sterile discitis causes less severe findings and resolved within a few months after the procedure. Infectious discitis is a bacterial infection mostly related to perioperative contamination. Infectious discitis causes destructive symptoms. Laser can cause thermal injury, and it may cause necrosis at the vascular plexus of the endplate and cause potential nutritional discitis [1]. Therefore, the high applied laser energy may cause discitis [6]. Discitis is identified with diagnostic tools such as enhanced MRI scans, laboratory findings, and needle aspiration or open biopsy. To prevent discitis, the surgical field should be kept clean and

J. H. Choi (✉)
Department of Neurosurgery, Chungdam Wooridul Spine Hospital, Seoul, Republic of Korea
e-mail: cjh77@wooridul.co.kr

J. Bae, S.-H. Lee (eds.), *Laser Spine Surgery*, https://doi.org/10.1007/978-981-16-2206-9_21

moist because water can immediately absorb laser energy. In addition, be careful not to use excessive amount of laser for reducing thermal injury at the surrounding tissue.

21.3 Nerve Root and Dural Sac Injury

Direct nerve root and dural sac injury or thermal neural injury can occur due to poor orientation of the laser tip or excessive use of the laser. These result in new radicular symptom or remnant symptom. Sometimes, even when the patient is conscious, inappropriate use of laser and thermal injury to neural tissues may not be detected [7]. If any painless muscle twitching is detected during the procedure, the surgeon must stop the procedure immediately and adjust the orientation of the laser beam [7]. This injury can be avoided by careful use of the laser, paying attention to laser tip orientation, use of the laser with appropriate energy, and continuous or frequent irrigation when using the laser to adjacent neural tissue.

21.4 Hemorrhage: Retroperitoneal/Epidural and Paraspinal

Hemorrhage into the retroperitoneal or paraspinal musculature is usually the result of aggressive approach at the foraminal and extraforaminal space. It is more frequent in patients with preexisting bleeding disorders. The surgeon must consider vascular application to the foraminal and extraforaminal areas because the terminal branches of the segmental lumbar artery could have been bleeding focus [8]. Excessive exploration of the foraminal and extraforaminal space might damage the arterial branches. Ventral epidural vessel injury of laser and inappropriate hemostasis result in epidural hematoma. Appropriate and gentle endoscopic approach, careful protection of the vascular structure when using the laser, and conscious hemostasis are effective in preventing hemorrhagic complications.

21.5 Thermal Injury of the Vertebral Body and Underlying Bone Marrow

Direct thermal trauma to an adjacent vertebral endplate and the underlying bone marrow is possible when using side-firing laser system. Excessive use or high energy of the side-firing laser and malposition of the side-firing laser are the causes of this complication. This injury can cause discitis. The surgeon should pay attention to the end of the laser point toward the right target, use the laser with appropriate energy, and keep constant irrigation to decrease thermal injury.

21.6 Abdominal Vessel and Visceral Injury

It is an important issue in using laser beam. In the case of CO_2 laser discectomy, excessive use of laser may puncture the anterior annulus and injure a major vessel or the bowel [4, 9]. The laser is used with caution and the surgical field is kept moist to absorb the laser energy. The surgeon must know the amount of laser energy and anatomical location of the end of laser beam.

21.7 Summary

The surgeon must recognize the physical capabilities of the laser and pay attention in using it, such as use with appropriate energy, must have accurate anatomical knowledge and location of the pathology, and keep moist the surgical field. The complications of laser spine surgery are preventable. Safe laser surgery has much benefit to spine surgery, such as precision, delicateness, minimal tissue manipulation, less bleeding, less swelling, less trauma, and less pain.

References

1. Singh V, Derby R. Percutaneous lumbar disc decompression. Pain Phys. 2006;9(2):139–46.
2. Farrar MJ, Walker A, Cowling P. Possible salmonella osteomyelitis of spine following laser disc decompression. Eur Spine J. 1998;7(6):509–11.
3. Choy DS. Percutaneous laser disc decompression (PLDD): twelve years' experience with 752 procedures in 518 patients. J Clin Laser Med Surg. 1998;16(6):325–31.
4. Choy DS. Percutaneous laser disc decompression: a 17-year experience. Photomed Laser Surg. 2004;22(5):407–10.
5. Hellinger J. Complications of non-endoscopic percutaneous laser disc decompression and nucleotomy with the neodymium: YAG laser 1064 nm. Photomed Laser Surg. 2004;22(5):418–22.
6. Grasshoff H, Mahlfeld K, Kayser R. Complications of percutaneous laser disc decompression. Lasers in the musculoskeletal system. Heidelberg: Springer; 2001. p. 343–4.
7. Ahn Y, Lee U. Use of laser in minimally invasive spine surgery. Expert Rev Med Devices. 2018;15(6):423–33.
8. Ahn Y, Kim JU, Lee BH. Postoperative retroperitoneal hematoma following transforaminal percutaneous endoscopic lumbar discectomy. J Neursurg Spine. 2009;10:595–602.
9. Jeong SH, Lee SH, Choi WC. Iliac artery perforation following lumbar discectomy with microsurgical carbon dioxide laser: a report of a rare case and discussion of the treatment. Spine (Phila Pa 1976). 2007;32(3):E124–5.

22 Future Technologies of Laser Spine Surgery

Young-jin Kim and Junseok Bae

Abstract

Laser technology is one of the powerful tools that enable surgical procedures through tiny incision in the era of minimally invasive surgery. The current use of laser technology in spine surgery can be divided into two categories—percutaneous endoscopic laser surgery and open microsurgery with laser. Many minimally invasive surgeries applied to medicine rely upon research and development of robot engineering, computer, and software science. Along with advance of surgical instruments, laser technologies also have been enormously developed and applied to various medical procedures since its first use. It is anticipated that grafting laser technology onto the robotic system will replace many conventional procedures in spine surgery. And laser technology itself will be advanced to take over its preexisting limitations. In this chapter, we will describe the technological future of laser in spine surgery—automated laser system and double shot irradiation system.

Keywords

Laser · Automated laser system · Double shot irradiation · Spine surgery · Minimally invasive surgery · Discectomy

Y.-j. Kim · J. Bae (✉)
Department of Neurosurgery, Chungdam Wooridul Spine Hospital, Seoul, Republic of Korea

22.1 Introduction

For decades, conventional surgery has been substituted by minimally invasive surgery due to the development of surgical instruments such as navigation system, laparoscope, endoscope, and microscope as well. In the era of minimally invasive surgery, surgeons perform surgical procedure through smaller incision instead of large incision which may induce more pain and complications to patients. And laser technology is one of the powerful tools which enables surgical procedures through tiny window.

Along with advance of surgical instruments, laser technologies also have been enormously developed and applied to various medical procedures since its first use. Since the American dermatologist and surgeon Leon Goldman used laser to removed tattoos in 1962, laser has been widely applied to a variety medical fields accompanied with the development of laser technology—including angioplasty, cancer diagnosis, cancer treatment, lithotripsy, laser mammography, medical imaging, microscopy, ophthalmology, optical coherence tomography, prostatectomy, plastic surgery, laser liposuction, surgery, and cosmetic procedures [1].

The history of laser use in spine surgery began with spinal tumor removal using CO2 laser by Ascher in 1978. However, in spine surgery, laser has been most widely applied to disc decompression [2]. The current use of laser technology in spine surgery can be divided into two catego-

J. Bae, S.-H. Lee (eds.), *Laser Spine Surgery*, https://doi.org/10.1007/978-981-16-2206-9_22

ries—percutaneous endoscopic laser surgery and open microsurgery with laser. Apart from surgical procedures, photobiomodulation therapy in chronic nonspecific low back pain is another use of laser in spine diseases.

In this chapter, we will describe the technological future of laser in spine surgery. Multilateral collaborations among the industry, natural science, and other aspect of medicine could help to predict and make future technologies feasible.

22.2 Future Technologies of Laser Spine Surgery

Today, many minimally invasive surgeries applied to medicine rely upon research and development of robot engineering, computer, and software science. Especially, robot-assisted surgery has been the spotlight and has an important role in many surgical fields of medicine.

For example, the Zeus system (Computer Motion, Inc., Santa Barbara, CA) and the Da Vinci system (Intuitive Surgical, Inc., Mountain View) have been used by a variety of disciplines for laparoscopic surgeries, including cholecystectomies, mitral valve repairs, radical prostatectomies, and reversal of tubal ligations, in addition to many gastrointestinal surgeries, nephrectomies, and kidney transplants [3].

In the neurosurgical field, robotic devices are used to carry out precise procedures—stereotactic surgery for brain and instrumentation such as pedicle screw insertion to the spine. Supervised robots like the SpineAssist and Renaissance systems (Mazor Surgical Technologies, Caesarea, Israel) are now widely used in spinal instrumentation and, more recently, have been approved for use in the brain [4].

22.2.1 Automated Laser Surgery

Spine surgery relies upon fine motor skills to manipulate neural elements and a steady hand, often exploiting small working corridors utilizing exposures that minimize collateral damage. Additionally, the procedures may be long and arduous, predisposing the surgeon to both mental and physical fatigue. Therefore, spine surgery may actually be an ideal candidate for the integration of navigation and robot-assisted procedures [5]. In this light, it is anticipated that grafting laser technology onto the robotic system will replace many conventional procedures in spine surgery.

One example of future laser technique is the automated laser surgery. Up to now, direction of laser beam is controlled manually with joystick installed in the microscope or foot switch. And to perform safe and precise laser surgery manually, surgeons should be well-trained and experienced. Even for the skilled surgeons, it is still hard to manipulate laser within tiny surgical field. Thus, automated laser surgery has several advantages and could compensate the risk of surgeon's fault. Reproducible and consistent treatment is possible due to automation. And it is expected that robotic, computer-controlled laser beam can provide precision, and very brief laser-tissue interaction leads to minimal thermal damage which is a major complication of laser use. With robotic-controlled laser beam, safe and steady movement is possible by eliminating hand tremor impact. AcuPulse CO_2 laser with SurgiTouch automation system (Lumenis, Israel) is one of the automated and robotic laser surgery systems which enables speed, precision, and convenience levels unattainable by manual laser treatment (Fig. 22.1).

22.2.2 Double Shot Irradiation

Irregular motion of disc fragments under massive saline irrigation in the closed space is a barrier of endoscopic discectomy. Unexpected damage of normal tissue can occur due to irregular motion of disc materials during laser procedure. And there has been similar concerns in urology too. Long-pulse mode produces stone retropulsion during laser lithotripsy. Recently, there is a new technology developed for a high-power 120-W Ho:YAG (holmium:YAG) lithotripter, called the MOSES effect. The theory is that this lithotripsy mode emits a modulated laser pulse whose first part divides the water between the laser fiber tip

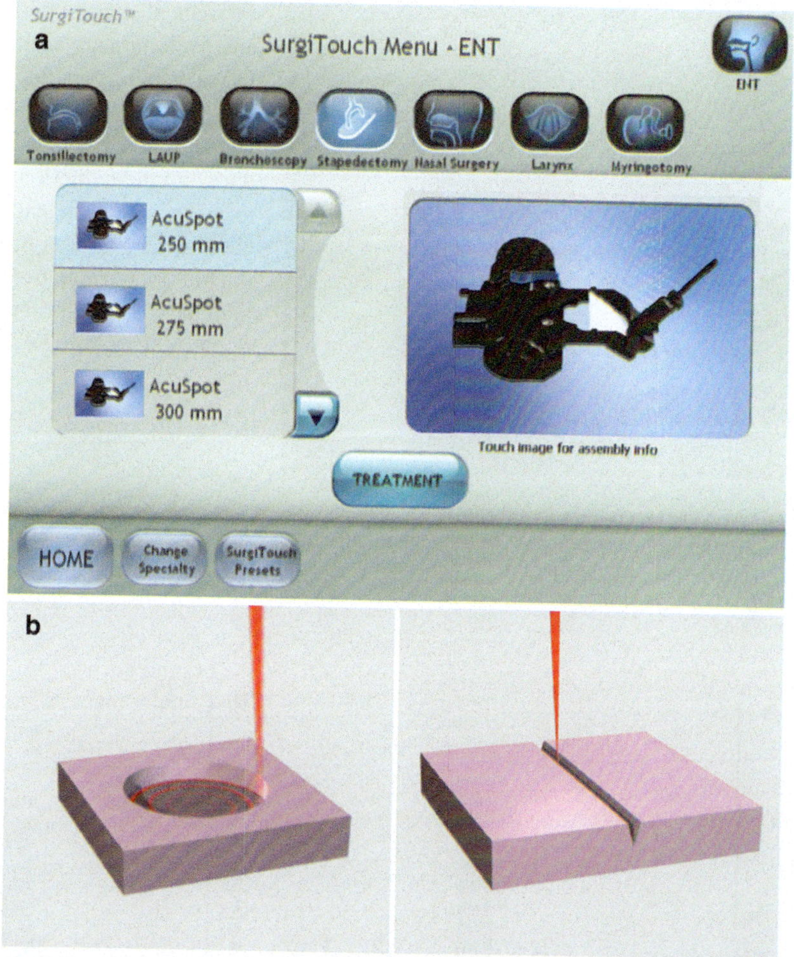

Fig. 22.1 (**a**) Application-guided user interface. Select specialty and application. (**b**) Automated ablation and incision through robotic SurgiTouch scanner

and the stone, allowing the second part of the pulse to hit the stone unobstructed, more efficiently, and with less retropulsion [6].

The MOSES laser system (Lumenis, Israel) irradiates two shots of laser in a moment, providing control of stone movement. The first shot of irradiation creates an air bubble. The bubble contraction produces power to attract the stone as shown in blue arrows, and the power is balanced by the second shot (Fig. 22.2). The MOSES laser system has two types of mode—contact mode and distance mode. Contact mode is used in near contact, basically used as the main mode. It has a weaker first shot to attract the stone or disc material and has a stronger second shot to fragment the stone or disc material. Distance mode is used if the fiber tip cannot reach the stone or disc material. Because the tip is far away from the stone or disc material, it has a stronger first shot to attract the stone or disc material and has a weaker second shot to fragment the stone or disc material (Fig. 22.3).

Ibrahim et al. studied and compared regular and MOSES modes of holmium laser lithotripsy. When compared with the regular mode, MOSES technology was associated with significantly lower fragmentation time (23.4 vs. 17.5 min, $p < 0.05$) and total procedural time (53 vs. 42.1 min, $p < 0.05$). MOSES technology was associated with significantly less retropulsion (mean grade was 1 vs. 0.4, $p < 0.05$) [7].

A preexisting laser device such as Ho:YAG has been used widely, but has several limitations too. Laser efficiency has been performed with the laser fiber in direct contact with the stone surface. It is supposed that the smaller the distance

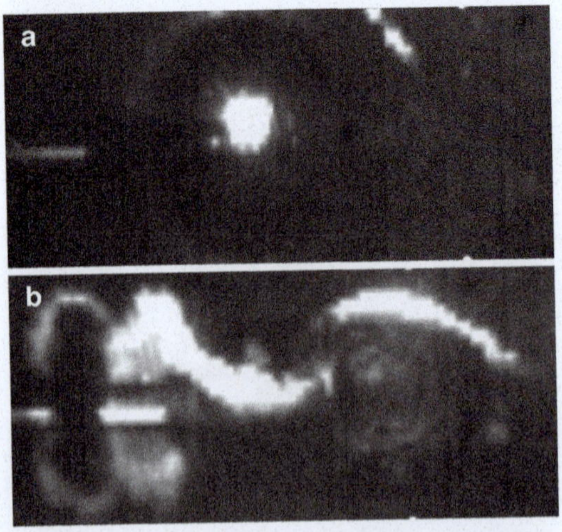

Fig. 22.2 In near contact to stone, (**a**) first shot: a bubble expands and contracts and the stone gets closer to the fiber tip, (**b**) second shot: another laser is irradiated before the stone hits the fiber tip, and the stone remains in the same position

between the laser fiber and the stone, the less energy is consumed during the formation of a vapor bubble and the greater amount of pulse energy remains for ablation [8]. In the same manner, during endoscopic laser discectomy procedure, irregular motion of disc fragments under massive saline irrigation in the closed space could reduce laser efficiency. It is anticipated that double shot irradiation mode of MOSES laser system will be helpful to get over those problems of preexisting laser devices.

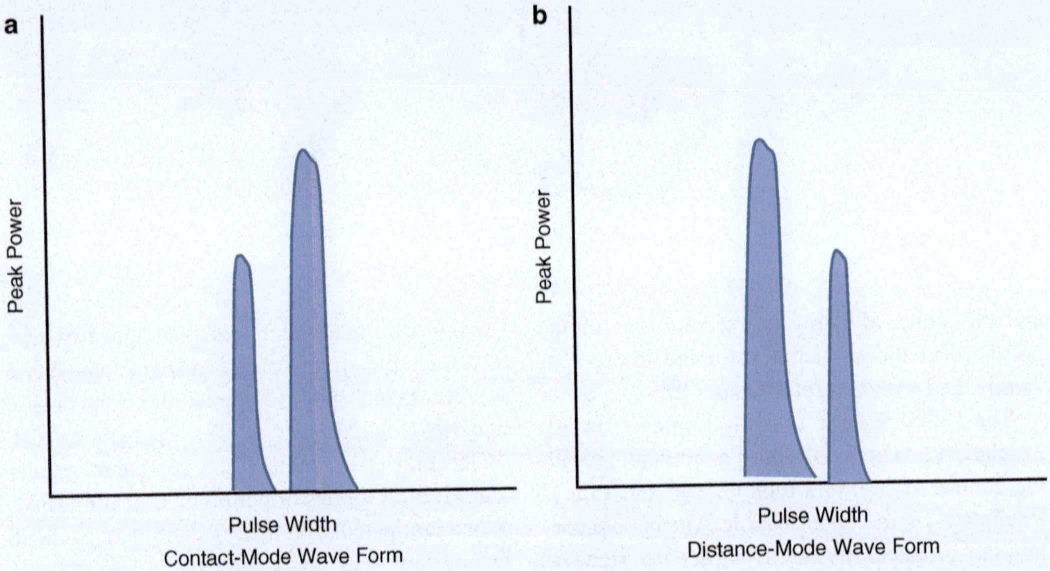

Fig. 22.3 (**a**) In contact mode, it has a weaker first shot to attract the stone (the bubble is small) and a stronger second shot to fragment the stone (the bubble is large). (**b**) In distance mode, it has a stronger first shot to attract the stone (the bubble is large) and a weaker second shot to fragment the stone (the bubble is small)

22.3 Summary

In tandem with advances in artificial intelligence, robotic science, and machine learning, laser technology in the spine surgery will also take a major step forward. And future laser technologies will eliminate mechanistic errors, reduce operating times, and provide the same or even greater resective margins with minimal-access surgery [4]. From this point of view, future laser technologies will make precise, elaborate, and safe surgery feasible which is the main concept and goal of minimally invasive spine surgery.

References

1. Song KU. Footprints in laser medicine and surgery: beginnings, present, and future. Med Lasers. 2017;6(1):1–4.
2. Ahn Y, Lee U. Use of lasers in minimally invasive spine surgery. Expert Rev Med Devices. 2018;15(6):423–33.
3. Lanfranco AR, et al. Robotic surgery: a current perspective. Ann Surg. 2004;239(1):14–21.
4. Bagga V, Bhattacharyya D. Robotics in neurosurgery. Ann R Coll Surg Engl. 2018;100(6):19–22.
5. Overley SC, et al. Navigation and robotics in spinal surgery: where are we now? Neurosurgery. 2017;80(3S):S86–99.
6. Kronenberg P, Somani B. Advances in lasers for the treatment of stones: a systematic review. Curr Urol Rep. 2018;19(6):45.
7. Ibrahim A, et al. PD53-04 double-blind prospective randomized clinical trial comparing regular and MOSES modes of holmium laser lithotripsy: preliminary results. J Urol. 2018;199:e1047.
8. De Coninck V, et al. Ho:YAG laser lithotripsy in non-contact mode: optimization of fiber to stone working distance to improve ablation efficiency. World J Urol. 2019;37(9):1933–9.

The manufacturer's authorised representative in the EU is Springer Nature Customer Service Centre GmbH, Europaplatz 3, 69115 Heidelberg, Germany. If you have any concerns regarding our products, please contact ProductSafety@springernature.com

Printed and bound by CPI Group (UK) Ltd, Croydon, CR0 4YY
30/07/2026
02182084-0001